Biological Protection With Prostaglandins

Volume I

Editor

Max M. Cohen, M.B., F.R.C.S., (Edin. + C.) F.A.C.S.
Associate Professor of Surgery
University of Toronto
Toronto, Ontario, Canada

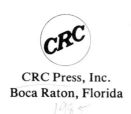

CRC Press, Inc.
Boca Raton, Florida

Library of Congress Cataloging in Publication Data
Main entry under title:

Biological protection with prostaglandins.

  Includes bibliographies and index.
  1. Prostaglandins--Physiological effect.
2. Prostaglandins--Therapeutic use--Evaluation.
I. Cohen, Max Mark.   [DNLM: 1. Prostaglandins.
QU 90 B615]
QP8012.P68B57   1985   615.7   85-5706
ISBN 0-8493-5962-7 (v. 1)
ISBN 0-8493-5963-5 (v. 2)

© 1985 by CRC Press, Inc.

International Standard Book Number 0-8493-5962-7 (Volume (I)
International Standard Book Number 0-8493-5963-5 (Volume (II)

Library of Congress Card Number 85-5706
Printed in the United States

PREFACE

Few areas of research have attracted more attention in recent years than the prosta-glandins. This is reflected by the enormous number of publications which appear each year on the subject and the fact that there are at least two journals devoted exclusively to the prostaglandins. It is becoming increasing difficult, even for the active investiga-tor, to keep abreast of all new developments.

The importance of the prostaglandins in medicine was acknowledged by the award of the Nobel prize in 1982 to three distinguished scientists (Drs. Bergstrom, Samuels-son, and Vane) who have made outstanding contributions to our understanding of the metabolism of prostaglandins and their biological role.

There have been many and diverse discoveries made concerning the physiology and pharmacology of the prostaglandins and the other products of the arachidonic acid cascade. One of the most dramatic is the phenomenon of protection against ulceration of the gastric mucosa by the prostaglandins. This exciting observation made by Robert in 1974 sparked an intensive search not only for its mechanism but also for evidence of biological protection by the prostaglandins in other organs.

No simple unifying concept has yet been proposed to explain the biological role of the eicosanoids. This book is an attempt to assemble most of the evidence available that suggests that the prostaglandins have a generally protective function. It is not intended as strong advocacy and, indeed, some of the contributors clearly do not view prostaglandins as protective agents. It is hoped that this will be of interest not only to investigators in this area but to all biologists and physicians.

There is inevitably some overlap between chapters, particularly in relation to the descriptions of synthesis, metabolism, and release of prostaglandins, and it is hoped that the reader will be tolerant of this. The critical reader will also detect some contra-dictions. The editor makes no apology for these; they reflect the lack of unanimity which exists and illustrate that our concepts of the biological role of the prostaglandins are still rather volatile. Some may consider, therefore, that this work is premature. That may prove to be true. My hope is that if it sparks new ideas or experiments, it would have proven timely.

THE EDITOR

Max M. Cohen, M.B., is Professor of Surgery at the University of Toronto and a General Surgeon on the staff of Mount Sinai Hospital, Toronto, Ontario, Canada.

Dr. Cohen graduated in medicine in 1963 from the University of Glasgow, Scotland, and obtained Fellowships in Surgery from the Royal College of Surgeons of Edinburgh in 1968, from the Royal College of Physicians and Surgeons of Canada in 1972 and from the American College of Surgeons in 1974. He was on the faculty of the University of British Columbia from 1972 until 1980 when he moved to Toronto.

Dr. Cohen is a member of many learned societies including: Canadian Association of Gastroenterology, Canadian Association of General Surgeons, American Gastroenterological Association, Society for Academic Surgery, Central Surgical Association, Society for Surgery of the Alimentary Tract and the Society of University Surgeons.

Dr. Cohen is a member of the Editorial Board of the Canadian Journal of Surgery. He has given numerous papers and lectures at national and international gastroenterological meetings and has published more than 100 research papers. His research interest is gastro-duodenal mucosal defense mechanisms with a major emphasis on the role of endogenous prostaglandins. His clinical interests are endoscopy and gastric, biliary, and pancreatic surgery.

CONTRIBUTORS

Adrian Allen
Medical School
University of Newcastle upon Tyne
Newcastle-upon-Tyne, England

Philippe Beau
University Hospital
Poitiers, France

Alan Bennett
King's College Hospital Medical School
London, England

Laszlo Z. Bito
College of Physicians and Surgeons
Columbia University
New York, New York

Pierre Borgeat
Laboratoire d'Endocrinologie
  Moléculaire
Le Centre Hospitalier de l'Université
  Laval
Quebec, Canada

Marie-Gilberte Borzeix
SIR International
Montrouge, France

Pierre Braquet
Georgetown University
Washington, D.C.

Shaun P. Brennecke
Queen Victoria Hospital
Adelaide, Australia

Jean Cahn
SIR International
Montrouge, France

Paul J. Cannon
Columbia University
New York, New York

Lars A. Carlson
King Gustav V Research Institute
Karolinska Institute
Stockholm, Sweden

Donald O. Castell
Bowman Gray School of Medicine
Winston-Salem, North Carolina

Peter Cervoni
American Cyanamid Company
Pearl River, New York

Peter S. Chan
American Cyanamid Company
Pearl River, New York

Heinrich Ditter
Justus-Liebig University
Giessen, West Germany

Lloyd N. Fleisher
North Carolina State University
Raleigh, North Carolina

Gunnar Flemström
Uppsala University Biomedical Center
Uppsala, Sweden

J. Raymond Fletcher
Saint Thomas Hospital
Nashville, Tennessee

Robert H. Gallavan, Jr.
College of Medicine
University of Cincinnati
Cincinnati, Ohio

Andrew Garner
ICI Pharmaceuticals Division
Macclesfield, Cheshire, England

Ryszard J. Gryglewski
N. Copernicus Academy of Medicine
Krakow, Poland

Friedrich W. Hehrlein
Justus-Liebig University
Giessen, West Germany

Dieter Heinrich
Justus-Liebig University
Giessen, West Germany

Barry H. Hirst
Medical School
University of Newcastle upon Tyne
Newcastle-Upon-Tyne, England

Kenneth V. Honn
Wayne State University
Detroit, Michigan

David F. Horrobin
Efamol Research Institute
Kentville, NS, Canada

Gabriel N. Hortobagyi
M. D. Anderson Hospital and Tumour
  Institute
Houston, Texas

Eugene D. Jacobson
College of Medicine
University of Cincinnati
Cincinnati, Ohio

Gordon L. Kauffman, Jr.
Wadsworth VA Medical Center
Los Angeles, California

Satoshi Kitamura
University of Tokyo
Tokyo, Japan

Eero Kivilaakso
University of Helsinki
Helsinki, Finland

Stanislaw J. Konturek
Institute of Physiology
Krakow, Poland

Moshe Ligumsky
Hadassah University Hospital
Jerusalem, Israel

F. Reinhard Matthias
Justus-Liebig University
Giessen, West Germany

Claude Matuchansky
University Hospital
Poitiers, France

Susan McQueen
Medical School
University of Newcastle upon Tyne
Newcastle-Upon-Tyne, England

David G. Menter
Wayne State University
Detroit, Michigan

Murray D. Mitchell
Department of Ophthalmology
UCSD Medical Center
San Diego, California

Anders G. Olsson
King Gustaf V Research Institute
Karolinska Institute
Stockholm, Sweden

James M. Onoda
Wayne State University
Detroit, Michigan

Wieslaw W. Pawlik
Medical Academy
Krakow, Poland

Louis M. Pelus
Sloan Kettering Institute
New York, New York

Daniel Rachmilewitz
Hadassah University Hospital
Jerusalem, Israel

Benjamin J. Reichstein
University of Health Sciences/The
  Chicago Medical School
North Chicago, Illinois

André Robert
Upjohn Company
Kalamazoo, Michigan

R. Paul Robertson
University of Colorado Health Sciences
  Center
Denver, Colorado

Marek Rola-Pleszcynski
University of Sherbrooke
Sherbrooke, PQ, Canada

Mary J. Ruwart
Upjohn Company
Kalamazoo, Michigan

Sheikh Arshad Saeed
Wellcome Research Labs
Karachi, Pakistan

John F. L. Shaw
Addenbrooke's Hospital
Cambridge, England

Dennis R. Sinar
East Carolina University School of
  Medicine
Greenville, North Carolina

Pierre Sirois
University of Sherbrooke
Sherbrooke, PQ, Canada

Bonnie F. Sloane
Wayne State University
Detroit, Michigan

Lynda A. Smeaton
Reckitt & Colman Plc.
Hull, England

Daniel M. Strickland
Wilford Hall Medical Center
San Antonio, Texas

Alan R. Tall
Columbia University College
New York, New York

John D. Taylor
Wayne State University
Detroit, Michcigan

Barry L. Tepperman
Health Sciences Centre
University of Western Ontario
London, ON, Canada

John L. Wallace
Wellcome Research Laboratories
Beckenham, Kent, England

Brendan J. R. Whittle
Wellcome Research Labs
Beckenham, Kent, England

Larry D. Witte
Columbia University
New York, New York

Armin Wollin
University of Sherbrooke
Sherbrooke, PQ, Canada

BIOLOGICAL PROTECTION WITH PROSTAGLANDINS

Volume I

Volume II

TABLE OF CONTENTS

Volume I

GENERAL CONSIDERATIONS, CANCER, AND THE IMMUNE SYSTEM

HEMOSTASIS AND THROMBOSIS AND OTHER SITES OF ACTION

To Rachel and Leah

General Considerations, Cancer, and the Immune System

Chapter 1

THE ARACHIDONIC ACID CASCADE

Max M. Cohen

TABLE OF CONTENTS

I. INTRODUCTION

The term "prostaglandin" (PG) was coined in 1935 by von Euler[1] to describe the component of human semen which he and Goldblatt[2] had independently found to be capable of stimulating smooth muscle contraction. This work was largely ignored and it was almost three decades later that the first PGs were isolated by investigators at the Karolinska Institute in Stockholm.[3,4] The PGs are synthesized from three separate fatty acids: dihomogammalinolenic acid, arachidonic acid, and eicosapentaenoic acid to give PGs of the 1, 2, and 3 series, respectively (Figure 1). These series are designated by the appropriate subscript numeral, e.g., PGE_1, PGE_2.

Arachidonic acid is the precursor of the 2-series of PGs, prostacyclin and the thromboxanes via the cyclooxygenase pathway; via the lipoxygenase pathway, it is the precursor of the leukotrienes. Arachidonic acid is present in the diet and can also be synthesized from dietary linoleic acid. The first step in the arachidonic acid cascade is the liberation of arachidonic acid from membrane phospholipids by phospholipase A_2. The capacity to synthesize PGs from arachidonic acid exists in almost all mammalian tissues. The term "eicosanoids" applies to all of the 20-carbon products of arachidonic acid; the term "prostanoids" applies to those based on prostanoic acid.

II. METABOLIC PATHWAYS

The steroidal anti-inflammatory agents such as glucocorticoids inhibit phospholipase A_2 activity,[5] possibly by inducing an endogenous inhibitor,[6] and thus inhibit the entire arachidonic acid cascade (Figure 2).

A. The Cyclooxygenase Pathway

The catecholamines, hydroquinone, L-tryptophan, and serotinin appear to be essential cofactors for the first biosynthetic step of conversion to the cyclic endoperoxides PGG_2 and PGH_2 by means of cyclooxygenase (Figure 3). It is this step which is inhibited by the nonsteroidal anti-inflammatory (NSAI) drugs such as aspirin, indomethacin, flurbiprofen, and ibuprofen. Thus, NSAI drugs prevent the formation not only of the PG, but also of the thromboxanes and prostacyclin; but they have no effect on the lipoxygenase pathway, except possibly to facilitate leukotriene formation by increasing the available arachidonic acid substrate (Figure 2).

1. Prostaglandins

The PGs (Figure 3) are not stored by cells but are rapidly synthesized on demand. Most cells appear to have the enzymatic capacity for this biosynthesis. Synthesis is stimulated under physiological conditions and in many pathological situations such as inflammation and neoplasm. The most trivial mechanical trauma is a potent stimulus for PG synthesis, perhaps by impairing membrane integrity. PGs have the classical "bobby-pin" configuration of prostanoic acid comprising a cyclopentane ring and two side chains for a total of 20 carbon atoms. PGs are designated A through F depending on the exact structure of the cyclopentane ring. The subscript number (e.g., 1, 2, or 3) denotes the number of double bonds in the side chains. The Greek letter that follows (either alpha or beta) describes the stereochemistry at the C9 position.

2. Thromboxanes

The enzyme that synthesizes thromboxane A_2 (TXA_2; Figure 4); from PGH_2 was first localized in platelets[7] and explains the origin of the name. The enzyme is found also in leukocytes, macrophages, and human lung fibroblasts. Organs shown to generate TXA_2 include spleen, lung, kidney, and stomach. It is not certain which cells in

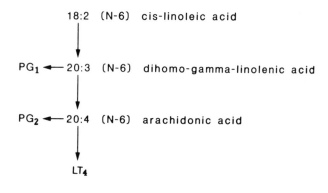

FIGURE 1. Formation of PGs of the 1, 2, and 3 series from fatty acids.

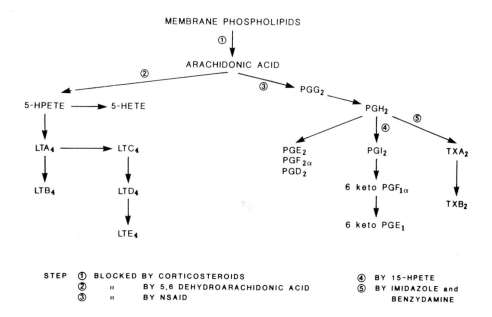

FIGURE 2. Diagram of the major metabolic synthetic pathways from arachidonic acid via the lipoxygenase and cyclooxygenase systems. The steps where synthesis can be blocked are shown.

these organs possess the thromboxane synthetase enzyme. The appearance of TXA_2 in platelets is accompanied by the appearance of malondialdehyde (MDA), and this has been used as a measure of thromboxane production. TXA_2 is a highly unstable metabolite which is a powerful platelet aggregator and will strongly constrict blood vessels. It is converted to the stable polar compound TXB_2. TXA_2 is a more potent stimulator of platelet aggregation than the PG endoperoxides; indeed it is likely that PGG_2 and PGH_2 must be converted to TXA_2 to aggregate platelets.

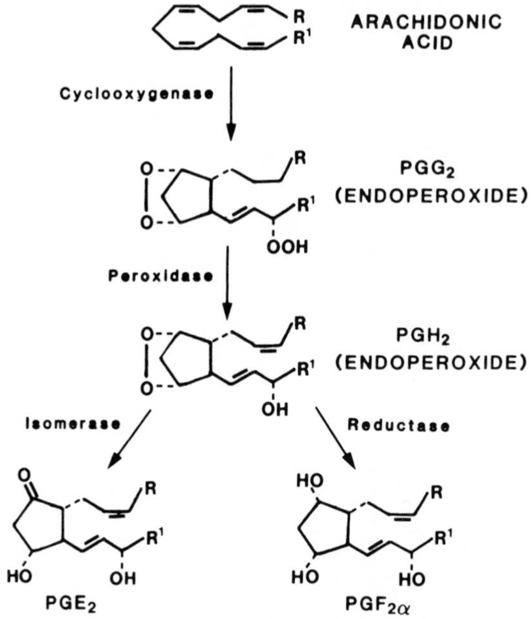

FIGURE 3.   Formation of the biologically active PGs from arachidonic acid via the cyclooxygenase pathway.

Imidazole[8] and dipyridamole[9] are relatively specific inhibitors of thromboxane synthetase (Figure 2). Both cyclic AMP (cAMP) and dibutyryl cAMP inhibit thromboxane synthesis by platelets. Zinc, cadmium, and even garlic[10] have been reported to inhibit thromboxane formation. Thromboxane formation is stimulated by the divalent cation ionophore A23187, suggesting that calcium ions are necessary for synthesis.[11]

3. Prostacyclin

Prostacyclin (PGI$_2$; Figure 4) has been assigned the approved name epoprostenol, but is widely known by its trivial name, which will be used throughout this volume. PGI$_2$ is generated from PGH$_2$ by blood vessel microsomes.[12] It has a half-life of only several minutes forming its stable metabolite 6-keto-PGF$_1\alpha$. PGI$_2$ synthetase is present mainly in the intima of arteries, but many tissues have been shown capable of synthesizing PGI$_2$ or 6-keto-PGF$_1\alpha$ (e.g., lung, heart, kidney, spleen, stomach, small intestine, uterus, placenta, and seminal vesicles). It is possible that at all of these sites the source of PGI$_2$ is vascular.

PGI$_2$ synthesis is inhibited by lipid peroxides[13] (Figure 2) and in the aortic microsomes, is stimulated by a soluble factor in the high speed supernatant that is nondialyzable and resistant to boiling.[14] PGI$_2$ is a powerful vasodilator and increases blood flow. It is the most potent inhibitor of platelet aggregation known.[15] PGI$_2$ has been clearly shown to be an important physiological anti-aggregation factor opposing the aggregatory effects of platelet thromboxanes.

B. The Lipoxygenase Pathway

Hypothesizing that there must be a pathway for arachidonic acid metabolism other than the cyclooxygenase to explain the very different effects of the steroids and the NSAI drugs, Samuelsson's group studied arachidonic acid metabolism in leukocytes from the rabbit peritoneal cavity and found that 5(S)-hydroxy-6,8,11,14-eicosatetraenoic acid (5-HETE) was the major product.[16] This led to the discovery of the lipoxy-

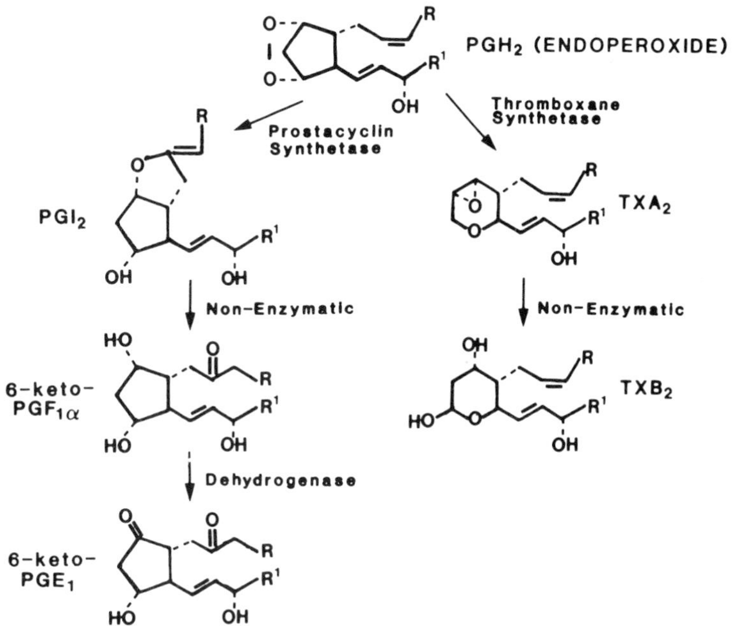

FIGURE 4.   Formation of prostacyclin and its metabolites, and the thromboxanes from the PG endoperoxide PGH_2.

genase pathway (Figure 5). Although the cyclooxygenase system has been identified in virtually all cells studied, the lipoxygenases have been identified only in platelets, leukocytes, endothelium, lung parenchyma, and the epicardium.

The term slow-reacting substance (SRS) was used to describe a smooth muscle factor which appeared in lung profusate after treatment with cobra venom.[17] It was subsequently shown to be a key mediator in asthma and other immediate hypersensitivity reactions.[18] It has now been clearly established that SRS of anaphylaxis (SRS-A) is a product of arachidonic acid synthesized via the 5-lipoxygenase pathway.[18] With their structural elucidation, the group of SRS' have been re-named leukotrienes.[19] The leukotrienes (LT) have three conjugated double bonds. Five LT have been identified and labeled LTA, LTB, LTC, LTD, and LTE. LTC, LTD, and LTE have been isolated from natural sources. SRS-A is thought to be a mixture of parent compound LTC and the metabolites LTD and LTE.

Since various precursors can be converted to leukotrienes containing three to five double bonds, a subscript to define this number is used (similar to PGs). Leukotriene A_4, for example, is the epoxy derivative of arachidonic acid which can be further transformed to LTB_4, LTC_4, LTD_4, and LTE_4. LTB_4 can cause increased capillary permeability[20] and is a powerful chemotactic agent for leukocytes.[21] The LT are powerful bronchoconstrictors.[22] These recent discoveries suggest that the LT may be of crucial importance as mediators of the inflammatory response and immediate sensitivity reactions.

The relationship between the lipoxygenase pathway and the cyclooxygenase pathway is shown in Figure 2. Steroidal anti-inflammatory agents prevent the release of arachidonic acid substrate from membrane phospholipids and block both pathways. NSAI drugs block only the cyclooxygenase pathway. Inhibition of leukotriene formation could explain some of the steriod effects which are not shared by the NSAI drugs. Other agents such as BW 755C (Wellcome) block both pathways to varying degrees and appear to have more organ specificity than do the steroids.

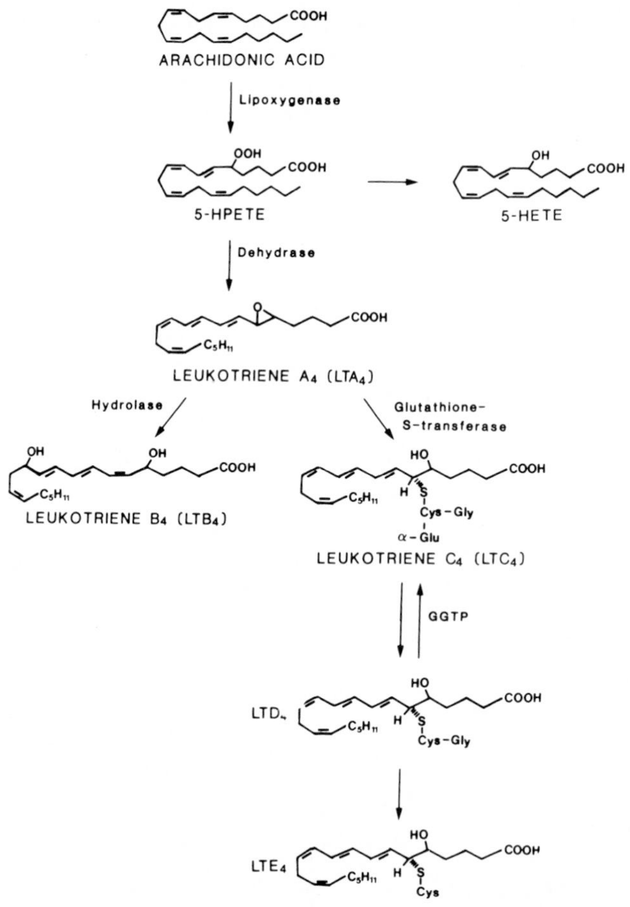

FIGURE 5. Formation of the leukotrienes from arachidonic acid via the lipoxygenase pathway.

III. MECHANISM OF BIOLOGICAL ACTIVITY

The products of the arachadonic acid cascade possess a bewildering array of biological and pharmacological activity. It is not the purpose of this chapter to review these actions. Many of them will be examined in depth in succeeding chapters. Little is known of the physiological role played by any of the eicosanoids, and even less is understood about their mechanism of cellular action.

A. Effect on Cyclic AMP

The PGs have been shown to inhibit ATPase of platelets and influence adenylate kinase.[23] PGs[24] and PGI$_2$,[25] stimulate the formation of intracellular cAMP, but little is known of their influence on cGMP. PG endoperoxide synthesis is inhibited by increased cAMP levels in human platelets.[26] These observations and the intrinsic lipid solubility of the PGs suggest that they may be capable of altering membrane fluidity.

B. Effect on Calcium Flux

Evidence is accumulating that the PGs are involved with the control of calcium ion movement acting as calcium ionophores. The relationship of calcium, hypercalcemia, and the PGs will be discussed further in Chapters 7 and 8. PGs have been shown to promote calcium efflux from mitochondria, and calcium stimulates the uptake of PGE$_1$,[27] suggesting that mitochondrial calcium may be regulated by PGs. It is well established that phospholipase is calcium dependent.[28] The configuration and small size of the eicosanoids are consistent with the theory that they act as calcium ionophores.[29]

C. Dual Mechanism of Action

Ramwell and Shaw[30] proposed in 1970 that all of the effects of PGs fell into the above two categories, interaction with adenylate cyclase or with calcium flux. More recent eicosanoid discoveries have allowed extension of this theory to the entire arachidonic acid cascade. Epithelial transport, gastric secretion, and lipolysis have all been shown to be affected by PGs and related alterations in the generation of cAMP. The effectiveness of prostanoids in contracting blood vessels appears to be related to their ability to utilize extracellular calcium,[31] in contrast to agents such as norepinephrine which use intracellular calcium. Adenylate cyclase can be inhibited by the influx of calcium ion. It is of interest then that the histamine-stimulated uptake of aminopyrine and the increased parietal cellular content of cAMP are both blocked by PG, suggesting that PG-induced inhibition of gastric acid secretion is mediated by inhibition of histamine-stimulated cAMP.[32] This effect may be due to a PG-mediated increase in calcium influx.

D. Receptors and Binding

One of the major sources of confusion in the field of PG research is that very similar PGs may have opposite effects on the same tissue and even different concentrations of the same prostanoid may have opposite effects. Examples of these phenomena exist in several tissues, e.g., intestinal smooth muscle and the umbilical artery, respectively. These apparently conflicting observations may be reconciled if there are several receptors on the same cell membrane either for different PGs or perhaps for each mechanism of cellular action. Thus it has been postulated that platelets have both a high-affinity receptor for PGI$_2$ and a low-affinity receptor for PGD$_2$ to explain the different effects of those metabolites on platelet aggregation.[33] Similarly, PGE$_1$ and PGE$_2$ may each have its own receptor on intestinal smooth muscle cells, allowing increased cAMP activity by one and increased calcium influx by the other.

Our understanding of PG receptors will be greatly enhanced by the development of specific antagonists. Specific inhibitors have so far been identified only for PGE, PGF, TXA$_2$, LTC$_4$, and LTD$_4$. None are yet generally available.

IV. CONCLUSIONS

Knowledge of the arachidonic acid cascade developed exponentially in the last few years. While less than 10 years ago only two biologically active products had been identified, the PGEs (mainly PGE$_2$) and the PGFs (mainly PGF$_2\alpha$), there are now known to be a large number of highly potent, but unstable metabolites that appear to play major roles not only in pathological conditions, but also perhaps in physiological homeostasis.

The cellular basis of action appears to be by two major mechanisms: regulation of intracellular cAMP and alteration of calcium movement across the cell membrane. The order of effectiveness of the arachidonic acid metabolites appears to be PGI$_2$, PGE$_2$, PGD$_2$, PGF$_2\alpha$, TXA$_2$, and LT$_4$.

This book is devoted to an exploration of the possible protective role played by these metabolites, and in particular the PGs, in biological systems. The great majority of the data supporting such a protective function comes from studies of the cyclooxygenase system. In the next chapter we look briefly at the lipoxygenase system before turning our attention to the other major pathway.

REFERENCES

1. von Euler, U. S., Kurze Wissenschaftlische mitteilungen — (uber die spezifische blut drucksenkende substanz des menschlichen prostata — und samenblasensekrets), *Klin. Wochenschr.*, 14, 1182, 1935.
2. Goldblatt, M. W., A depressor substance in seminal fluid, *J. Soc. Chem. Ind. London*, 52, 1056, 1933.
3. Bergstrom, S. and Sjovall, J., The isolation of prostaglandin F from sheep prostate glands, *Acta Chem. Scand.*, 14, 1693, 1960.
4. Samuelsson, B., The structure of prostaglandin E₃, *J. Am. Chem. Soc.*, 85, 1878, 1963.
5. Chang, J. A., Lewis, G. P., and Piper, P. J., Inhibition by glucocorticoids of prostaglandin release from adipose tissue in vitro, *Br. J. Pharmacol.*, 59, 425, 1977.
6. Flower, R. J. and Blackwell, G. J., Anti-inflammatory steroids induce biosynthesis of a phospholipase A₂ inhibitor which prevents prostaglandin generation, *Nature (London)*, 278, 456, 1979.
7. Moncada, S., Needleman, P., Bunting, S. et al., Prostaglandin endoperoxide and thromboxane generating systems and their selective inhibition, *Prostaglandins*, 12, 323, 1976.
8. Moncada, S., Bunting, S., Mullane, K. et al., Imidazole: a selective potent antagonist of thromboxane synthetase, *Prostaglandins*, 13, 611, 1977.
9. Ally, A. I., Manku, M. S., Horrobin, D. F. et al., Dipyridamole: a possible potent inhibitor of thromboxane A₂ synthetase in vascular smooth muscle, *Prostaglandins*, 14, 607, 1977.
10. Makheja, A. N., Vanderhoek, J. V., and Baily, J. M., Inhibition of platelet aggregation and thromboxane synthesis by onion and garlic, *Lancet*, 1, 781, 1979.
11. Knapp, H. R., Oelz, O. L., Roberts, J., Sweetman, B. J., Oates, J. A., and Reed, P. W., Ionophores stimulate prostaglandin and thromboxane biosynthesis, *Proc. Natl. Acad. Sci. U.S.A.*, 74, 4251, 1977.
12. Moncada, S., Gryglewski, R. J., Bunting, S., and Vane, J. R., An enzyme isolated from arteries transforms prostaglandin endoperoxides to an unstable substance that inhibits platelet aggregation, *Nature (London)*, 263, 663, 1976.
13. Moncada, S., Gryglewski, R. J., Bunting, S., and Vane, J. R., A lipid peroxide inhibits the enzyme in blood vessel microsomes that generates from prostaglandin endoperoxides the substance (prostaglandin X) which prevents platelet aggregation, *Prostaglandins*, 12, 715, 1976.
14. Wlodawer, P. and Hammarstrom, S., Some properties of prostacyclin synthase from pig aorta, *FEBS Lett.*, 97, 32, 1979.
15. Moncada, S. and Vane, J. R., Pharmacology and endogenous roles of prostaglandin endoperoxides, thromboxane A₂ and prostacyclin, *Pharmacol. Rev.*, 30, 293, 1979.
16. Borgeat, P., Hamberg, M., and Samuelsson, B., Transformation of arachidonic acid and homogamma-linolenic acid by rabbit polymorphonuclear leukocytes, *J. Biol. Chem.*, 251, 7816, 1976.
17. Feldberg, W. and Kellaway, C. H., Liberation of histamine and formation of lysolecithin-like substances by cobra venom, *J. Physiol. (London)*, 94, 187, 1938.
18. Murphy, R., Hammarstrom, S., and Samuelsson, B., Leukotriene C: a slow-reacting substance from murine mastocytoma cells, *Proc. Natl. Acad. Sci. U.S.A.*, 76, 4275, 1979.
19. Samuelsson, B., Borgeat, P., Hammarstrom, S., and Murphy, R. C., Introduction of a nomenclature: leukotrienes, *Prostaglandins*, 17, 785, 1979.
20. Eakins, K. E., Heggs, G. A., and Moncada, S., The effects of arachidonate lypoxygenase products on plasma exudation in rabbit skin, *J. Physiol. (London)*, 307, 71P, 1980.
21. Carr, S., Higgs, G., Salmon, J. et al., The effects of arachidonate lipoxygenase products on leukocyte migration in rabbit skin, *Br. J. Pharmacol.*, 73, 253P, 1981.
22. Dahlen, S.-E., Hedqvist, P., Hammarstrom, S., and Samuelsson, B., Leukotrienes are potent contrictors of human bronchi, *Nature (London)*, 288, 484, 1980.
23. Johnson, M. and Ramwell, P. W., Prostaglandin modification of membrane-bound enzyme activity: a possible mechanism of action? *Prostaglandins*, 3, 703, 1973.
24. Kuehl, F. A., Jr., Prostaglandins, cyclic nucleotides and cell function, *Prostaglandins*, 5, 325, 1974.
25. Lands, W. E. M., The biosynthesis and metabolism of prostaglandins, *Ann. Rev. Physiol.*, 41, 633, 1979.
26. Malstem, C., Granstrom, E., and Samuelsson, B., Cyclic-AMP inhibits the synthesis of prostaglandin endoperoxide (PGG₂) in human platelets, *Biochem. Biophys. Res. Commun.*, 68, 569, 1976.

27. Carafoli, E. and Crovelli, F., Interactions between PGE_1 and Ca^{2+} at the level of the mitochondrial membrane, *Arch. Biochem. Biophys.,* 154, 40, 1973.

28. Oelz, O., Knapp, H. R., Roberts, L. J., Oelz, R., Sweetman, B. J., Oates, J. A., and Reed, P. W., Calcium-dependent stimulation of thromboxane and prostaglandin biosynthesis by ionophores, in *Advances in Prostaglandin and Thromboxane Research,* Vol. 3, Galli, C., Galli, G., and Porcellati, G., Eds., Raven Press, New York, 1978, 147.

29. Gerrard, J. M., Butler, A. M., and Graff, G., Prostaglandin endoperoxides promote calcium release from a platelet membrane fraction in vitro, *Prostaglandins Med.,* 1, 373, 1978.

30. Ramwell, P. W. and Shaw, J. E., Biological significance of the prostaglandins, *Recent Progr. Hormone Res.,* 26, 139, 1970.

31. Loutzenhizer, R. and Van Breemen, C., The mechanism of activation of isolated rabbit aorta by the PGH_2 analog, U44069, *Am. J. Physiol.,* 241, C243, 1981.

32. Soll, A., Prostaglandin inhibition of histamine-stimulated aminopyrine uptake and cyclic AMP generation by isolated canine parietal cells, *Gastroenterology,* 72, 1146, 1978.

33. Harris, R. H., Ramwell, P. W., and Gilmer, P. J., Cellular mechanisms of prostaglandin action, *Ann. Rev. Physiol.,* 41, 653, 1979.

Chapter 2

LEUKOTRIENES AND INFLAMMATION

Pierre Borgeat, Pierre Sirois, Pierre Braquet, and Marek Rola-Pleszczynski

TABLE OF CONTENTS

I. INTRODUCTION

Leukotrienes (LTs) are novel eicosanoids recently discovered in the course of studies on the metabolism of arachidonic acid in rabbit peritoneal polymorphonuclear leukocytes (PMNL).[1,2] Figure 1 shows the structures and mechanism of synthesis of LTs. The biosynthesis of LTs is initiated in a lipoxygenase-type reaction leading to the 5S-hydroperoxy-eicosatetraenoic acid (5-HPETE), which is in turn transformed into leukotriene A_4 (LTA$_4$), an unstable allylic epoxide (the key compound in the leukotriene pathway). LTA$_4$ is the precursor of leukotriene B_4 (LTB$_4$) and of leukotriene C_4 (LTC$_4$); a hydrolase catalyzes the conversion of LTA$_4$ into LTB$_4$. LTC$_4$ is formed by the action of a glutathione transferase on LTA$_4$. Peptidases transform LTC$_4$ successively into leukotriene D_4 (LTD$_4$) and leukotriene E_4 (LTE$_4$) (loss of the glycyl residue).[3]

Shortly after the discovery of the leukotriene pathway in leukocytes, these novel transformations of arachidonic acid raised enormous interest among scientists involved in allergy and inflammation research when the biologically active components of different preparations of slow-reacting substances (SRS) and SRS of anaphylaxis (SRS-A) were identified as mixtures of LTC$_4$, LTD$_4$, and LTE$_4$ in variable proportions.[4,5] LTs were rapidly available from chemical synthesis and studies of their pharmacological properties on smooth muscle preparations of human (and other animal species) revealed potent bronchoconstrictor effects in vitro and in vivo.[6,7] These data, together with the observations that LTs are released from lungs and leukocytes upon immunological stimulation, supported the hypothesis that LTs (SRS and SRS-A) are involved in the pathophysiology of hypersensitivity reactions.[8,9]

LTB$_4$ was the first leukotriene discovered;[10] it is a dihydroxylated derivative of arachidonic acid and thus differs substantially from LTC$_4$, D$_4$, and E$_4$, all of which contain a peptidic moiety (Figure 1). Although LTB$_4$ is released by anaphylactic guinea pig lung (unpublished data) and shows some myotropic activity on human and guinea pig lung parenchymal strips (it is less potent than LTC$_4$ and D$_4$ in this respect),[7] it is not a component of classical SRS or SRS-A preparations. Investigation of the pharmacological properties of LTB$_4$ were performed and a number of recent studies clearly suggested a role for the substance (and other LTs) in inflammatory processes. In the following pages, we shall briefly summarize the present knowledge on the inflammatory properties of LTs, the synthsesis of LTs by the cellular mediators of inflammation, the stimulation of leukotriene synthesis by inflammatory stimuli, and the immunoregulatory properties of LTB$_4$.

II. THE INFLAMMATORY PROPERTIES OF LEUKOTRIENES

A. Vascular Effects

LTB$_4$, C$_4$, D$_4$, and E$_4$ exhibit biological activities on the microvasculature. Although experiments were carried out using a number of different experimental models, a relatively clear picture of the vascular effects of LTs, especially in the hamster cheek pouch and the guinea pig skin, has recently emerged. When applied topically on hamster cheek pouch preparations, LTC$_4$ and D$_4$ (but not LTB$_4$) cause intense and short-lived constrictions of arterioles, being in this respect equipotent to angiotensin. The vasoconstriction induced by LTC$_4$ or D$_4$ was followed by an increase in vascular permeability and extravasation of macromolecules. LTC$_4$ and D$_4$ were more potent than LTB$_4$ and about 1000-fold more active than histamine in increasing vascular permeability in the hamster cheek pouch model.[11] Similarly, LTC$_4$ D$_4$, and E$_4$ also increased vascular permeability in guinea pig skin[12,13] and trachea,[14] whereas LTB$_4$ showed little activity.[15]

However, in association with PGE$_1$ or PGE$_2$ (potent vasodilators), LTB$_4$ did cause

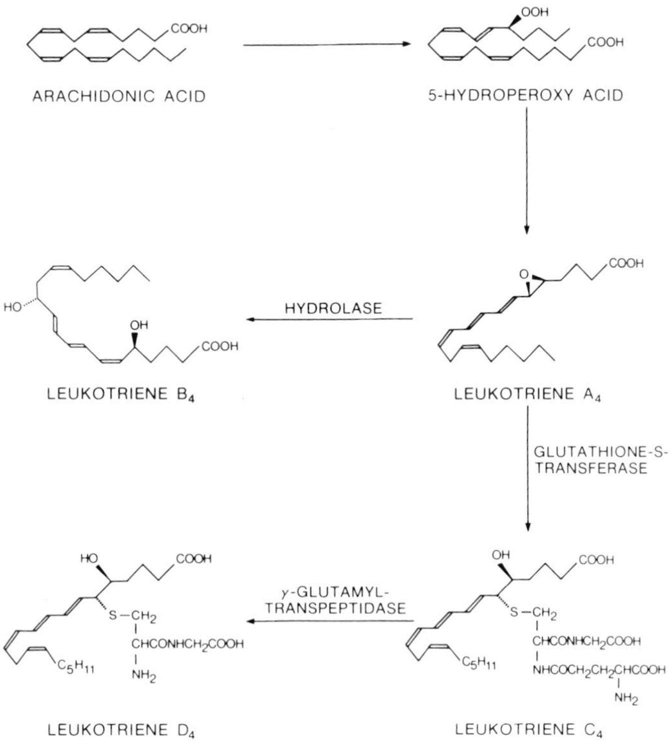

FIGURE 1. Partial scheme of the metabolism of arachidonic acid through the 5-lipoxygenase pathway. These compounds have recently been obtained by chemical synthesis and the stereochemistry of the bioactive leukotrienes A_4, B_4, C_4, and D_4 as well as the reaction steps depicted have been confirmed.

macromolecule leakage in rabbit or guinea pig skin.[15] PGE_1 and PGE_2 also potentiated the permeability increasing activity of LTC_4 and D_4 in the guinea pig skin.[12,13] Interestingly, evidence was obtained that PMNL (neutrophils) play a role in the permeability increase evoked by LTB_4 in the hamster cheek pouch.[16] It is noteworthy that considerable variations were noted with respect to vascular effects of LTs in different animal species.[17]

These in vivo observations strongly suggest that LTs are potential mediators of vascular permeability in inflammation.

B. Chemokinetic and Chemotactic Properties

Chemotactic activity was the first biological activity attributed to LTB_4 and has remained an exclusive feature of the dihydroxy acid (LTC_4, D_4, and E_4 are not chemoattractant).

Early studies with biosynthetic LTB_4 have indeed revealed that the substance is a potent stimulator of phagocyte locomotion in vitro, being a chemokinetic and chemotactic agent for PMNL (neutrophils and eosinophils), monocytes, and macrophages from various animal species, including man.[18-22] The chemokinetic activity of LTB_4 in vitro was comparable to that of other recognized potent agents such as the complement fragment C5a and the chemotactic peptide formyl-methionyl-leucyl-phenylalanine (f-MLP).[18,23] These effects of LTB_4 were stereospecific, as related HETEs and stereoisomeric dihydroxy acids, as well as the products of the ω-oxidation of LTB_4, exhibited much reduced activity.[18,19,23-25]

Specific receptors for LTB$_4$ have been recently characterized in human PMNL.[26] In parallel to chemokinetic properties of LTB$_4$, a number of investigators have observed that the compound also produces the aggregation of PMNL[18,20,24,27-29] (an effect shared with other chemoattractants such as C5a and f-MLP). The biological significance of this in vitro effect of LTB$_4$ on PMNL is not clear, but it indicates that LTB$_4$ alters some properties of the cell membrane and certainly its adhesiveness.

The chemotactic activity of LTB$_4$ was also demonstrated in several systems in vivo. Intraperitoneal injection of LTB$_4$ caused the accumulation of macrophages and PMNL in rat peritoneal cavity.[22] Injection of LTB$_4$ into the interior chamber of rabbit eye and intradermal injections also produced neutrophil accumulation at the site of administration.[27,30] Similar effects of LTB$_4$ were observed using skin chamber techniques on the rabbit back and the human forearm.[31] Elegant experiments were performed to directly observe (microscopy) the effects of LTB$_4$ on leukocytes and microvasculature in hamster cheek pouch or rabbit mesentery preparations. Topical applications of solutions of LTB$_4$ (nanomolar) were shown to rapidly cause the adherence of PMNL to vascular cells in exposed postcapillary venules and their progressive migration (diapedesis) into extravascular tissues.[11,16,31] The adhesion of PMNL to endothelial cells was rapid and reversible (within minutes) upon withdrawal of LTB$_4$ stimulation; it lasted longer if a higher dose of LTB$_4$[31] was used. The migration of PMNL into interstitial spaces was apparent 20 min after treatment of rabbit mesentery with LTB$_4$.[31]

When injected intravenously into rabbits, LTB$_4$ caused acute and reversible neutropenia with accumulation of PMNL in lung vascular bed.[31,32] This phenomenon is consistent with the effect of LTB$_4$ observed in vitro on PMNL aggregation and is likely related to increased adhesiveness of the cells to the vascular endothelium. These in vivo observations are of considerable significance and support a role for LTB$_4$ in acute inflammatory responses.

C. Secretory Activity

In addition to its effects on vascular permeability and chemotaxis, LTB$_4$ is also a secretagogue in PMNL and stimulates the release of granule-bound enzymes.[33-36] Its secretagogue activity is characterized by a high degree of specificity. Analogous dihydroxy acids and monohydroxy acids as well as ω-oxidized metabolites of LTB$_4$ exhibit little secretory activity.[35-37] Pretreatment of PMNL with LTB$_4$ induced a persistent and specific desensitization of the cells which retain responsiveness to other secretory stimuli, indicating a different mechanism of action for the fatty acid.[38] However, the secretory activity of LTB$_4$ on PMNL is dependent on cytochalasin B treatment of the cells,[34,35,37-39] and the secretion evoked by LTB$_4$ under optimal conditions is of smaller amplitude than that induced by other secretagogues (C5a, f-MPL).[33,34,37] It is also noteworthy that the LTB$_4$ concentration required for secretory activity in PMNL is higher than that required for expression of chemotactic activity or aggregation.[33,35,39]

D. Modulation of Ca^{++} Homeostasis in PMNL

It is not in the scope of this chapter to discuss all of the biochemical processes underlying the biological activities of LTs. It seems essential, however, to mention that LTB$_4$ has been shown to alter calcium metabolism in PMNL. As shown in extensive studies, LTB$_4$ evokes influx of extracellular Ca^{++} and redistribution of intracellular pools (membrane bound Ca^{++});[40] LTB$_4$ is active at 10^{-8} to 10^{-7} M and exhibits stereospecificity, as shown by the decreased activity or lack of activity of analogous substances.[41] Interestingly, it was recently found that LTB$_4$ exerts specific ionophoretic activity for Ca^{++}, as shown by translocation of the divalent cation into preformed liposomes.[42] The capacity of LTB$_4$ to alter Ca^{++} fluxes in PMNL is likely related to the various biological effects of the compounds (on PMNL) described above.

III. THE SYNTHESIS OF LEUKOTRIENES BY THE CELLULAR
MEDIATORS OF INFLAMMATION

A. General Comments on Leukotriene Synthesis

The concept that the formation of the various arachidonic acid metabolites is dependent on substrate availability is well established and the addition of arachidonic acid to cells and tissues in vitro usually results in conversions into prostaglandins (PGs), thromboxanes, or hydroxy acids. The concentration of free arachidonic acid in cells under normal conditions is low (as compared to the total amount of the fatty acid present in the form of esters).[43] The formation of cyclooxygenase and lipoxygenase products is thus initially controlled by the activity of the various lipases that make arachidonic acid available to metabolizing enzymes.[44,45] The effects of the divalent cation ionophore A23187, which nonspecifically stimulates the release of arachidonic acid (likely through stimulation of Ca^{2+}-dependent phospholipase A_2) and the synthesis of cyclooxygenase and lipoxygenase products in a variety of systems, support this concept.[46]

The synthesis of 5-HETE and LTs also depends on substrate availability. The addition of arachidonic acid to suspensions of rabbit peritoneal PMNL (glycogen-induced) results in an immediate formation of 5-HETE and LTB_4.[10,47] However, in other systems, such as in human blood PMNL (neutrophils or eosinophils) and guinea pig lungs, the 5-lipoxygenase will not readily transform exogenous arachidonic acid (or only to a small extent), whereas incubation of these cells or tissues in the presence of the ionophore A23187 leads to synthesis of substantial amounts of 5-HETE and LTB_4 from endogenous arachidonic acid (unpublished data).[48,49] These observations were of primary importance since they clearly indicated that the ionophore not only causes the release of arachidonic acid, but also activates the 5-lipoxygenase (Ca^{2+}-dependent enzyme)[50] involved in the further transformation of the fatty acid. Thus, the 5-lipoxygenase shows a low basal activity in several of the systems so far investigated and unlike other known dioxygenases, must be activated to transform arachidonic acid.

B. The Synthesis of Leukotrienes by Phagocytes

Among the cells involved in host defense mechanisms, phagocytes and more particularly PMNL are better characterized with regard to leukotriene production. Human peripheral blood (PMNL) suspensions (containing 5% or less eosinophils) release approximately 200 ng of LTB_4 and 300 ng of 5-HETE from endogenous arachidonic acid per 10×10^6 cells during 5 min stimulation with the ionophore A23187 (2 μM). The ω-hydroxy-LTB_4, which forms rapidly under these in vitro conditions, is also present in considerable amounts ($\sim$100 ng), whereas the synthesis of LTC_4 reaches only $\sim$10% of that of LTB_4 (Figure 2). The release of LTB_4 and LTC_4 by human PMNL has been reported by other investigators.[51,52]

Human PMNL suspensions prepared from the blood of donors with eosinophilia were also investigated for leukotriene synthesis. A major difference was observed with the PMNL fraction from normal donor. Indeed, in eosinophil-rich (25 to 50%) PMNL fractions, the synthesis of LTB_4 was lower, whereas the synthesis of LTC_4 was strikingly important, being up to 10 times that of LTB_4 (unpublished observations). These data are in agreement with results reported by other investigators on the synthesis of LTB_4 and LTC_4 in horse eosinophils.[53]

Human alveolar macrophages obtained by bronchoalveolar lavage from normal volunteers were tested for 5-lipoxygenase activity. As with neutrophils PMNL the major metabolites formed were 5-HETE and LTB_4. The synthesis of LTC_4 was not detectable in the experimental conditions used (as described in Figure 2 legend, except that cell concentration was 1×10^6/mℓ).[100] The synthesis of LTB_4 in human alveolar macro-

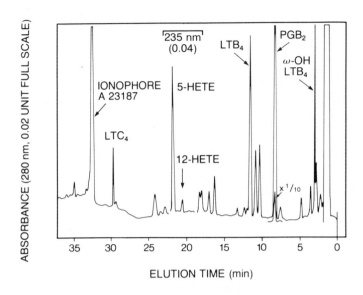

FIGURE 2.   Reversed-phase high pressure liquid chromatography (RP-HPLC) analysis of the products generated upon incubation of human blood PMNL with the ionophore A23187. Citrated blood was treated with dextran and the remaining red cells were eliminated by ammonium chloride lysis; PMNL and mononuclear cells were separated by centrifugation on Ficoll-Paque® (Pharmacia).[16] PMNL (10×10^6 in 1 ml of Dulbecco's phosphate buffered saline) were incubated 5 min at 37°C in the presence of the ionophore (2 μM) before addition of 1 ml of methanol (to stop the reaction) containing 200 ng of PGB_2 as internal standard. The sample was centrifuged to remove precipitated material, acidified, and injected (injection volume, 2 ml) without further treatment. The column was a Radial Pak C18®, 8 × 100 mm, 5 μm particles (Waters Assoc.), the compounds were eluted using gradients of organic solvents (methanol and acetonitrile in water), and a pH gradient (details of the chromatographic procedures will be reported separately).

phages was reported recently.[54] Interestingly, another group reported the formation of LTD_4 by cultured (24 hr) human alveolar macrophages.[55] In our experiments, alveolar macrophages were washed once (centrifuged and resuspended) and incubated immediately (not cultured), which might explain the difference in 5-lipoxygenase product profiles. The synthesis of LTC_4 by mouse peritoneal macrophages has also been conclusively shown.[56,57]

Recent studies from our laboratory have shown that human blood mononuclear leukocytes, i.e., lymphocytes and monocytes, do not release detectable amounts of 5-, 12-, or 15-lipoxygenase products (data not shown). These studies do not rule out that LTs or other lipoxygenase products might have been released in small amounts below the detection limit or our analytical procedure. They do, however, clearly indicate that, on a per cell basis, lymphocytes or monocytes show much lower lipoxygenase activity (5% or less) than either PMNL or alveolar macrophages. These results come into conflict with data from another group, who reported considerable lipoxygenase activity and LTB_4 synthesis in human lymphocytes.[58] The reasons for this discrepancy are unknown.

Nevertheless, the synthesis of LTs by phagocytes that have central roles in host defense against infection, namely the polymorphonuclear neutrophil and the macrophage, has clearly been demonstrated.

C. Leukotriene Synthesis by Inflammatory Stimuli

As mentioned above, in several systems studied so far the 5-lipoxygenase required activation in order to actively metabolize arachidonic acid. The divalent cation ionophore A23187, which was initially recognized as a potent activator of SRS and SRS-A synthesis, is currently used to trigger the synthesis of 5-HETE and LTs in PMNL and other cells and tissues. It is believed to exert its stimulatory activity by causing Ca^{++} influx or redistribution on intracellular pools (the 5-lipoxygenase is Ca^{++}-dependent).[50] The ionophore A23187 was an aid for biochemical studies on leukotriene synthesis and indicated the importance of Ca^{++} in 5-lipoxygenase activation, but its action has no physiological significance; however, some recent observations from a number of laboratories indicated that biological stimuli could also induce the synthesis of LTs. Most interestingly, it was shown that phagocytic stimuli induce leukotriene synthesis. Ingestion of zymosan particles causes the release of LTC_4 and LTB_4 from mouse peritoneal macrophages.[59,60] Mouse and rabbit pulmonary macrophages were also reported to release LTC_4 and LTB_4, respectively, in response to phagocytic stimulation with zymosan.[61,62] Data on the effect of phagocytic stimulation (opsonized zymosan) of human PMNL on the synthesis of LTs are contradictory. In some studies, zymosan did not cause the release of labeled 5-HETE or LTB_4 from PMNL radiolabeled with [^{3}H] arachidonic acid,[63,64] whereas in another study, it induced the synthesis of LTB_4 from PMNL as measured by HPLC.[65] The discrepancy might be explained by the different experimental procedures used. In the former situation, the synthesis of LTB_4 may have occurred from an unlabeled pool of arachidonic acid upon zymosan stimulation.

Chemotactic factors activate phagocytes and constitute important inflammatory stimuli. The synthetic peptide f-MLP is a potent chemotactic agent for PMNL and macrophages.[66] f-MLP also causes aggregation and degranulation in PMNL.[67,68] f-MLP has recently been shown to stimulate the synthesis of 5-HETE and LTB_4 (ω-hydroxy-LTB_4) in PMNL,[69-71] indicating that chemotactic stimulation also triggers the transformation of endogenous arachidonic acid into 5-lipoxygenase products. The platelet-activating factor, 1-0-alkyl-2-0-acetyl-sn-glycero-3-phosphocholine (PAF or AAGPC) is also a potent chemical mediator. It is released by PMNL and other cells and stimulates various platelet and leukocyte functions.[72] PAF induces the release of [^{3}H] arachidonic acid from prelabeled PMNL (rabbit) and the concomitant formation of 5-HETE and LTB_4.[73] The release of LTB_4 from human PMNL stimulated with PAF was also demonstrated by HPLC analysis and evidence was obtained that the amount of LTB_4 produced upon PAF stimulation could account for several effects of this mediator on PMNL.[74]

There is increasing evidence that platelets, in addition to their function in hemostasis, play some role in inflammation and allergy.[75] In agreement with this concept, it was recently reported that a product of the oxidative metabolism of arachidonic acid in human platelets, the 12S-hydroxy-5,8,10,14-eicosatetraenoic acid (12-HPETE), which is formed in platelets during thrombin- or collagen-induced aggregation, is a potent activator of human PMNL 5-lipoxygenase.[49] Indeed, addition of the labile 12-HPETE to a suspension of human PMNL leads to the activation of the 5-lipoxygenase up to levels obtained upon stimulation of the cells with the ionophore A23187. Similar activation of the 5-lipoxygenase was observed when human PMNL and platelets were co-incubated and stimulated with arachidonic acid. These data suggested that platelet-leukocyte interactions may constitute a mechanism for the activation of granulocyte 5-lipoxygenase. Another recent report supported cell-cell interactions via the lipoxygenase pathways in PMNL and platelets.[76]

It is certainly noteworthy that several inflammatory stimuli evoke a common biochemical response, i.e., the synthesis of LTs, in phagocytes in vitro. The biological properties of LTB_4 (especially its chemotactic activity for PMNL and macrophages and its ability to induce adhesion of PMNL to vascular endothelium), together with these observations, are highly suggestive of a triggering role of the substance in the inflammatory process. Hypothetically, tissue macrophages and PMNL present at the site of injury would be activated by phagocytic and chemotactic stimuli and by mediators released by aggregating platelets. LTB_4 would then be released and act as chemoattractant to stimulate the migration of PMNL at the site of injury, thus accelerating the development of the inflammatory reaction.

IV. LEUKOTRIENES AS MODULATORS OF THE IMMUNE RESPONSE

In view of the very powerful activity of LTB_4 on several neutrophil functions and their suggested involvement in inflammatory processes, LTs were also studied on human lymphocytes and were shown to have immunoregulatory functions.

A. Induction of Suppressor Lymphocytes

When LTB_4, and to a lesser extent, LTD_4 were added to human peripheral blood mononuclear leukocyte (PBML) cultures stimulated with the mitogens concanavalin A (ConA) or phytohemagglutin (PHA), significant inhibition of the lymphoproliferative response was observed at concentrations as low as 10^{-14} M.[77] Similar findings were also reported for LTD_4 and LTE_4[78] and for 15-HETE[79] in mice. These initial observations suggested the possibility that suppressor cell activation could be involved in these responses. Suppressor cells can be generated in vitro by preincubating lymphocytes with mitogens such as ConA,[80,81] antigens,[82,83] or histamine.[84,85] Their suppressive activity can be subsequently tested by adding them to fresh PBML cultures stimulated with mitogens or antigens and measuring the reduction in the proliferative responsiveness of the latter. Using such a co-culture system, normal human PBML were preincubated for 24 hr with various concentrations of LTB_4. A significant suppressor cell activity was generated at concentrations of LTB_4 ranging from 10^{-10} M to 10^{-14} M.[77] LTD_4 induced no significant suppressor activity. The magnitude of the suppressor cell activity generated by LTB_4 was comparable to that seen with ConA or histamine, but the concentrations at which it occurred were far lower than those seen with histamine (10^{-3} M to 10^{-5} M).[85] Although a 24 hr preincubation with LTB_4 was optimal, as little as 3 hr were sufficient for generating suppressor activity. LTB_4-induced suppressor cells were shown to be T-lymphocytes that did not require proliferation to exert their activity, as mitomycin C treatment of preincubated cells before addition to the fresh PBML cultures did not affect the suppressor function. In contrast, irradiation with 2000 rad abolished all suppressor activity.[77] This also suggested that carryover of LTB_4 on the surface of preincubated lymphocytes was not responsible for the subsequent supression. These findings have recently been corroborated by Payan et al.[86] who also showed that LTB_4 suppressed lymphokine production.

Although T cells were the main cell type affected by LTB_4 during preincubation, the suppressor effect required adherent cells to be manifested.[87] In addition, cyclooxygenase products were also involved in the responder cell culture as indomethacin blocked the observed suppressor cell effect.[87] More recently, phospholipids, namely phosphatidylethanolamine and phosphatidylinositol, were also shown to induce suppressor cell function and to specifically bind to $OKT8^+$ suppressor T cells.[88]

Phospholipid metabolism and leukotriene (particularly LTB_4) synthesis and release may thus play a potentially important role in immune or nonimmune inflammatory reactions by inducing or activating nonspecific suppressor cells. This in turn may serve as a crucial feedback mechanism for down regulating the immune response.

B. Augmentation of Natural Cytotoxicity

Suppressor cells can be generated concomitantly with cytotoxic effector cells[83] and both types of cells share some membrane markers.[89] We investigated whether LTB$_4$ would also be involved in the activation of natural cytotoxic cell activity. PBML-mediated killing of target cells infected with herpes simplex virus type 1 (HSV) during a 5-hr co-culture was used as a model of natural cytotoxicity (NC). There are several reports in the literature indicating that PGEs are inhibitory for cytotoxic effector cells,[90,92] and indomethacin at low concentrations causes an augmentation of NC activity.[90,93] In contrast, we found the lipoxygenase inhibitor nordihydroguaiaretic acid (NDGA) to inhibit NC activity by more than 80%.[93] This was also the case when natural killing was measured using the K562 erythroleukemia cells as targets.[94] Furthermore, some involvement of thromboxanes in NC activity was suggested by our findings that the thromboxane synthetase inhibitor OKY-1581 abolished greater than 60% of NC activity.[93]

When LTB$_4$ was added to the PBML-target cell co-culture, a significant augmentation of NC activity was observed, ranging from 60 to 280%.[93] This augmentation was not significantly modified when indomethacin was added, suggesting that a plateau was being reached in boostable NC activity. The magnitude of this augmentation was similar to that reported for interferon or interleukin-2.[95] On the other hand, the inhibition of NC activity by NDGA could be significantly reversed by LTB$_4$, indicating that exogenous lipoxygenase products could compensate for endogenous lipoxygenase inhibition.[93] The abrogation of NC activity by OKY-1581, however, was not influenced by exogenous LTB$_4$.

The recent findings described above all point to a central and potentially important role for lipoxygenase products, and in particular LTB$_4$, in immune modulation. The concomitant induction of cytotoxic and suppressor cell activities by LTB$_4$ may constitute part of the initial mechanisms for defense against foreignness (induction or augmentation of natural cytotoxicity) as well as for regulation of the immune response via a negative feedback (induction of suppressor cells) as illustrated in Figure 3.

V. CONCLUSIONS

Several features support a role of LTs as mediators of inflammatory reactions. Firstly, LTs are formed in PMNL and macrophages (among other sources), and were found in inflammatory exudates, e.g., in the synovial fluid of rheumatoid arthritis (RA) patients[97,98] and in the sputum of patients with cystic fibrosis.[99]

Secondly, LTs show inflammatory properties. Indeed LTs augment vascular permeability, an effect potentiated by E-type PGs. Exogenous LTs also stimulate the more subtle events of inflammation described above, for instance, the migration of phagocytes and the release of their enzyme content. LTs may also fulfill a third criterion for their mediator role in inflammation since their formation is likely inhibited by steroid anti-inflammatory drugs. Indeed, corticosteroids are believed to inhibit the whole arachidonic acid cascade, whereas NSAI drugs are inhibitors of the formation of the cyclooxygenase products only. Corticosteriods were shown to induce in various cells and tissues the formation of proteins called macrocortin, renocortin, and lipomodulin, three closely related (if not identical) substances that inhibit phospholipase A$_2$, the enzyme which acts as a gate for arachidonic acid mobilization (Figure 4). Thus, this newly reported effect of corticosteroids on arachidonic acid metabolism is in agreement with their efficacy in asthma as well as in inflammatory reactions since the reduction of arachidonic acid available should also lower the formation of bronchoconstrictor and inflammatory LTs. This expected inhibition of leukotriene synthesis has, however, not yet been rigorously demonstrated.

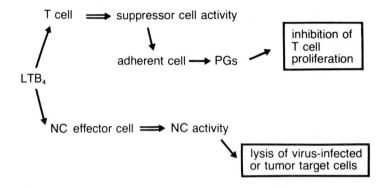

FIGURE 3.   The immunoregulatory properties of LTB_4.

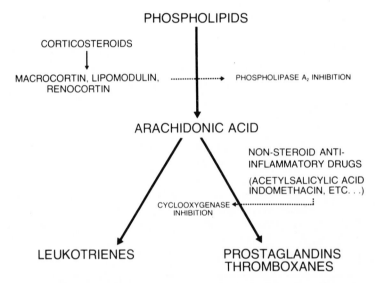

FIGURE 4.   Sites of action of anti-inflammatory drugs on the arachidonic acid cascade.

Evidence now supports an integrated role for PGs and LTs in inflammatory reactions. Together, they contribute to produce the series of subtle biochemical events underlying host defense mechanisms. The inhibition of some events (fever, pain, edema, erythema) by aspirin-like drugs probably accounts for the clear beneficial effect of these drugs in inflammatory reactions. On the other hand, the concomitant inhibition of the two families of mediators derived from arachidonic acid, i.e., the PGs and the LTs, by corticosteroids may account for the more profound anti-inflammatory and therapeutic actions of these drugs.

The measurement of LTs in various pathological conditions as well as the synthesis of leukotriene inhibitors and antagonists, and structure-activity studies will most likely help to define the contribution of LTs to inflammatory and hypersensitivity reactions and hopefully lead to the development of novel and more specific anti-inflammatory drugs.

REFERENCES

1. Borgeat, P. and Samuelsson, B., Metabolism of arachidonic acid in polymorphonuclear leukocytes: unstable intermediate in formation of dihydroxy acids, *Proc. Natl. Acad. Sci. U.S.A.*, 76, 3213, 1979.
2. Samuelsson, B., Borgeat, P., Hammarstrom, S., and Murphy, R. C., Introduction of a nomenclature: leukotrienes, *Prostaglandins*, 17, 785, 1979.
3. Sirois, P. and Borgeat, P., Leukotrienes: a new approach to the biochemistry of hypersensitivity, *Surv. Immunol. Res.*, 1, 279, 1982.
4. Murphy, R. C., Hammarstrom, S., and Samuelsson, B., Leukotriene C: a slow-reacting substance from murine mastocytoma cells, *Proc. Natl. Acad. Sci. U.S.A.*, 76, 4275, 1979.
5. Morris, H. R., Taylor, G. W., Piper, P. J., Samhoun, M. N., and Tippins, J. R., Slow reacting substances (SRSs): the structure identification of SRSs from rat basophil leukaemia (RBL-1) cells, *Prostaglandins*, 19, 185, 1980.
6. Drazen, J. M., Austen, K. F., Lewis, R. A., Clark, D. A., Goto, G., Marfat, A., and Corey, E. J., Comparative airway and vascular activities of leukotrienes C-1 and D in vivo and in vitro, *Proc. Natl. Acad. Sci. U.S.A.*, 77, 4354, 1980.
7. Sirois, P., Roy, S., Tétrault, J. P., Borgeat, P., Picard, S., and Corey, E. J., Pharmacological activity of leukotrienes A_4, B_4, C_4, and D_4 on selected guinea-pig, rat, rabbit and human smooth muscles, *Prostaglandins Med.*, 7, 327, 1981.
8. Samuelsson, B., The leukotrienes, highly biologically active substances involved in allergy and inflammation, *Angew. Chem. Int. Ed. Engl.*, 21, 902, 1982.
9. Sirois, P. and Borgeat, P., Mediators of immediate hypersensitivity, in *Immunopharmacology*, Sirois, P. and Rola-Pleszczynski, M., Eds., Elsevier/North-Holland, Amsterdam, 1982, 201.
10. Borgeat, P. and Samuelsson, B., Transformation of arachidonic acid by rabbit polymorphonuclear leukocytes: formation of a novel dihydroxy-eicosatetraenoic acid, *J. Biol. Chem.*, 254, 2643, 1979.
11. Dahlén, S. E., Bjork, J. Hedqvist, P., Arfors, K. E., Hammarstrom, S., Lindgren, J. A., and Samuelsson, B., Leukotrienes promote plasma leakage and leukocyte adhesion in post-capillary venules: *in vivo* effects with relevance to the acute inflammatory response, *Proc. Natl. Acad. Sci. U.S.A.*, 78, 3887, 1981.
12. Williams, T. J. and Piper, P. J., The action of chemically pure SRS-A on the microcirculation *in vivo*, *Prostaglandins*, 19, 779, 1980.
13. Peck, M. J., Piper, P. J., and Williams, T. J., The effect of leukotrienes C_4 and D_4 on the microvasculature of guinea-pig skin, *Prostaglandins*, 21, 315, 1981.
14. Woodward, D. F., Weichman, B. M., Gill, C. A., and Wasserman, M. A., The effect of synthetic leukotrienes on tracheal microvascular permeability, *Prostaglandins*, 25, 131, 1983.
15. Bray, M. A., Cunningham, F. M., Ford-Hutchinson, A. W., and Smith, M. J. H., Leukotriene B_4: a mediator of vascular permeability, *Br. J. Pharmacol.*, 72, 483, 1981.
16. Björk, J., Hedqvist, P., and Arfors, K. E., Increase in vascular permeability induced by leukotriene B_4 and the role of polymorphonuclear leukocytes, *Inflammation*, 6, 189, 1982.
17. Ueno, A., Tanaka, K., Katori, M., Hayashi, M., and Arai, Y., Species difference in increased vascular permeability by synthetic leukotriene C_4 and D_4, *Prostaglandins*, 21, 637, 1981.
18. Ford-Hutchinson, A. W., Bray, M. A., Doig, M. V., Shipley, M. E., and Smith, M. J. H., Leukotriene B, a potent chemokinetic and aggregating substance released from polymorphonuclear leucocytes, *Nature (London)*, 286, 264, 1980.
19. Palmer, R. M. J., Stepney, R. J., Higgs, G. A., and Eakins, K. E., Chemokinetic activity of arachidonic acid lipoxygenase products on leukocytes of different species, *Prostaglandins*, 20, 411, 1980.
20. Doig, M. V. and Ford-Hutchinson, A. W., The production and characterization of products of the lipoxygenase enzyme system released by rat peritoneal macrophages, *Prostaglandins*, 20, 1007, 1980.
21. König, W., Kroegel, C., Kunau, H. W., and Borgeat, P., Comparison of the eosinophil chemotactic factor (ECF) with endogenous hydroxyeicosatetraenoic acids of leukocytes, *Int. Arch. Allergy Appl. Immunol.*, 66, 165, 1981.
22. Smith, M. J. H., Ford-Hutchinson, A. W., and Bray, M. A., Leukotriene B: a potential mediator of inflammation, *J. Pharm. Pharmacol.*, 32, 517, 1980.
23. Palmblad, J., Malmsten, C. L., Udén, A. M., Radmark, O., Engstedt, L., and Samuelsson, B., Leukotriene B_4 is a potent stereospecific stimulator of neutrophil chemotaxis and adherence, *Blood*, 58, 658, 1981.
24. Camp, R. D. R., Woollard, P. M., Mallet, A. I., and Funcham, N. J., Neutrophil aggregating and chemokinetic properties of a 5,12,20-trihydroxy-6,8,10,14-eicosatetraenoic acid isolated from human leukocytes, *Prostaglandins*, 23, 631, 1982.
25. Ford-Hutchinson, A. W., Rackham, A., Zamboni, R., Rokach, J., and Roy, S., Comparative biological activities of synthetic leukotriene B_4 and its ω-oxidation products, *Prostaglandins*, 25, 29, 1983.

26. Goldman, D. W. and Goetzl, E. J., Specific binding of leukotriene B_4 to receptors on human poly-morphonuclear leukocytes, *J. Immunol.*, 129, 1600, 1982.

27. Flaherty, J. T., Hammett, M. J., Shewmake, T. B., Wykle, R. L., Love, S. H., McCall, C. E., and Thomas, M. J., Evidence for 5,12-dihydroxy-6,8,10,14-eicosatetraenoate as a mediator of human neutrophil aggregation, *Biochem. Biophys. Res. Commun.*, 103, 552, 1981.

28. Cunningham, F. M., Carter, H. R., Smith, M. J. H., Ford-Hutchinson, A. W., and Bray, M. A., Aggregation of polymorphonuclear leucocytes (PMNs) by leukotriene B_4: effects of cyclooxygenase products and metabolic inhibitors, *Agents Actions*, 11, 583, 1981.

29. Cunningham, F. M. and Smith, M. J. H., Leukotriene B_4: biological activities and the cytoskeleton, *Br. J. Pharmacol.*, 75, 383, 1982.

30. Bhattacherjee, P., Hammond, B., Salmon, J. A., Stepney, R., and Eakins, K. E., Chemotactic re-sponse to some arachidonic acid lipoxygenase products in the rabbit eye, *Eur. J. Pharmacol.*, 73, 21, 1981.

31. Bray, M. A., Ford-Hutchinson, A. W., and Smith, M. J. H., Leukotriene B_4: an inflammatory mediator in vivo, *Prostaglandins*, 22, 213, 1981.

32. O'Flaherty, J. T., Thomas, M. J., Cousart, S. L., Salzer, W. L., and McCall, C. E., Neutropenia induced by systemic infusion of 5,12-dihydroxy-6,8,10,14-eicosatetraenoic acid, *J. Clin. Invest.*, 69, 993, 1982.

33. Rae, S. A. and Smith, M. J. H., The stimulation of lysosomal enzyme secretion from human poly-morphonuclear leukocytes by leukotriene B_4, *J. Pharm. Pharmacol.*, 33, 616, 1981.

34. O'Flaherty, J. T., Wykle, R. L., Lees, C. J., Shewmake, T., McCall, C. E., and Thomas, M. J., Neutrophil-degranulating action of 5-12-dihydroxy-6,8,10,14-eicosatetraenoic acid and 1-0-alkyl-2-0-acetyl-sn-glycero-3-phosphocholine, *Am. J. Pathol.*, 105, 264, 1981.

35. Serhan, C. N., Radin, A., Smolen, J. E., Korchak, H., Samuelsson, B., and Weissman, G., Leuko-triene B_4 is a complete secretagogue in human neutrophils: a kinetic analysis, *Biochem. Biophys. Res. Commun.*, 107, 1006, 1982.

36. Showell, H., Naccache, P., Borgeat, P., Picard, S., Vallerand, P., Becker, E., and Sha'afi, R., Characterization of the secretory activity of leukotriene B_4 towards rabbits neutrophils, *J. Immunol.*, 128, 811, 1982.

37. Hafstrom, I., Palmblad, J., Malmsten, C. L., Radmard, O., and Samuelsson, B., Leukotriene B_4 - a stereospecific stimulator for release of lysosomal enzymes from neutrophils, *FEBS Lett.*, 130, 146, 1981.

38. O'Flaherty, J. T., Wykle, R. L., McCall, C. E., Shewmake, T. B., Lees, C. J., and Thomas, M., Desensitization of the human neutrophil degranulation response: studies with 5,12-dihydroxy-6,8,10,14-eicosatetraenoic acid, *Biochem. Biophys. Res. Commun.*, 101, 1290, 1981.

39. Rollins, T. E., Zanolari, B., Springer, M. S., Guindon, Y., Zamboni, R., Lau, C.-K., and Rokach, J., Synthetic leukotriene B_4 is a potent chemotaxin but a weak secretagogue for human PMN, *Prostaglandins*, 25, 281, 1983.

40. Sha'afi, R. I., Naccache, P. H., Molski, T. F., Borgeat, P., and Goetzl, E, J., Intracellular role of leukotriene B_4: its effects on cation homeostasis in rabbit neutrophils, *J. Cell. Physiol.*, 108, 401, 1981.

41. Naccache, P. H., Molski, T. F. P., Becker, E. L., Borgeat, P., Picard, S., Vallerand, P., and Sha'afi, R. I., Specificity of the effect of lipoxygenase metabolites of arachidonic acid on calcium homeostasis in neutrophils: correlation with functional activity, *J. Biol. Chem.*, 257, 8608, 1982.

42. Serhan, C. N., Fridovich, J., Goetzl, E. J., Dunham, P. B., and Weissmann, G., Leukotriene B_4 and phosphatidic acid are calcium ionophores. Studies employing arsenazo III in liposomes, *J. Biol. Chem.*, 257, 4746, 1982.

43. Ramwell, P. W., Leovey, E. M. K., and Sintetos, A. L., Regulation of the arachidonic acid cascade, *Biol. Reprod.*, 16, 70, 1977.

44. Irvine, R. F., How is the level of free arachidonic acid controlled in mammalian cells? *Biochem. J.*, 204, 3, 1982.

45. Lapetina, E. G., Regulation of arachidonic acid production: role of phospholipases C and A_2, *Trends Pharmacol. Sci.*, 3, 115, 1982.

46. Knapp, H. R., Oelz, O., Roberts, J., Sweetman, B. J., Oates, J. A., and Reed, P. W., Ionophores stimulate prostaglandin and thromboxane biosynthesis, *Proc. Natl. Acad. Sci. U.S.A.*, 74, 4251, 1977.

47. Borgeat, P., Hamberg, M., and Samuelsson, B., Transformation of arachidonic acid and homo-γ-linolenic acid in rabbit polymorphonuclear leukocytes, *J. Biol. Chem.*, 252, 8772, 1977.

48. Borgeat, P. and Samuelsson, B., Metabolism of arachidonic acid in polymorphonuclear leukocytes. Effects of the ionophore A23187, *Proc. Natl. Acad. Sci. U.S.A.*, 76, 2148, 1979.

49. Maclouf, J., Fruteau de Laclos, B., and Borgeat, P., Stimulation of leukotriene biosynthesis in hu-man blood leukocytes by platelet-derived 12-hydroperoxy-icosatetraenoic acid, *Proc. Natl. Acad. Sci. U.S.A.*, 79, 6042, 1982.

50. Parker, C. W. and Aykent, S., Calcium stimulation of the 5-lipoxygenase from RBL-1 cells, *Biochem. Biophys. Res. Commun.*, 109, 1011, 1982.
51. Aehringhaus, U., Wölbling, R. H., König, W., Patrono, C., Peskar, B. M., and Peskar, B. A., Release of leukotriene C_4 from human polymorphonuclear leucocytes as determined by radioimmunoassay, *FEBS Lett.*, 146, 111, 1982.
52. Hansson, G. and Radmark, O., Leukotriene C_4: isolation from human polymorphonuclear leukocytes, *FEBS Lett.*, 122, 87, 1980.
53. Jörg, A., Henderson, W. R., Murphy, R. C., and Klebanoff, S. J., Leukotriene generation by eosinophils, *J. Exp. Med.*, 155, 390, 1982.
54. Fels, A. O., Pawlowski, N. A., Cramer, E. B., King, T. K. C., Cohn, Z. A., and Scott, W. A., Human alveolar macrophages produce leukotriene B_4, *Proc. Natl. Acad. Sci. U.S.A.*, 79, 7866, 1982.
55. Damon, M., Chavis, C., Godard, Ph., Michel, F. B., and Crastes de Paulet, A., Purification and mass spectrometry identification of leukotriene D_4 synthesized by human alveolar macrophages, *Biochem. Biophys. Res. Commun.*, 111, 518, 1983.
56. Rankin, J. A., Hitchcock, M., Merrill, W., Bach, M. K., Brashler, J. R., and Askenase, P. W., IgE-dependent release of leukotriene C_4 from alveolar macrophages, *Nature (London)*, 297, 329, 1982.
57. Scott, W. A., Rouzer, C. A., and Cohn, Z. A., Leukotriene C release by macrophages, *Fed. Proc. Fed. Am. Soc. Exp. Biol.*, 42, 129, 1983.
58. Goetzl, E. J., Selective feedback inhibition of the 5-lipoxygenation of arachidonic acid in human T-lymphocytes, *Biochem. Biophys. Res. Commun.*, 101, 344, 1981.
59. Humes, J. L., Sadowski, S., Galavage, M., Goldenberg, M., Subers, E., Bonney, R. J., and Kuehl, F. A., Jr., Evidence for two sources of arachidonic acid for oxidative metabolism by mouse peritoneal macrophages, *J. Biol. Chem.*, 257, 1591, 1982.
60. Scott, W. A., Pawlowski, N. A., Murray, H. W., Andreach, M., Zrike, J., and Cohn, Z. A., Regulation of arachidonic acid metabolism by macrophage activation, *J. Exp. Med.*, 155, 1148, 1982.
61. Rouzer, C. A., Scott, W. A., Hamill, A. L., and Cohn, Z. A., Synthesis of leukotriene C and other arachidonic acid metabolites by mouse pulmonary macrophages, *J. Exp. Med.*, 155, 720, 1982.
62. Hsueh, W. and Sun, F. F., Leukotriene B_4 biosynthesis by alveolar macrophages, *Biochem. Biophys. Res. Commun.*, 106, 1085, 1982.
63. Walsh, C. E., Waite, B. M., Thomas, M. J., and DeChatelet, L. R., Release and metabolism of arachidonic acid in human neutrophils, *J. Biol. Chem.*, 256, 7228, 1981.
64. Walsh, C. E., Dechatelet, L. R., Thomas, M. J., O'Flaherty, J. T., and Waite, M., Effect of phagocytosis and ionophores on release and metabolism of arachidonic acid from human neutrophils, *Lipids*, 16, 120, 1981.
65. Claesson, H. E., Lundberg, U., and Malmsten, C., Serum-coated zymosan stimulates the synthesis of leukotriene B_4 in human polymorphonuclear leukocytes. Inhibition by cyclic AMP, *Biochem. Biophys. Res. Commun.*, 99, 1230, 1981.
66. Shiffmann, E., Corcoran, B. A., and Wahl, S. M., N-formylmethionyl peptides as chemoattractants for leucocytes, *Proc. Natl. Acad. Sci. U.S.A.*, 72, 1059, 1975.
67. O'Flaherty, J. T., Showell, H. J., Ward, P. A., and Becker, E. L., A possible role of arachidonic acid in human neutrophil aggregation and degranulation, *Am. J. Pathol.*, 96, 799, 1979.
68. Naccache, P. H., Showell, H. J., Becker, E. L., and Sha'afi, R. I., Arachidonic acid induced degranulation of rabbit peritoneal neutrophils, *Biochem. Biophys. Res. Commun.*, 87, 292, 1979.
69. Bokoch, G. M. and Reed, P. W., Stimulation of arachidonic acid metabolism in the polymorphonuclear leukocyte by an N-formylated peptide. Comparison with ionophore A23187, *J. Biol. Chem.*, 255, 10223, 1980.
70. Bonser, R. W., Siegel, M. I., McConnell, R. T., and Cuatrecas, P., Chemotactic peptide stimulated endogenous arachidonic acid metabolism in HL60 granulocytes, *Biochem. Biophys. Res. Commun.*, 102, 1269, 1981.
71. Jubiz, W., Radmark, O., Malmsten, C., Hansson, G., Lindgren, J. A., Palmblad, J., Udén, A. M., and Samuelsson, B., A novel leukotriene produced by stimulation of leukocytes with formylmethionylleucylphenylalanine, *J. Biol. Chem.*, 257, 6106, 1982.
72. Benveniste, J., Jouvin, E., Pirotzky, E., Arnoux, B., Mencia-Huerta, J. M., Roubin, R., and Vargaftig, B. B., Platelet-activating factor (PAF-acether): molecular aspects of its release and pharmacological actions, *Int. Arch. Allergy Appl. Immunol.*, 66(Suppl. 1), 121, 1981.
73. Chilton, F. H., O'Flaherty, J. T., Walsh, C. E., Thomas, M. J., Wykle, R. L., DeChatelet, L. R., and Waite, B. M., Stimulation of the lipoxygenase pathway in polymorphonuclear leukocytes by 1-0-alkyl-2-0-acetyl-SN-glycero-3-phosphocholine, *J. Biol. Chem.*, 257, 5402, 1982.
74. Lin, A. H., Morton, D. R., and Gorman, R. R., Acetyl glyceryl ether phosphorylcholine stimulates leukotriene B_4 synthesis in human polymorphonuclear leukocytes, *J. Clin. Invest.*, 70, 1058, 1982.
75. Vargaftig, B. B., Chignard, M., Lefort, J., and Benveniste, J., Platelet-tissue interaction: role of platelet-activating factor (PAF-acether), *Agents Actions*, 10, 502, 1980.

76. Marcus, A. J., Broekman, M. J., Safier, L. B., Ullman, H. L., Islam, N., Serhan, C. N., Rutherford, L. E., Korchak, H. M., and Weissmann, G., Formation of leukotrienes and other hydroxy acids during platelet-neutrophil interactions *in vitro, Biochem. Biophys. Res. Commun.,* 109, 130, 1982.

77. Rola-Pleszczynki, M., Borgeat, P., and Sirois, P., Leukotriene B$_4$ induces human suppressor lymphocytes, *Biochem. Biophys. Res. Commun.,* 108, 1531, 1982.

78. Webb, D. R., Nowowiejski, I., Healy, C., and Rogers, T. J., Immunosuppressive properties of leukotrienes D$_4$ and E$_4$ *in vitro, Biochem. Biophys. Res. Commun.,* 104, 1617, 1982.

79. Bailey, J. M., Bryant, R. W., Low, C. E., Pupilla, M. B., and Vanderhoeck, J. Y., Regulation of T-lymphocyte mitogenesis by the leucocyte product, 15-HETE, *Cell, Immunol.,* 67, 112, 1982.

80. Shou, L., Schwartz, S. A., and Good, R. A., Suppressor cell activity after concanavalin A treatment of leucocytes from normal donors, *J. Exp. Med.,* 143, 1100, 1976.

81. Rola-Pleszczynski, M. and Blanchard, R., Suppressor cell function in respiratory allergy, *Int. Arch. Allergy Appl. Immunol.,* 64, 361, 1981.

82. Haynes, B. F. and Fauci, A. S., Activation of human B-lymphocytes, *J. Immunol.,* 121, 559, 1978.

83. Rola-Pleszczynski, M. and Lieu, H., Concomitant induction of cytotoxic and suppressor cells: modulation by theophylline, *Cell. Immunol.,* 65, 13, 1981.

84. Rocklin, R. E., Breard, J., Gupta, S., Good, R. A., and Melmon, K. L., Characterization of the human blood lymphocytes that produced a histamine-induced suppressor factor (HSS), *Cell. Immunol.,* 51, 226, 1980.

85. Rocklin, R. E. and Haberk-Davidson, A., Histamine activates suppressor cells *in vitro* using a co-culture technique, *J. Clin. Immunol.,* 1, 73, 1981.

86. Payan, D. G., Valone, S. H., and Goetzl, E. J., Leukotriene modulation of human T-lymphocyte function, *Fed. Proc. Fed. Am. Soc. Exp. Biol.,* 42, 444, 1983.

87. Rola-Pleszczynski, M. and Sirois, P., Leukotrienes as immunoregulators, in *Leukotrienes and Other Lipoxygenase Products,* Piper, P. J., Ed., John Wiley & Sons, London, in press.

88. Wadee, A. A. and Rabson, A. R., Binding of phosphatidyl-ethanolamine and phosphatidylinositol to OKT8$^+$ lymphocytes activates suppressor cell activity, *J. Immunol.,* 130, 1271, 1983.

89. Reinherz, E. and Scholssman, S. F., The differentiation and function of human T lymphocytes, *Cell,* 19, 821, 1980.

90. Kohl, S., Jansen, D. M., and Loo, L. S., Indomethacin enhancement of human natural killer cytotoxicity to herpes simplex virus infected cells *in vitro* and *in vivo, Prostaglandins Leukotrienes Med.,* 9, 159, 1982.

91. Bankhurst, A. D., The modulation of human natural killer cell activity by prostaglandins, *J. Clin. Lab. Immunol.,* 7, 85, 1982.

92. Koren, H. S. and Leung, K. M., Modulation of human NK cells by interferon and prostaglandin E$_1$, *Mol. Immunol.,* 19, 1341, 1982.

93. Rola-Pleszczynski, M., Gagnon, L., and Sirois, P., Leukotriene B$_4$ augments human natural cytotoxic cell activity, *Biochem. Biophys. Res. Commun.,* in press.

94. Seaman, W. E., Natural killer cell activity reversibly inhibited by inhibitors of lipoxygenase, *Fed. Proc. Fed. Am. Soc. Exp. Biol.,* 42, 1379, 1983.

95. Henney, C. S., Kuribayashi, K., Kern, D. E., and Gillis, S., Interleukin-2 augments natural killer cell activities, *Nature (London),* 291, 335, 1981.

96. Rola-Pleszczynski, M., Gagnon, L., Rudzinska, P., Borgeat, P., and Sirois, P., Human natural cytotoxic cell activity: enhancement by leukotrienes (LT) A$_4$, B$_4$ and D$_4$ but not by stereoisomers of LTB$_4$ or HETEs, *Prostaglandins Leukotrienes Med.,* in press.

97. Klickstein, L. B., Shapleigh, C., and Goetzl, E. J., Lipoxygenation of arachidonic acid as a source of polymorphonuclear leukocyte chemotactic factors in synovial fluid and tissue in rheumatoid arthritis and spondyloarthritis, *J. Clin. Invest.,* 66, 1166, 1980.

98. Davidson, E. M., Rae, S. A., and Smith, M. J. H., Leukotriene B$_4$ in synovial fluid, *J. Pharm. Pharmacol.,* 34, 410, 1982.

99. Cromwell, O., Walport, M. J., Morris, H. R., Taylor, G. W., Hodson, M. E., Batten, J., and Kay, A. B., Identification of leukotrienes D and B in sputum from cystic fibrosis patients, *Lancet,* July 25, p. 164, 1981.

100. Borgeat, P. and Laviolette, M., Unpublished data.

Chapter 3

ARACHIDONIC ACID METABOLISM IN THE FETUS AND NEONATE

Murray D. Mitchell, Shaun P. Brennecke, Sheikh A. Saeed, and Daniel M. Strickland

TABLE OF CONTENTS

I. INTRODUCTION

The human fetus exists in an environment in which there is an apparent over-abundance of prostaglandins (PGs). This is true also, to some extent, of the neonate. Since both the fetus and neonate have a significant potential for PG catabolism, it may be inferred that some benefits accrue from a PG-rich environment. Hence, it is reasonable to assume that PGs are serving important roles in both intrauterine and early extrauterine life. PGs are formed from nonesterified arachidonic acid by the action of fatty acid cyclooxygenase. Arachidonic acid may be metabolized also by way of lipoxygenase enzyme pathways. Little information is available concerning these pathways in fetal and neonatal tissues. Significantly, products of the lipoxygenase pathways are known to modulate PG biosynthesis. In this chapter it is our intent to describe the results of studies designed to evaluate arachidonic acid metabolism in the fetus and neonate. We will focus attention also on arachidonic acid metabolism in uterine and intrauterine tissues since the products of such metabolism are almost certainly of great importance for normal fetal growth and development. For the purposes of this review we will concentrate exclusively on the human fetus and neonate.

II. CONCENTRATIONS OF EICOSANOIDS IN PLASMA

A. Fetal Circulation

Information on the concentrations of hormones in the plasma of human fetuses has been limited to that obtained from measurements in umbilical plasma obtained at delivery. Recently, however, blood samples have been obtained by fetoscopy from human fetuses at 16 to 20 weeks of gestation and PG concentrations determined.[1] The PGs measured in the study were PGE_2, $PGF_{2\alpha}$, and 6-keto-$PGF_{1\alpha}$. 6-Keto-$PGF_{1\alpha}$ is the nonenzymatically formed product of prostacyclin (PGI_2) degradation.[2] Concentrations of PGs in fetal plasma are greater than concentrations of the same PGs in maternal peripheral plasma. Strikingly, the concentrations of 6-keto-$PGF_{1\alpha}$ in fetal plasma are many-fold greater than concentrations in the maternal circulation. These findings suggest that PGI_2 may serve an important role in the fetus during early pregnancy. Whether PGI_2 circulating in the fetus is acting to influence fetal organogenesis or is exerting a tonic effect on the placental vascular bed is uncertain. PGI_2 is potently inhibitory of platelet aggregation and also is a highly active vasodilatory agent.[3] Hence it is not unreasonable to propose that high concentrations of PGI_2 circulating in the fetus, which are reflected by plasma concentrations of 6-keto-$PGF_{1\alpha}$, are part of a biological protection mechanism for the fetus (PGI_2 being protective of umbilical-placental blood flow and aiding maintenance of adequate oxygenation and nutrition for the fetus).

B. Umbilical Circulation

Concentrations of PGE_2, $PGF_{2\alpha}$, and 13,14-dihydro-15-keto-$PGF_{2\alpha}$ (PGFM, the major circulating metabolite of $PGF_{2\alpha}$ in umbilical plasma are greater than those in maternal plasma[4-6] (Table 1), whereas maternal and fetal plasma concentrations of 6-keto-$PGF_{1\alpha}$ and thromboxane (TX)B_2 (TXB_2, the degradation product formed from TXA_2) are similar.[7,8] Concentrations of PGE, PGF, and PGFM are all significantly raised in umbilical plasma obtained after the onset of labor,[6,9] indicating that labor is a stimulus to PG production by the feto-placental unit. Umbilical plasma concentrations of 6-keto-$PGF_{1\alpha}$ and TXB_2, however, are unaffected by labor. A significant arterio-venous difference exists across the umbilical circulation for PGE_2, with higher concentrations in venous plasma. This arterio-venous difference exists both before and after the onset of labor.[6,9] Similar arterio-venous plasma differences cannot be demonstrated for

Table 1

PGs IN THE MATERNAL AND UMBILICAL
CIRCULATIONS AT TERM[5,6]

	Maternal circulating		Umbilical (spontaneous labor)	
	Late pregnancy n = 13	Labor; cervix, 5—8 cm n = 5	Artery n = 12	Vein n = 12
PGE	4.8 ± 1.0	5.4 ± 2.2	109.3 ± 26.9	241.9 ± 24.9
PGF	6.2 ± 0.5	12.4 ± 3.5	79.7 ± 10.4	87.8 ± 11.1
PGFM	59.0 ± 7.8	282.7 ± 55.3	639.9 ± 180.2	630.8 ± 107.3

Note: All values are given as pg/mℓ mean ± SEM.

PGF, PGFM, 6-keto-PGF$_{1\alpha}$, or TXB$_2$. The finding that PGE concentrations are higher in umbilical venous blood than in umbilical arterial blood has been considered as suggestive that PGE in the fetal circulation is, at least partly, placental in origin. This proposition is consistent with the results of studies in sheep in which the fetal placenta appears to be a major source of PGE.[10,11] The elegant studies of Coceani and Olley[12] and Elliott and Starling[13,14] have clearly indicated that PGE maintains the patency of the ductus arteriosus in utero in experimental animals and this is likely the case in the human fetus. Hence, the high PGE concentration in the umbilical circulation at birth reflects an intrauterine environment in which patency of the ductus arteriosus would be maintained with PGE being dominant over PGF. It should be noted that the possibility has been raised that products of arachidonate lipoxygenase action may play a part in the mechanism of ductal closure.[15] However, strong evidence has been presented[16] that lipoxygenase-derived products of arachidonic acid do not play a role in closure of the ductus arteriosus.

C. Neonatal Circulation

The first report describing plasma PG levels in the neonatal period came from Siegler and co-workers,[17] who measured PGE in cord blood after term delivery and in peripheral plasma at 2 to 3 days of age and throughout childhood. The plasma level of PGE was found to be significantly lower at 2 to 3 days of age compared with values in cord blood but then increased continuously thereafter until adult life. The authors speculated that low levels of PGE may reflect functional peculiarities of the immature kidney. These results must be interpreted with caution since the adult plasma levels of PGE described were approximately 10-fold greater than accepted values. In a study of the possible relationship between PGs and respiratory distress syndrome Friedman and Demers[18] measured plasma levels of PGE and PGF in a control group of infants over the first 10 days of life following preterm delivery. No difference was found in circulating levels of either PGE or PGF between the first and tenth day after delivery. The authors did not comment on the sustained high levels of PGE and PGF during the period of ductal closure when enhanced PG catabolism would be expected. Using highly sensitive radioimmunoassay methods[5] that can accurately determine adult plasma concentrations, consistent with accepted values, we have found that circulating concentrations of PGE in neonates born at term are significantly reduced by the sixth day of extrauterine life compared with levels at birth.[19] Mean concentrations of PGF and PGFM also are lowered in the first week of life, although not to the same extent. Quite a different pattern obtains for circulating concentrations of 6-keto-PGF$_{1\alpha}$ and TXB$_2$ in the perinatal period.[20] By 6 days after vaginal delivery at term, neonates have higher circulating levels of both 6-keto-PGF$_{1\alpha}$ and TXB$_2$ than at birth. Infants born

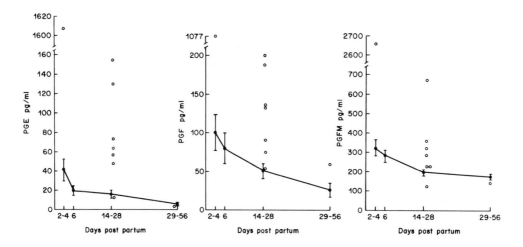

FIGURE 1.   Concentrations of PGs (mean ± SEM, n = 6) in plasma from normal preterm infants (•) compared with concentrations in plasma from infants with patent ductus arteriosus (o). (From Lucas, A. and Mitchell, M. D., *Lancet,* 2, 130, 1978. With permission.)

before term, but uncomplicated by major disease, have plasma concentrations of PGE, PGF, and PGFM on the sixth day of life, similar to those of infants born at term. Delivery before term is not therefore associated with obvious differences in capacity for PG biosynthesis or metabolism in the neonatal period. It has been found that PG concentrations in the plasma of preterm infants are raised above those of adults for at least 60 days (Figure 1). Significantly, concentrations of PGE in neonatal plasma decline more rapidly than concentrations of other PGs, and this reduction may play an active or facilitatory role in closure of the ductus arteriosus. It should be noted that PGI_2 and TXA_2 have little action on the ductus arteriosus.[21]

D. Neonatal Diseases

Infants with a patent ductus arteriosus have been shown to have excessively high circulating concentrations of PGE, PGF, and PGFM,[22] the elevation in PGE concentrations being particularly impressive (Figure 1). This finding has been disputed by Friedman and Demers[18] who reported that concentrations of PGF fall and levels of PGE rise shortly before the appearance of clinical symptoms of patent ductus arteriosus in neonates. In another study[23] concentrations of both PGE and PGF were found to be elevated shortly before clinical symptoms of patent ductus arteriosus were noted; however, it was found that the PGE to PGF ratio increased markedly at the same time. PGE_2 has been used to maintain the ductus arteriosus patent in neonates with certain forms of congenital cyanotic heart disease in whom oxygenation is dependent upon a patent ductus arteriosus.[24,25]

Constriction of the ductus arteriosus of human fetuses by the maternal administration of an inhibitor of PG synthesis has been demonstrated.[26] In a proportion of neonates born to mothers who have ingested such drugs persistent pulmonary hypertension of the newborn has been diagnosed[27] and drastically reduced plasma PGE concentrations have been reported.[28] Persistent pulmonary hypertension of the newborn is a potentially life-threatening disease. Hence one may safely suggest that since PGE_2 in the fetal circulation is of critical importance for maintaining the patency of the ductus arteriosus, then maintenance of high circulating levels of PGE_2 constitutes a biological protection mechanism. Medical management of patent ductus arteriosus with PG synthetase inhibitors, e.g., indomethacin, while consistently lowering PG concentrations in plasma does not always result in ductal closure.[22] Moreover, surgical ligation of the ductus arteriosus does not immediately reduce circulating PG concentrations.[22]

Friedman and Demers[18] have suggested that neonates who develop respiratory distress syndrome have raised plasma levels of PGE and PGF. The authors' own study[29] of infants with hyaline membrane disease was indicative that plasma concentrations of PGE are normal in such infants, although we also found significantly increased levels of PGF. Furthermore, plasma concentrations of PGFM were raised several-fold over control values, and this increase was disproportionate to the increase in PGF levels. Whether treatment with PG synthetase inhibitors to reduce the increased biosynthesis of PGF may be of some benefit to infants with hyaline membrane disease remains an open question.

III. METABOLISM OF ARACHIDONIC ACID IN TISSUES

A. Fetal Tissues
1. Cyclooxygenase Pathway

The potential for prostanoid (essentially PG and TX) biosynthesis by human fetal tissues has only recently been evaluated in detail.[30] Human fetal tissues were obtained from pregnancies in the first and second trimesters of gestation. Tissues were minced into small pieces and then superfused. The method of tissue superfusion allows prostanoids, formed acutely due to the traumatization of tissues, to be removed before commencing timed collections under steady-state conditions. The results of the study are presented diagrammatically in Figure 2. The rate of formation of 6-keto-PGF$_{1\alpha}$ by all tissues studied was generally greater than the rate of formation of PGF$_{2\alpha}$ or PGE$_2$. The highest rate of formation of 6-keto-PGF$_{1\alpha}$ was by aorta. It is not surprising that PGI$_2$ formation was greatest in a vascular tissue since the intimal lining of vascular tissue is considered to be a major site of PGI$_2$ biosynthesis.[31] Furthermore, vascular tissue from fetuses of other animal species has been shown to produce predominantly PGI$_2$.[32,33] PGI$_2$ so formed is undoubtedly protective of the vasculature and serves to prevent platelet adhesion and clumping. Intriguingly, the highest rate of formation of 6-keto-PGF$_{1\alpha}$ by a fetal tissue, excluding aorta, was by stomach. In adult tissue, it is thought that PGI$_2$ may act in the stomach to have a cytoprotective effect.[34] The fetal lung and adrenal also produce PGI$_2$, although at lower rates. The adult lung has been thought to be a major source of PGI$_2$.[35,36] Formation of PGI$_2$ by the human fetal adrenal is of interest since PGI$_2$ is a potent stimulant of adenylate cyclase activity[37] and hence may be of importance as a regulator of steroid hormone formation. In general, in the other tissues investigated, the rate of production of PGF$_{2\alpha}$ was greater than that of PGE$_2$. This finding is consistent with the results of studies by Pace-Asciak[38] using fetal tissues from sheep early in gestation. Pace-Asciak reported that the ratio of PGF$_{2\alpha}$ to PGE$_2$ formation was reversed closer to delivery. Such data obviously are unavailable for human fetal tissues.

2. Lipoxygenase Pathways

The first detailed evaluation of arachidonic acid metabolism by way of lipoxygenase pathways in human fetal tissues has been conducted recently.[39] Human fetal tissues were obtained after voluntary termination of pregnancy between 12 and 18 weeks of gestational age. Tissues were minced and homogenized prior to incubation with radiolabeled arachidonic acid. Following incubation of homogenates with radiolabeled arachidonic acid, the radiolabeled products were extracted and subjected to thin layer chromatography (TLC). The various lipoxygenase products, separated by TLC mobilities, were determined and are shown in Figure 3. All tissues investigated formed lipoxygenase derivatives of arachidonic acid. The extent of conversion of arachidonic acid

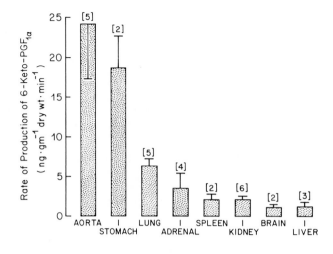

A

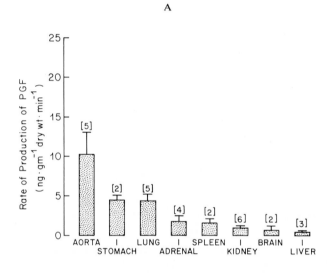

B

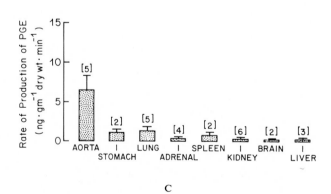

C

FIGURE 2.   Rates of production of PGs [(A) 6-keto-PGF$_{1a}$; (B) PGF$_{2a}$; (C) PGE$_2$] by human fetal tissues superfused in vitro.

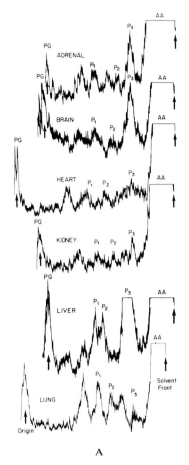

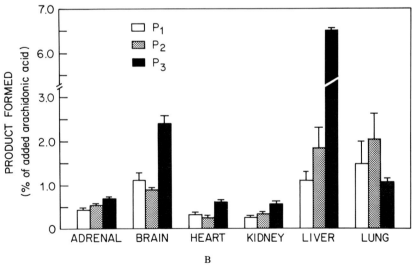

FIGURE 3.   (A) Radiochromatograms of the products formed upon incubation of homogenates of human fetal tissues with [^{14}C] arachidonic acid. PG: prostaglandin; P_{1-3}: lipoxygenase products; AA: arachidonic acid. (Modified from Saeed, S. A. and Mitchell, M. D., *Biochem. Med.*, 30, 322, 1983.) (B) Conversion of [^{14}C] arachidonic acid to radiolabeled lipoxygenase products (P_{1-3}) by homogenates of human fetal tissues. Results are presented as means ± SEM of three determinations. (From Saeed, S. A. and Mitchell, M. D., *Biochem. Med.*, 30, 322, 1983. With permission.)

Table 2
RATES OF PRODUCTION OF PROSTANOIDS BY HUMAN INTRAUTERINE TISSUES SUPERFUSED IN VITRO[8,46,47]

| | Prostanoid | Production of prostanoid (ng/min/g dry wt) | | | |
		Amnion	Chorion	Decidua	Placenta
Tissues obtained after	PGE	13.17 ± 2.21	2.89 ± 0.46	1.72 ± 0.24	2.02 ± 0.38
spontaneous vaginal	PGF	0.83 ± 0.19	0.51 ± 0.12	0.49 ± 0.09	0.66 ± 0.13
delivery	TXB_2	1.59 ± 0.37	0.61 ± 0.19	2.13 ± 0.38	4.94 ± 0.39
	6-Keto-$PGF_{1\alpha}$	6.31 ± 2.40	2.43 ± 0.64	1.46 ± 0.43	1.33 ± 0.39
Tissues obtained at	PGE	9.62 ± 1.62	3.13 ± 0.59	2.50 ± 0.57	2.84 ± 0.47
elective Caesarean	PGF	0.74 ± 0.19	0.76 ± 0.20	0.80 ± 0.25	0.82 ± 0.24
section	TXB_2	2.42 ± 0.79	0.88 ± 0.26	2.76 ± 1.09	4.84 ± 1.05
	6-Keto-$PGF_{1\alpha}$	2.37 ± 0.65	1.76 ± 0.40	1.41 ± 0.38	1.11 ± 0.21

Note: Values are means $\pm$ S.E.M. for 10 individual determinations.

to the various lipoxygenase derivatives is given in Figure 3B. As can be readily observed the liver was a major source of lipoxygenase metabolites. The high rates of conversion of arachidonic acid to lipoxygenase metabolites by the human fetal liver are similar to the high rates of formation of such metabolites in adult rat liver.[40]

Although absolute identification of the products formed is not available, P2 and P3 have chromatographic mobilities identical with (5S) 5-hydroxy-6,8,11,14-eicosatetraenoic acid (5-HETE) and 12-HETE, respectively. It should be noted that the formation of 5-HETE reflects the biosynthesis of the precursor 5-HPETE, which is an essential intermediate in the formation of leukotrienes.[41] Both 12-HPETE and 15-HPETE have been shown to inhibit PGI_2 formation[42,43] and hence the production of 12-HETE by tissues may well form part of a self-regulatory mechanism of arachidonic acid metabolism; however, the rate of formation of PGI_2 also has been shown to be enhanced by certain leukotrienes.[44,45] The relative rates of formation of different lipoxygenase derivatives may therefore be of signal importance in the regulation of PGI_2 formation by fetal tissues.

B. Uterine and Intrauterine Tissues
1. Cyclooxygenase Pathway

Using the technique of tissue superfusion described earlier, a concerted series of experiments have been performed to evaluate the production of prostanoids by uterine and intrauterine tissues. The results of such studies[8,46,47] have been drawn together in Table 2. Amnion is a significant source of PGE_2 and indeed PGE_2 is the major prostanoid synthesized by most tissues. Substantial formation of TXB_2, however, occurs in decidua vera and placenta. The mean rate of formation of PGE_2 by amnion tissue after labor in one study[46] was almost 50% higher than before labor, although the difference was not statistically significant. Subsequently Okazaki et al.[48] have demonstrated that there is a significant increase in PG synthase activity in amnion during labor. It is widely considered that the biosynthesis of PGE_2 by fetal membranes, and in particular amnion, is of signal importance in the events culminating in the onset and maintenance of labor. The low rates of formation of $PGF_{2\alpha}$ by the tissues are consistent with an environment in which the production of substances with vasoconstrictor activity should be minimized. PGI_2 formation by the various intrauterine tissues may act as a tonic stimulus to utero-placental blood flow and hence be protective of fetal development. Data are also available suggestive that the cervix is a major source of PGs, particularly of the E series, and it has been hypothesized that softening and dilation of

Table 3

RATES OF PRODUCTION OF PGD₂ BY HUMAN INTRAUTERINE TISSUES
SUPERFUSED IN VITRO

Tissues obtained[a]	Rate of production of PGD_2 (mean ± SEM; ng/g dry wt/min)			
	Placenta	Amnion	Chorion laeve	Decidua vera
1. Cesarean section before labor (n = 4)	8.16 ± 1.71	2.36 ± 0.65	2.09 ± 0.62	1.43± 0.48
2. Vaginal delivery after spontaneous labor (n = 4)	10.49 ± 3.37	3.22 ± 0.88	3.58 ± 0.98	3.06 ± 1.17
1 and 2 combined[b] (n = 8)	9.32 ± 1.80	2.79 ± 0.53	2.83 ± 0.61	2.25 ± 0.66
	(a)	(b)	(c)	(d)

Note: Statistical differences: (a) vs. (b) (c) (d) $p < 0.01$; all others $p > 0.1$.

[a] For further details see text.
[b] For all tissues 1 and 2 were not significantly different ($p > 0.1$).

From Mitchell, M. D., Kraemer, D. L., and Strickland, D. M., *Prostaglandins, Leukotrienes Med.*, 8, 383, 1982. With permission.

the cervix at term are dependent upon locally formed PGs.[49,50] Such an action is a protective mechanism for the fetus, since without cervical softening and dilatation, the onset of labor would result in contractions during which the fetus would be pressed against an inflexible structure. PG formation has also been demonstrated in myometrium. Recently, we have obtained evidence that the placenta is a major source of PGD_2[51] (Table 3). This observation may be of great significance for fetal well-being since it has been shown that in sheep, PGD_2 is a potent dilator of the utero-placental vascular bed.[52] We have hypothesized that reduced secretion of PGD_2 may play a role in the morbidity associated with pregnancy-induced hypertension. It should be noted that PGD_2 is also an inhibitor of platelet aggregation,[53] therefore, its properties mimic those of PGI_2, although PGD_2 is known to have its own receptor.[54]

2. Lipoxygenase Pathways

Human uterine and intrauterine tissues have the potential to form lipoxygenase metabolites of arachidonic acid.[55] The major lipoxygenase product formed by human amnion, decidua vera, and placenta is 12-HETE with smaller amounts of 5-HETE also formed (Figure 4). Chorion laeve produces only a trace amount of 12-HETE. It has been postulated that since various HETEs are potent chemotactic agents for human neutrophils, eosinophils, and macrophages (see Chapter 2) production of these metabolites by human intrauterine tissues may serve to regulate leukocyte and/or macrophage infiltration during pregnancy and parturition.[56] Such infiltration occurs in cervical tissue during cervical ripening,[57] and it has been demonstrated that the cervix produces lipoxygenase derivatives of arachidonic acid.[58] Arachidonate lipoxygenase activities are resident also in myometrium.[56] Again, the balance between potential leukotriene stimulation of prostanoid formation and the potential inhibition of PGI_2 formation by 12-HPETE and 15-HPETE may be of crucial importance to normal physiological function or the production of a pathophysiological state. The biosynthesis of lipoxygenase derivatives of arachidonic acid by placental tissue may be of critical importance in the maintenance of fetal homeostasis since changes in formation of PGI_2 and/or other prostanoids in this tissue could lead directly to a change in utero-placental blood flow and hence to oxygenation of the fetus. The arachidonate lipoxygenase

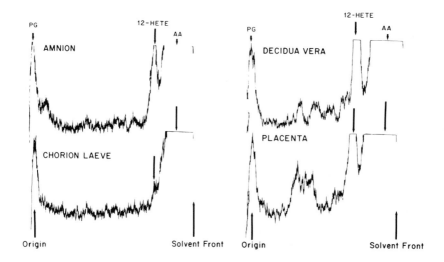

FIGURE 4.   Radiochromatograms of the products formed upon incubation of homogenates of human intrauterine tissues with [^{14}C] arachidonic acid. PG: prostaglandin; 12-
HETE: 12-L-hydroxy-5,8,10,14-eicosatetraenoic acid; AA: arachidonic acid. (From Saeed,
S. A. and Mitchell, M. D., *Prostaglandins, Leukotrienes Med.*, 8, 635, 1982. With permission.)

products formed in other uterine and intrauterine tissues may serve important functions in the mechanisms of the onset of labor at term. Once again, any alteration in
the normal progression of labor would result in deleterious effects on the fetus, and
hence the production of lipoxygenase metabolites in these tissues may be considered
important for fetal well-being.

IV. REGULATION OF THE METABOLISM OF ARACHIDONIC ACID

A. Inhibitory Factors
1. Inhibition of Prostanoid Biosynthesis

In 1977, Saeed and co-workers[59] demonstrated the existence of a circulating inhibitor
of PG synthesis. This substance they named EIPS (endogenous inhibitor of PG synthesis; Figure 5). EIPS activity in the plasma of pregnant women has been demonstrated[60] and the activity is thought to fall to a small but significant, extent during the
third trimester of pregnancy.[61] Recently, however, a significant fall during labor in the
activity of EIPS in amniotic fluid has been demonstrated (Figure 6).[62] This is a key
observation since amniotic fluid is the fluid that bathes the amnion, which as we have
already suggested, is a key structure in the mechanisms of the onset of human labor
through its production of PGE$_2$. Hence it is possible that the biosynthesis of PGs is
tonically inhibited throughout pregnancy and that such inhibition is withdrawn at the
onset of labor. This inhibition of PG biosynthesis is undoubtedly of benefit to the fetus
since it prevents labor before term and may reduce excessive PG formation near the
utero-placental vascular bed, which could lead to vascular constriction. The fetus has
less EIPS activity in its plasma than the adult; this is true both in sheep and in man.[63]
Umbilical plasma has less EIPS activity than adult plasma although no aterio-venous
differences have been found. EIPS concentrations in the neonate increase gradually
during the first month of life to reach adult levels by 1 to 2 months of life. Interestingly, this is just the opposite of circulating PG levels, which decline to those of the
adult during the same time period.

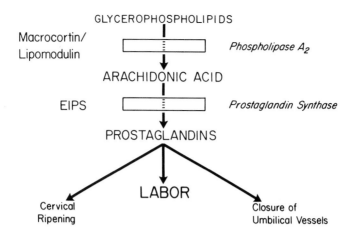

FIGURE 5. A simplified representation of some aspects of arachidonic acid metabolism.

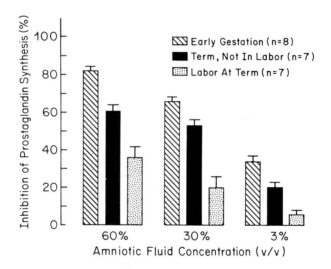

FIGURE 6. The inhibition of PG synthesis by human amniotic fluid in relation to gestation and labor. Results are presented as means ± SEM inhibitory activities for amniotic fluid (at three concentrations) obtained in early gestation (15 to 17 weeks), term gestation, and term gestation in spontaneous labor. (From Saeed, S. A., Strickland, D. M., Young, D., Dang, A., and Mitchell, M. D., *J. Clin. Endocrinol. Metab.,* 55, 801, 1982. With permission.)

2. Inhibition of Lipoxygenase Activities

An endogenous inhibitor of lipoxygenase activity has been described.[64] No substantial information is available on such activity during pregnancy and parturition, although we have recently obtained results suggesting that such an inhibitor is present in human amniotic fluid. If this inhibitor does circulate in pregnant women, it may serve to regulate lipoxygenase activities and hence may be important in preventing the potential deleterious effects of 12-HPETE and 15-HPETE on PGI_2 formation within the uterus.

3. Inhibition of Phospolipase Activities

The elegant studies of Flower and Blackwell[65,66] and Hirata and colleagues[67] have

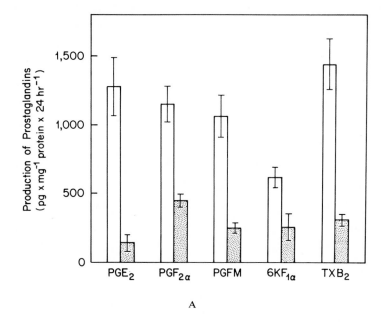

A

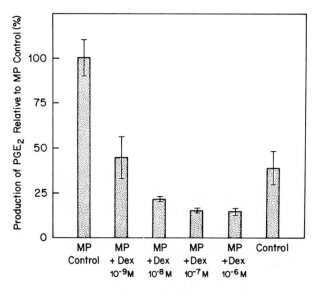

B

FIGURE 7.   (A) Effect of corticotropin$_{1-24}$ on rates of production of prostanoids by human fetal adrenal tissue, control (open bars), 4 μM corticotropin$_{1-24}$ (hatched bars). Results are presented as means ± SEM from media of 4 replicate dishes. (B) Effect of dexamethasone (Dex) at various concentrations on the rate of secretion of PGE$_2$. MP: metyrapone, to inhibit endogenous cortisol formation. Results are presented as means ± SEM from media of 5 replicate dishes. (From Mitchell, M. D., Carr, B. R., Mason, J. I., and Simpson, E. R., *Proc. Natl. Acad. Sci., USA*, 79, 7547, 1982. With permission.)

suggested that glucocorticosteroids act to inhibit PG formation by inhibition of phospholipase activities. The mediator of this effect has been named macrocortin or lipomodulin (Figure 5). In a recent study, human fetal adrenal tissue has been shown to respond to glucocorticosterioids by inhibition of PG formation in a manner consistent with the formation of lipomodulin by this tissue (Figure 7).[68] This finding may be of importance for our understanding of the regulation of adrenal growth and the secretion of steroid hormones by the tissue. Moreover, it may be of importance in our understanding of the regulation of regression of the fetal zone of the adrenal during early neonatal life. The suppression of PGs that have vasodilatatory properties could provide a mechanism whereby the blood supply to the inner fetal zone of the adrenal was reduced or completely abolished and hence the fetal zone would regress rapidly. We have been unable to demonstrate an action of glucocorticosteroids on PG formation by human amnion cells in monolayer culture or by endometrial stromal cells in monolayer culture.[69] Interestingly, human myometrial cells in monolayer culture do respond to glucocorticosteroids by reduced formation of PG.[69] The latter observation is particularly interesting since the major PG formed by the myometrium is PGI_2,[70] a PG that has been shown to be inhibitory of uterine activity in sheep.[71] Hence, an increased rate of glucocorticosteroid biosynthesis during labor may act to reduce the rate of biosynthesis of a uterine relaxant and thus allow the effects of uterotonic PGs to be dominant. The presence of glucocorticosteroid-sensitive tissues within the fetal and uterine environments provides another regulator mechanism for prostanoid formation during pregnancy and parturition.

B. Stimulatory Factors
1. Circulating Substances

A variety of substances found in the maternal circulation have been reported to stimulate prostanoid formation. The substances include oxytocin, bradykinin, and estrogens.[72-75] Whether the substances have tonic effects on PG biosynthesis by uterine tissues is unknown. It seems somewhat unlikely that such substances would play a major role in maintaining fetal homeostasis since the stimulation of any prostanoid by these substances would occur not only within the uterus, but also in other maternal tissues.

2. Substances in Uterine and Intrauterine Tissues

There is exciting evidence that uterine and intrauterine tissues contain cytosolic factors that cause a stimulation of PG biosynthesis.[76] The stimulation of biosynthesis is different not only for different PGs, but also between different uterine tissues. Indeed the nature of the stimulation is also different (Figure 8). At present no data are available concerning the presence of such stimulants in fetal tissues; however, the potential for stimulation of PG biosynthesis within intrauterine tissues may provide yet another regulatory mechanism for arachidonic acid metabolism. It should be noted that a specific stimulant of PGI_2 formation has been described previously[77] and its activity is thought to be reduced in cases of placental insufficiency. Since PGI_2 biosynthesis is increased enormously during pregnancy, it is likely that a specific stimulant of PGI_2 formation is present within intrauterine tissues.

It would then seem possible that a reduced activity of such a stimulant could lead to a chronic reduction in utero-placental blood flow and thence lead to growth retardation and other diseases such as pregnancy-induced hypertension. Given the multitude of effects of PGI_2 within the body, the finding of a potential stimulant of PGI_2 biosynthesis within intrauterine tissues has wider significance since the characterization of such a substance may eventually permit clinical treatment with the substance.

V. FINAL COMMENTS

It is apparent from the foregoing sections that the regulation of arachidonic acid metabolism within the uterus and by the fetus is an extremely complex event. It likely

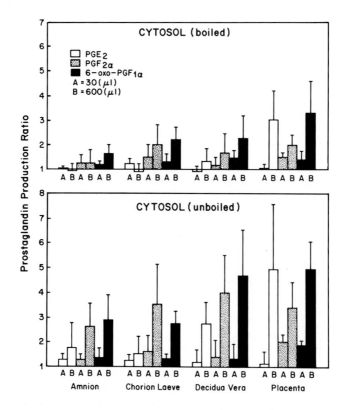

FIGURE 8.   Stimulation of PG biosynthesis by cytosolic fractions from various intrauterine tissues. Results are presented (means ± SEM, n = 5) as PG production ratio, which is the ratio of PG produced in the presence of test cytosol to that produced in its absence. (From Saeed, S. A. and Mitchell, M. D., *Prostaglandins,* 24, 475, 1982. With permission.)

involves a series of inhibitory and stimulatory factors that include a combination of the different products of arachidonic acid metabolism. Hence products of lipoxygenase action on arachidonic acid metabolism may influence the direction of cyclooxygenase pathways of arachidonic acid metabolism. Complexity of the interactions will make future investigations extremely difficult. However, given the clinical importance of PG formation by the fetus and within the uterus it is of signal importance that such studies are conducted. Which, if any, of the factors is the ultimate regulator of PG formation is at present unknown and may remain so for many years. However, our ability to modulate the formation of various arachidonic metabolites during pregnancy will have major clinical implications since PGs do have several protective actions on the uterus, and in particular on the fetus and on the neonate. On the other hand it should be recognized that interference with the normal pattern of arachidonic acid metabolism could also have disastrous consequences. Hence there is a strong rationale for extensive basic scientific studies to be conducted before clinical trials of any of the substances described in this review are considered.

REFERENCES

1. MacKenzie, I. Z., MacLean, D. A., and Mitchell, M. D., Prostaglandins in the human fetal circulation in mid-trimester and term pregnancy, *Prostaglandins,* 20, 649, 1980.
2. Johnson, R. A., Morton, D. R., Kinner, J. H., Gorman, R. R., McGuire, J. R., Sun, F. F., Whittaker, N., Bunting, S., Salmon, J., Moncada, S., and Vane, J. R., The chemical structure of prostaglandin X (prostacyclin), *Prostaglandins.* '2, 915, 1976.
3. Moncada, S., Gryglewski, R., Bunting, S., and Vane, J. R., An enzyme isolated from arteries transforms prostaglandin endoperoxides to an unstable substance that inhibits platelet aggregation, *Nature (London),* 263, 663, 1976.
4. Craft, I. L., Scrivener, R., and Dewhurst, C. J., Prostaglandin F_{2o} in the maternal and fetal circulations in late pregnancy, *J. Obstet. Gynaecol. Br. Commonw.,* 80, 616, 1973.
5. Mitchell, M. D., Flint, A. P. F., Bibby, J., Brunt, J., Arnold, J. M., Anderson, A. B. M., and Turnbull, A. C., Plasma concentrations of prostaglandins during late human pregnancy: influence of normal and pre-term labor, *J. Clin. Endocrinol. Metab.,* 46, 947, 1978.
6. Mitchell, M. D., Brunt, J., Bibby, J., Flint, A. P. F., Anderson, A. B. M., and Turnbull, A. C., Prostaglandins in the human umbilical circulation at birth, *Br. J. Obstet. Gynaecol.,* 85, 114, 1978.
7. Mitchell, M. D., Sellers, S. M., Jamieson, D. R. S., and Turnbull, A. C., 6-Keto-PGF_{1o}: concentrations in human umbilical plasma and production by umbilical vessels, in *Advances in Prostaglandin and Thromboxane Research,* Vol. 7, Samuelsson, B., Ramwell, P. W., and Paoletti, R., Eds., Raven Press, New York, 1980, 1401.
8. Mitchell, M. D., Bibby, J. G., Hicks, B. R., Redman, C. W. G., Anderson, A. B. M., and Turnbull, A. C., Thromboxane B_2 and human parturition: concentrations in the plasma and production in vitro, *J. Endocrinol.,* 78, 435, 1978.
9. Bibby, J. G., Brunt, J. D., Hodgson, H., Mitchell, M. D., Anderson, A. B. M., and Turnbull, A. C., Prostaglandins in umbilical plasma at elective caesarean section, *Br. J. Obstet. Gynaecol.,* 86, 282, 1979.
10. Mitchell, M. D. and Flint, A. P. F., Concentrations of prostaglandins in intrauterine tissues from late-pregnant sheep before and after labour, *Prostaglandins,* 14, 563, 1977.
11. Mitchell, M. D. and Flint, A. P. F., Prostaglandin production by intrauterine tissues from periparturient sheep: use of a superfusion technique, *J. Endocrinol.,* 76, 111, 1978.
12. Coceani, F. and Olley, P. M., The response of the ductus arteriosus to prostaglandins, *Can. J. Physiol. Pharmacol.,* 51, 220, 1973.
13. Elliott, R. B. and Starling, M. B., The effect of prostaglandin F_{2o} in the closure of the ductus arteriosus, *Prostaglandins,* 2, 399, 1972.
14. Starling, M. B. and Elliott, R. B., The effects of prostaglandins, prostaglandin inhibitors, and oxygen on the closure of the ductus arteriosus, pulmonary arteries, and umbilical vessels in vitro, *Prostaglandins,* 8, 187, 1974.
15. Needleman, P., Holmberg, S., and Mandelbaum, B., Ductus arteriosus closure may result from suppression of prostacyclin synthetase by an intrinsic hydroperoxy fatty acid, *Prostaglandins,* 22, 675, 1981.
16. Coceani, F., Jhamandas, V. M., Bodach, E., Labuc, J., Olley, P. M., and Borgeat, P., Evidence against a role for lipoxygenase-derived products of arachidonic acid in the lamb ductus arteriosus, *Can. J. Physiol. Pharmacol.,* 60, 345, 1982.
17. Siegler, R. L., Walker, M. B., Crouch, R. H., Christenson, P., and Jubiz, W., Plasma prostaglandin E concentrations from birth throughout childhood, *J. Pediatr.,* 91, 734, 1977.
18. Friedman, Z. and Demers, L., Essential fatty acids, prostaglandins and respiratory distress syndrome of the newborn, *Pediatrics,* 61, 341, 1978.
19. Mitchell, M. D., Lucas, A., Etches, P., Brunt, J., and Turnbull, A. C., Plasma prostaglandin levels during early neonatal life following term and pre-term delivery, *Prostaglandins,* 16, 319, 1978.
20. Mitchell, M. D., Sellers, S. M., Menchini, M., Aynsley-Green, A., and Turnbull, A. C., 6-Keto-prostaglandin F_{1o} and thromboxane B_2 in the human umbilical and neonatal circulations, *IRCS J. Med. Sci.,* 9, 222, 1981.
21. Coceani, F. and Olley, P. M., Role of prostaglandins, prostacyclin, and thromboxanes in the control of prenatal patency and postnatal closure of the ductus arteriosus, *Semin. Perinatol.,* 4, 109, 1980.
22. Lucas, A. and Mitchell, M. D., Plasma prostaglandins in pre-term neonates before and after treatment for patent ductus arteriosus, *Lancet,* 2, 130, 1978.
23. Lucas, A. and Mitchell, M. D., Prostaglandins in patent ductus arteriosus, *Lancet,* 1, 937, 1978.
24. Noah, L., Use of prostaglandin E_1 for maintaining the patency of the ductus arteriosus, in *Advances in Prostaglandin and Thromboxane Research,* Vol. 4, Coceani, F. and Olley, P. M., Eds., Raven Press, New York, 1979, 355.

25. Silove, E. D., Coe, J. Y., Shiu, M. F., Brunt, J. D., Page, J. F., Singh, S. P., and Mitchell, M. D., Oral prostaglandin E_2 in ductus dependent pulmonary circulation, *Circulation*, 63, 682, 1981.

26. Levin, D. L., Fixler, D. E., Morriss, F. C., and Tyson, J., Morphological analysis of the pulmonary vascular bed in infants exposed in utero to prostaglandin synthetase inhibitors, *J. Pediatr.*, 92, 478, 1978.

27. Manchester, D., Margolis, H. S., and Sheldon, R. E., Possible association between maternal indomethacin therapy and primary pulmonary hypertension in the newborn, *Am. J. Obstet. Gynecol.*, 126, 467, 1976.

28. Wilkinson, A. R., Aynsley-Green, A., and Mitchell, M. D., Persistent pulmonary hypertension and abnormal prostaglandin E levels in premature infants after maternal treatment with naproxen, *Arch. Dis. Child.*, 54, 942, 1979.

29. Mitchell, M. D., Lucas, A., Whitfield, M., Brunt, J. D., and Turnbull, A. C., Selective elevation of circulating prostaglandin concentrations in hyaline membrane disease in pre-term infants, *Prostaglandins Med.*, 1, 207, 1978.

30. Strickland, D. M. and Mitchell, M. D., Production of prostaglandins by human fetal tissues, Proc. Annu. Meet. Endocrine Soc., Abstr. 1034, San Francisco, 1982, 338.

31. Moncada, S., Herman, A. G., Higgs, E. A., and Vane, J. R., Differential formation of prostacyclin (PGX or PGI_2) by layers of the arterial wall. An explanation for the anti-thrombotic properties of vascular endothelium, *Thromb. Res.*, 11, 323, 1977.

32. Powell, W. S. and Solomon, S., Biosynthesis of prostaglandins and thromboxanes in fetal tissues, in *Advances in Prostaglandin and Thromboxane Research*, Vol. 4, Coceani, F. and Olley, P. M., Eds., Raven Press, New York, 1978, 61.

33. Terragno, N. A. and Terragno, A., Prostaglandin metabolism in the fetal and maternal vasculature, *Fed. Proc. Fed. Am. Soc. Exp. Biol.*, 38, 75, 1979.

34. Robert, A., Prostaglandins and digestive diseases, in *Advances in Prostaglandin and Thromboxane Research*, Vol. 8, Samuelsson, B., Ramwell, P. W., and Paoletti, R., Eds., Raven Press, New York, 1980, 1533.

35. Gryglewski, R. J., Korbut, R., and Ocetkiewicz, A. C., Generation of prostacyclin by lungs in vivo and its release into the arterial circulation, *Nature (London)*, 273, 765, 1978.

36. Moncada, S., Korbut, R., Bunting, S., and Vane, J. R., Prostacyclin is a circulating hormone, *Nature (London)*, 273, 767, 1978.

37. Gorman, R. R., Bunting, S., and Miller, O. V., Modulation of human platelet adenylate cyclase by prostacyclin (PGX), *Prostaglandins*, 13, 377, 1977.

38. Pace-Asciak, C. R., Prostaglandin biosynthesis and catabolism in several organs of developing fetal and neonatal animals, in *Advances in Prostaglandin and Thromboxane Research*, Vol. 4, Coceani, F. and Olley, P. M., Eds., Raven Press, New York, 1978, 45.

39. Saeed, S. A. and Mitchell, M. D., Conversion of arachidonic acid to lipoxygenase products by human fetal tissues, *Biochem. Med.*, 30, 322, 1983.

40. Capdevila, J., Chacos, N., Werringloer, J., Prough, R. A., and Estabrook, R. W., Liver microsomal cytochrome P-450 and the oxidative metabolism of arachidonic acid, *Proc. Natl. Acad. Sci. U.S.A.*, 78, 5362, 1981.

41. Samuelsson, B., Borgeat, P., Hammarstrom, S., and Murphy, R. C., Leukotrienes: a new group of biologically active compounds, in *Advances in Prostaglandin and Thromboxane Research*, Vol. 6, Samuelsson, B., Ramwell, P. W., and Paoletti, R., Eds., Raven Press, New York, 1980, 1.

42. Moncada, S., Gryglewski, R. J., Bunting, S., and Vane, J. R., A lipid peroxide inhibits the enzyme in blood vessel microsomes that generates from prostaglandin endoperoxides the substance (prostaglandin X) which prevents platelet aggregation, *Prostaglandins*, 12, 715, 1976.

43. Turk, J., Wyche, A., and Needleman, P., Inactivation of vascular prostacyclin synthetase by platelet lipoxygenase products, *Biochem. Biophys. Res. Commun.*, 95, 1628, 1980.

44. Omini, C., Folco, G. C., Vigano, T., Rossoni, G., Brunelli, G., and Berti, F., Leukotriene C_4 induces generation of PGI_2 and TXA_2 in guinea-pig in vivo, *Pharmacol. Res. Commun.*, 13, 633, 1981.

45. Serhan, C. N., Fridovich, J., Goetzl, E. J., Dunham, P. B., and Weissman, G., Leukotriene B_4 and phosphatidic acid are calcium ionophores. Studies employing arsenazo III in liposomes, *J. Biol. Chem.*, 257, 4746, 1982.

46. Mitchell, M. D., Bibby, J., Hicks, B. R., and Turnbull, A. C., Specific production of prostaglandin E_2 by human amnion in vitro, *Prostaglandins*, 15, 377, 1978.

47. Mitchell, M. D., Bibby, J. G., Hicks, B. R., and Turnbull, A. C., Possible role for prostacyclin in human parturition, *Prostaglandins*, 16, 931, 1978.

48. Okazaki, T., Casey, M. L., Okita, J. R., MacDonald, P. C., and Johnston, J. M., Initiation of human parturition. XII. Biosynthesis and metabolism of prostaglandins in human fetal membranes and uterine decidua, *Am. J. Obstet. Gynecol.*, 139, 373, 1981.

49. Ellwood, D. A., Mitchell, M. D., Anderson, A. B. M., and Turnbull, A. C., Oestrogens, prostaglandins and cervical ripening, *Lancet*, 1, 376, 1979.

50. Ellwood, D. A., Mitchell, M. D., Anderson, A. B. M., and Turnbull, A. C., *In vitro* production of prostanoids by the human cervix during pregnancy: preliminary observations, *Br. J. Obstet. Gynaecol.*, 87, 210, 1980.

51. Mitchell, M. D., Kraemer, D. L., and Strickland, D. M., The human placenta: a major source of prostaglandin D_2, *Prostaglandins, Leukotrienes Med.*, 8, 383, 1982.

52. Clark, K. E., Austin, J. E., and Stys, S. J., Effect of bisenoic prostaglandins on the uterine vasculature of the nonpregnant sheep, *Prostaglandins*, 22, 333, 1981.

53. Smith, J. B., Silver, M. J., Ingerman, C. M., and Kocsis, J. J., Prostaglandin D_2 inhibits the aggregation of human platelets, *Thromb. Res.*, 5, 291, 1974.

54. Siegl, A. M., Smith, J. B., and Silver, M. J., ^{3}H-PGD$_2$ binding by intact human platelets, in *Advances in Prostaglandin and Thromboxane Research*, Vol. 6, Samuelsson, B., Ramwell, P. W., and Paoletti, R., Eds., Raven Press, New York, 1980, 395.

55. Saeed, S. A. and Mitchell, M. D., Formation of arachidonate lipoxygenase metabolites by human fetal membranes, uterine decidua vera and placenta, *Prostaglandins, Leukotrienes Med.*, 8, 635, 1982.

56. Mitchell, M. D., Strickland, D. M., Brennecke, S. P., and Saeed, S. A., New aspects of arachidonic acid metabolism and human parturition, in Proc. Ross Conf. Obstet. Res., Initiation of Parturition: Prevention of Prematurity, Porter, J. C., Eds., Ross, Columbus, In press, 1983.

57. Liggins, G. C., Cervical ripening as an inflammatory reaction, in *The Cervix in Pregnancy and Labour*, Ellwood, D. A. and Anderson, A. B. M., Eds., Churchill Livingstone, Edinburgh, 1981, 1.

58. Saeed, S. A. and Mitchell, M. D., New aspects of arachidonic acid metabolism in human uterine cervix, *Eur. J. Pharmacol.*, 81, 515, 1982.

59. Saeed, S. A., McDonald-Gibson, W. J., Cuthbert, J., Copas, J. L., Schneider, C., Gardiner, P. J., Butt, N. M., and Collier, H. O. J., Endogenous inhibitor of prostaglandin synthetase, *Nature (London)*, 270, 32, 1977.

60. Mitchell, M. D., Brennecke, S. P., Denning-Kendall, P. A., McDonald-Gibson, W. J., Saeed, S. A., and Collier, H. O. J., Comparisons between the abilities of various human and ovine plasmas to inhibit prostaglandin synthesis, *Prostaglandins Med.*, 6, 495, 1981.

61. Brennecke, S. P., Bryce, R. L., Turnbull, A. C., and Mitchell, M. D., The prostaglandin synthase inhibiting ability of maternal plasma and the onset of human labour, *Eur. J. Obstet. Gynaecol. Reprod. Biol.*, 14, 81, 1982.

62. Saeed, S. A., Strickland, D. M., Young, D., Dang, A., and Mitchell, M. D., Inhibition of prostaglandin synthesis by human amniotic fluid: acute reduction in inhibitory activity of amniotic fluid obtained during labor, *J. Clin. Endocrinol. Metab.*, 55, 801, 1982.

63. Brennecke, S. P., Kirkham, F. J., Morton, K. E., Wilkinson, A. R., and Mitchell, M. D., Ontogeny and neonatology of circulating endogenous inhibitor(s) of prostaglandin synthase in the human, Submitted for publication.

64. Saeed, S. A., Drew, M., and Collier, H. O. J., Endogenous inhibitors of lipoxygenase, *Eur. J. Pharmacol.*, 67, 169, 1980.

65. Flower, R. J. and Blackwell, G. J., Anti-inflammatory steroids induce biosynthesis of a phospholipase A_2 inhibitor which prevents prostaglandin generation, *Nature (London)*, 278, 456, 1979.

66. Blackwell, G. F., Carnuccio, R., DiRosa, M., Flower, R. J., Parente, L., and Persico, P., Macrocortin: a polypeptide causing the anti-phospholipase effect of glucocorticoids, *Nature (London)*, 287, 147, 1980.

67. Hirata, F., Schiffmann, E., Venkatasubramanian, K., Salomon, D., and Axelrod, J., A phospholipase A_2 inhibitory protein in rabbit neutrophils induced by glucocorticoids, *Proc. Natl. Acad. Sci. U.S.A.*, 77, 2533, 1980.

68. Mitchell, M. D., Carr, B. R., Mason, J. I., and Simpson, E. R., Prostaglandin biosynthesis in the human fetal adrenal: regulation by glucocorticosteroids, *Proc. Natl. Acad. Sci. U.S.A.*, 79, 7547, 1982.

69. Casey, M. L., MacDonald, P. C., and Mitchell, M. D., In preparation.

70. Abel, M. H. and Kelly, R. W., Differential production of prostaglandins within the human uterus, *Prostaglandins*, 18, 821, 1979.

71. Lye, S. J. and Challis, J. R. G., Inhibition by PGI-2 of myometrial activity in vivo in non-pregnant ovariectomized sheep, *J. Reprod. Fertil.*, 66, 311, 1982.

72. Barcikowski, B., Carlson, J. C., Wilson, L., and McCracken, J. A., The effects of endogenous and exogenous estradiol-17β on the release of prostaglandin $F_{2\alpha}$ from the ovine uterus, *Endocrinology*, 95, 1340, 1974.

73. Mitchell, M. D., Flint, A. P. F., and Turnbull, A. C., Stimulation by oxytocin of prostaglandin F levels in uterine venous effluent in pregnant and puerperal sheep, *Prostaglandins*, 9, 47, 1975.

74. Whalley, E. T., The action of bradykinin and oxytocin on the isolated whole uterus and myometrium of the rat in oestrous, *Br. J. Pharmacol.*, 64, 21, 1978.

75. Williams, K. I. and El-Tahir, K. E. H., Effects of uterine stimulant drugs on prostacyclin production by the pregnant rat myometrium. I. Oxytocin, bradykinin and $PGF_{2\alpha}$, *Prostaglandins,* 19, 31, 1980.
76. Saeed, S. A. and Mitchell, M. D., Stimulants of prostaglandin biosynthesis in human fetal membranes, uterine decidua vera and placenta, *Prostaglandins,* 24, 475, 1982.
77. Remuzzi, G., Zoja, C., Marchesi, D., Schieppati, A., Mecca, G., Misiani, R., Donati, M. B., and De Gaetano, G., Plasmatic regulation of vascular prostacyclin in pregnancy, *Br. Med. J.,* 282, 512, 1981.

Chapter 4

PROSTAGLANDIN E: BIPHASIC CONTROL OF HEMATOPOIESIS*

Louis M. Pelus

TABLE OF CONTENTS

*   Supported by Grant CA-33225 awarded by the National Cancer Institute, D.H.H.S., and the Gar Reich-
    man Foundation. Dr. Pelus is a Scholar of the Leukemia Society of America.

I. INTRODUCTION

Blood cell production is regulated by complex homeostatic mechanisms which act to maintain cell numbers within narrowly defined ranges, yet permit the capacity to respond rapidly to a variety of immunological and hematologic insults requiring enhanced cell production. The development of in vitro bone marrow semi-solid matrix culture systems that support the proliferation and differentiation of bone marrow multipotential stem cells[1-4] and lineage-restricted progenitor cells[5-7] have facilitated the investigation of mechanisms that control normal cell production and protect against loss of normal regulatory controls. With respect to granulocyte and macrophage production, marrow culture studies have demonstrated that the proliferation of bipotentially committed progenitor cells that give rise solely to granulocytes and macrophages, CFU-GM, can be directly modulated by both negative and positive regulators,[5,8-10] and furthermore, that abnormalities in these control mechanisms may underlie the pathophysiology of myeloid leukemias.[11-13]

This chapter will describe recent studies on the control of normal myeloid cell differentiation, particularly as they relate to the expression of HLA-DR, Ia-like antigens, and mechanisms for modulating antigen expression as a means to control normal and abnormal granulocyte and macrophage production.

II. EFFECTS OF PROSTAGLANDIN E ON CFU-GM

Prostaglandins (PGs) of the E series have been shown to inhibit the proliferation of normal CFU-GM in a dose-dependent fashion when added directly to agar cultures over a concentration range of 10^{-5} M through 10^{-12} M,[9] with an $ID_{50} = 10^{-7}$ M on total CFU-GM and 5×10^{-9} M on those CFU-GM committed solely to monocytoid differentiation.[9,14,15] The preferential effect of PGE on monocyte-macrophage restricted colony forming cells (M-CFC) was established by morphological analysis of *in situ* clones. The dose-dependent effect of PGE noted in vitro most likely results as a consequence of chemical instability, and in this regard, in vivo evidence using the stable PG analog 16,16 dimethyl PGE_2[44] suggests a plateau inhibitory effect on CFU-GM over a range of 10^{-5} M to 10^{-11} M in intact mice. Furthermore, the preferential effect of PGE on monocytoid committed CFC could also be duplicated and confirmed in vivo.

Analysis of PGE sensitivities of CFU-GM from patients with leukemia indicate that abnormal regulatory responses characterize most forms of leukemia.[11,13,16,17] In patients with acute (n = 34) or chronic (n = 40) myeloid leukemia, their CFU-GM are virtually insensitive to the inhibitory effects of PGE, with concentrations of greater than 10^{-5} M required for 50% inhibition[11,13,18] of CFU-GM proliferation. In 13 patients with preleukemia, including refractory anemia with excess of blasts (RAEB) and chronic myelomonocytic syndrome (CMMS), an overall heterogeneity of response was observed. However, in 3 patients (2 RAEB, 1 CMMS) whose CFU-GM initially displayed normal or near normal sensitivity to inhibition by PGE, subsequent loss of CFU-GM sensitivity was observed coinciding with clinical progression to acute leukemia. Loss of CFU-GM sensitivity to PGE occurred 1.2, 2.5, and 2.8 months prior to clinical onset of acute leukemia.[19] The progressive loss of PGE sensitivity in patients developing leukemia may indicate a state of "clonal competition" with the progressive development of a malignant clone insensitive to normal humoral regulators. The insensitivity of leukemic clones to normal regulation appears to characterize the overtly leukemic phenotype, and most likely provides a significant growth advantage to the abnormal clone. In this regard, mechanisms that might alter regulatory phenotype would have important clinical applications in controlling leukemic onset and progression.

III. SUBPOPULATION SPECIFICITY OF PROSTAGLANDIN E

Investigations into the mechanism of action of PGE on CFU-GM using high specific activity ^{3}H-thymidine (^{3}H-Tdr) and treatment with mouse anti-human monoclonal antibodies plus complement indicate a selective of PGE on those CFU-GM which are in S-phase of the cell cycle and express HLA-DR, Ia-like antigen preferentially or perhaps at higher density relative to S-phase of the cell cycle.[13,20,21]

The expression of Ia-antigen by human CFU-GM appears necessary for regulation of cell proliferation, at least in vitro. Furthermore, CFU-GM Ia-antigen must be expressed in a particular quantitative pattern (plateau 50% over 3 log dilution of antibody)[13,20,21] consistent with cycle-related antigen expression. This requirement is particularly significant with respect to patients with chronic myeloid leukemia, whereas in most patients, absent or reduced expression of Ia-antigens on leukemic CFU-GM occurs coincidently with CFU-GM insensitivity to PGE (Tables 1 and 2). In two patients, higher levels of Ia-antigen expression by CFU-GM were observed, and occurred coincident with considerable, albeit abnormal, sensitivity to inhibition by PGE (Table 2). Furthermore, the degree of CFU-GM sensitivity to PGE observed in these two patients was lost following treatment with anti-HLA-DR antibody plus complement, again indicating the requirement of CFU-GM Ia-antigen expression for appropriate growth regulation.

In vivo, the human CFU-GM population is in a dynamic process of differentiation and clonal expansion. Pulse treatment with ^{3}H-Tdr or anti-HLA-DR antibody plus complement in vitro will define only that subpopulation of CFU-GM in S-phase and Ia-antigen positive at the time of pulse treatment. This subpopulation does not represent the total population of CFU-GM that has the capacity to ultimately enter S-phase and express Ia-antigen. In agar culture, colony, and cluster formation, the measure of CFU-GM proliferation is asynchronous, with differentiation and proliferation occurring throughout the 7-day culture period. Thus, all CFU-GM and their progeny with the capacity to differentiate will enter S-phase, presumably express Ia-antigen, and should be sensitive to growth inhibition by PGE. This is not the case, however, the degree of inhibition usually observed being equivalent to the number of S-phase, Ia-antigen positive CFU-GM which can be quantitated at culture initiation. The lack of total population sensitivity to inhibition by PGE does not result as a consequence of rapid metabolism of PG, as determined by delayed and multiple time additions. Rather, analysis of human CFU-GM Ia-antigen expression over time indicates a transient expression.[13,20,21] Loss of CFU-GM Ia-antigen detection occurs within 3 to 6 hr at 37°C. Coincidently, CFU-GM sensitivity to PGE inhibition is also lost. In contrast, CFU-GM Ia-antigen expression and sensitivity to PGE was maintained in cells kept at 4°C for up to 48 hr. This phenomenon may underlie the subpopulation effects of PGE. In addition, membrane turnover/shedding of CFU-GM Ia-antigen may represent a mechanism whereby limitation of myeloid cell clonal expansion can occur only if inhibitory regulators are present at precise times or maintained in elevated amounts for extended times.

IV. EFFECTS OF PROSTAGLANDIN E ON CFU-GM CELL CYCLE AND HLA-DR ANTIGEN EXPRESSION

The transitory nature of CFU-GM Ia-antigen expression and its importance to hemopoietic regulation led us to ask if CFU-GM Ia-antigen expression could be modulated, and if so, does this coincide with equivalent changes in the sensitivity of these cells to inhibition by PGE. Several studies have demonstrated that in vitro pulse exposure to PGE elevates the fraction of murine and human stem cells in S-phase of the cell

Table 1
Ia$^+$ CFU-GM IN NORMAL DONORS AND PATIENTS WITH CML

Source of bone marrow cells	$\bar{x}$% Ia-antigen positive CFU-GM[a]			
	Anti-Ia-antibody dilution[b]			
	1:100	1:250	1:500	1:1000
Normal (n = 7)	52 ± 2	46 ± 3	49 ± 3	47 ± 2
CML (n = 13)	18 ± 5[c]	10 ± 5[c]	18 ± 4[c]	4 ± 2[c]

[a] Data are expressed as the mean percent Ia$^+$-CFU-GM (colonies plus clusters) determined from quadruplicate cultures for each normal donor and patient with CML.

[b] Mouse anti-human HLA-DR antibody (NEI-011), New England Nuclear Corp., Boston.

[c] $P < 0.0005$.

Table 2
PG RESPONSIVENESS AND Ia EXPRESSION IN PATIENTS WITH CHRONIC MYELOID LEUKEMIA

Molar PGE conc.	% Inhibition of CFU-GM[a]					
	CML (n = 11)		K.P. (□)[b]		C.R. (●)[c]	
	C'	αIa[d] + C'	C'	αIa + C'	C'	αIa + C'
10^5 M	16 ± 4	12 ± 4(14 ± 5%)[e]	54 ± 5	0 (46%)	62 ± 6	15 (36 ± 2%)
10^6 M	3 ± 2	1 ± 2	34 ± 1	—	46 ± 3	0
10^7 M	0 ± 3	0 ± 1	16 ± 4	—	32 ± 2	—
10^8 M	—	—	10 ± 4	—	12 ± 1	—
10^9 M	—	—	2 ± 3	—	2 ± 2	—
10^{10} M	—	—	0 ± 1	—	0 ± 1	—

[a] Inhibition of CFU-GM (colonies and clusters) per 10^5 low density (<1.074 g/mℓ) bone marrow cells.

[b] The PG responsiveness of this patient was analyzed on 3 separate occasions over an 18-month period. Quantitation of the number of Ia-antigen positive CFU-GM was performed only once.

[c] The presence of Ia-antigens and PG responsiveness in this patient was analyzed on 2 separate occasions during a 6-month period.

[d] Anti-Ia-antibody (NEI-011) was used at a 1/100 dilution.

[e] Percentage of Ia-antigen positive CFU-GM detected.

From Pelus, L. M., Gold, E., Salatan, S., Coleman, M., *Blood,* 62, 158, 1983. With permission.

cycle.[22,23] The relationship between CFU-GM S-phase, Ia-antigen expression, and sensitivity to growth inhibition observed in vitro suggested that PGE might be used to investigate events associated with the control of CFU-GM differentiation/proliferation.

In order to investigate the mechanisms of action associated with modulation of CFU-GM proliferation, a liquid preculture system was developed (Figure 1). The response of marrow CFU-GM to inhibition by PGE is determined prior to the suspension culture, as is the total proportion of CFU-GM in S-phase and expressing Ia-antigen. The appropriate treated groups (usually media, ^{3}H-Tdr, C, and αIa + C') are then placed in suspension culture in the absence and presence of PGE for various time periods. Following suspension culture, each individual group is retreated to quantitate

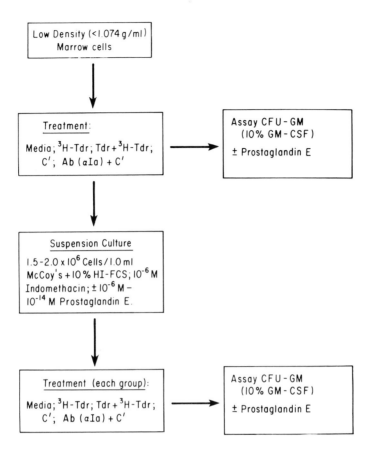

FIGURE 1.   Schematic representation of liquid preculture assay system.

the fraction of CFU-GM in S-phase and Ia-antigen positive at the end of the suspension culture. In addition, the sensitivity of each group of CFU-GM to inhibition by PGE in agar culture is analyzed. In this fashion, the effects of PGE present during the suspension culture, on cell cycle, Ia-antigen expression, and sensitivity to growth regulation can be determined.

As previously described, human CFU-GM Ia-antigen expression is transient and cannot be detected beyond 3 hr when CFU-GM are maintained at 37°C (Table 3). Coincidently, loss of CFU-GM sensitivity to inhibition by PGE is observed. Analysis of cell cycle indicated that the loss of Ia-antigen positive CFU-GM observed did not result from a loss of S-phase CFU-GM. In contrast, while the addition of PGE to the suspension culture did not prevent the loss of CFU-GM Ia-antigen seen at 6 hr of culture, CFU-GM Ia-antigen was detected after 24 hr of culture. Coincident with the re-expression of CFU-GM Ia-antigen, CFU-GM sensitivity to inhibition by PGE was also detected. CFU-GM Ia-antigen expression and sensitivity to growth regulation was not observed by cells maintained in the absence of PG.

The detection of Ia-antigen positive CFU-GM following suspension culture with PGE could be shown to occur by two mechanisms: (1) induction of the differentiation of new Ia-antigen positive, S-phase CFU-GM from a noncycling Ia-antigen negative cell compartment, and (2) restoration of antigen expression by Ia-antigen negative S-phase CFU-GM (Table 4). In those groups of cells treated to remove S-phase and Ia-

Table 3

PGE MEDIATED EXPRESSION OF CFU-GM Ia-ANTIGEN IN SUSPENSION CULTURE

Present throughout suspension culture	Time in suspension culture (hr)	% of CFU-GM		% Inhibition by $10^{-7} M$ PGE$_1$
		Ia$^+$	S-phase	
	0	48 ± 3	49 ± 6	52 ± 6
Media	3	56 ± 6	54 ± 3	52 ± 4
$10^{-8} M$ PGE$_1$	3	53 ± 5	50 ± 4	53 ± 2
Media	6	2 ± 2	48 ± 3	2 ± 2
$10^{-8} M$ PGE$_1$	6	11 ± 7	50 ± 2	0 ± 2
Media	24	4 ± 3	48 ± 1	0 ± 1
$10^{-8} M$ PGE$_1$	24	55 ± 2	57 ± 3	50 ± 6

Note: Data are from five experiments.

Table 4

CFU-GM CELL CYCLE STATUS, Ia-ANTIGEN EXPRESSION, RESPONSE TO INHIBITION BY PGE AFTER SUSPENSION CULTURE

Treatment prior to suspension culture	Present throughout suspension culture	% of CFU-GM		% Inhibition by $10^{-7} M$ PGE$_1$
		Ia$^+$	S-phase	
Media	Media	4 ± 1	39 ± 1	0 ± 1
	$10^{-8} M$ PGE$_1$	48 ± 4	52 ± 2	49 ± 3
^{3}H-Tdr	Media	0 ± 2	0 ± 0	0 ± 2
	$10^{-8} M$ PGE$_1$	32 ± 4	38 ± 3	36 ± 2
Ia + C'[a]	Media	3 ± 1	2 ± 1	4 ± 1
	$10^{-8} M$ PGE$_1$	35 ± 1	39 ± 3	36 ± 1

[a] Monoclonal mouse anti-human HLA-DR antibody (NEI-011) used at a final dilution of 1:250.

antigen positive CFU-GM prior to suspension culture both Ia-antigen positive and S-phase CFU-GM could be detected in a one to one relationship following culture with PGE, but not in control cultures. Under these conditions, the S-phase Ia-antigen positive CFU-GM detected appear to have been induced from a population of noncycling Ia-antigen negative cells (perhaps earlier myeloid stem cells) which give rise to CFU-GM as a consequence of the addition of PGE. Responsiveness of these CFU-GM to inhibition by PGE in agar culture appears to be a direct consequence of Ia-antigen expression by these CFU-GM. In control untreated cultures incubated with PGE an increase in the proportion of S-phase is observed, as is the detection of Ia-antigen positive CFU-GM equal to the number of S0-phase CFU-GM, and the restoration of responsiveness of these CFU-GM to inhibition by PGE. The majority of S-phase, Ia-antigen positive CFU-GM detected probably derive from noncycling cells induced by PGE; however, since no Ia-antigen positive CFU-GM are detected in control cultures despite the presence of S-phase CFU-GM (whereas following culture with PGE both are present to an equivalent degree), it appears that Ia-antigen was re-expressed on those Ia-antigen negative S-phase CFU-GM detected in control cultures. The two mechanisms whereby PGE modulates CFU-GM Ia-antigen expression and cell cycle are diagrammed schematically in Figure 2. The capacity of PGE to mediate these effects was observed to occur in plateau fashion over the concentration range of $10^{-6} M$

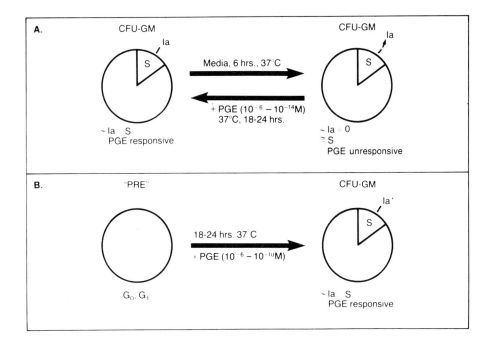

FIGURE 2. Mechanism(s) of action by which PGE modulates CFU-GM Ia antigen expression and regulatory response. $\sim$Ia = s indicates that the proportion of Ia + CFU-GM is equal to the number of S-phase CFU-GM. $\sim$Ia = 0 denotes absence of Ia^{+}-CFU-GM despite the detection of S-phase CFU-GM equivalent in number ($\cong$S) to that found prior to the suspension culture.

to 10^{-10} *M* PGE, and to a lesser but still significant degree with as little as 10^{-12} *M* to 10^{-14} *M* PGE concentrations.[20]

Kinetic experiments indicate that in order to observe CFU-GM Ia-antigen re-expression after 24 hr in the suspension preculture system described, the presence of PGE was required early (within the first 3 hr of culture), and that the effects of PGE were long-lived, resulting in the differentiation/renewal of Ia-antigen positive CFU-GM for at least 7 days.[24] Since PGE production by monocytic cells in vitro is usually not detected during the first 3 hr of liquid culture,[25] the lack of constitutive Ia-antigen re-expression or differentiation of new Ia-antigen positive CFU-GM in vitro may be related to the absence of endogenously produced PGE during this critical period. This is supported by the lack of constitutive Ia-antigen expression in this system regardless of the absence or presence of indomethacin in the suspension culture.[20]

V. MODULATION OF LEUKEMIC PHENOTYPE BY PROSTAGLANDIN E

The lack of or diminished expression of Ia-antigens on CFU-GM from patients with chronic myelogenous leukemia (CML) has been associated with the lack of regulatory sensitivity simultaneously observed in these patients.[13] In order to further define the role of Ia-antigen expression as a principal factor involved in the abnormal regulatory phenotype observed, the capacity to modulate leukemic CFU-GM Ia-antigen expression as a means to alter regulatory response was investigated[26] (Table 5). In contrast to CML CFU-GM tested prior to suspension culture, which were essentially Ia-antigen negative and unresponsive to PGE, those CMNL CFU-GM detected following culture with PGE for 24 hr displayed regulatory sensitivity equivalent to normal CFU-GM. Furthermore, culture of CML-CFU-GM with PGE results in the detection of a quan-

Table 5

MODULATION OF Ia-ANTIGEN EXPRESSION AND
REGULATORY RESPONSE OF CFU-GM FROM PATIENTS WITH
CML FOLLOWING CULTURE WITH PGE

Time in suspension culture (hr)	Present during suspension culture	% of CFU-GM		% Inhibition by 10^{-7} M PGE$_1$
		S-phase	Ia$^+$	
0	—	45 ± 3	2 ± 2	1 ± 1
24	Media	52 ± 6	1 ± 1	2 ± 1
24	10^{-8} M PGE$_1$	48 ± 1	45 ± 3	40 ± 5

Note: Average data from 6 patients with chronic phase CML.

titatively normal pattern of Ia-antigen expression. Thus, phenotypically, those CML CFU-GM detected following culture with PGE for 24 hr can no longer be distinguished from normal CFU-GM.

Analysis of human CFU-GM Ia-antigen expression using different monoclonal anti-human HLA-DR antibodies or rabbit alloantisera has resulted in differences with respect to the proportion of CFU-GM that can be shown to be Ia-antigen positive.[13,20,21,27-30] In this regard, heterogeneity of Ia-antigen expression,[31] changes in HLA-DR antigen density[32] relative to cell cycle, and the recognition by different antibodies of HLA-DR epitopes[33-36] have been documented. As a consequence, different monoclonal anti-HLA-DR antibodies may recognize different Ia-antigens or epitopes which may or may not be cycle related, and may or may not be involved in the control of cellular proliferation. In patients with CML, the inability to detect quantitatively normal Ia-antigen expression, even with antibodies which detect all normal CFU-GM, may relate to any of these possibilities or may relate to altered or unique Ia-antigenic structures. Recent biochemical characterization of HLA-DR antigens on leukemic cells suggests the preservation of qualitatively normal gene expression and cell surface antigen on leukemic cells.[37] The capacity to restore a normalized growth responsiveness associated with a quantitatively normal pattern of Ia-antigen expression to CML CFU-GM by culture with PGE supports the hypothesis that Ia-antigen expression by CFU-GM from these patients is altered, rather than replaced by unique leukemic antigens.

These studies suggest that a population of CFU-GM with the capacity to express a normal regulatory phenotype in vitro is present in the marrow of patients with CML, but cannot be detected in primary agar culture. Two possible explanations may account for this effect: (1) the CFU-GM detected in CML patients following culture with PGE are in fact residual normal CFU-GM, and (2) preculture with PGE results in a phenotypic reversion in a population of leukemic CFU-GM. Cytogenetic analysis of proliferating clones indicates that all metaphases detected both before and after suspension culture with PGE were Philadelphia chromosome (Ph^1) positive and therefore members of the neoplastic clone.[26] Although under conditions of aggressive chemotherapy, nonclonal and presumably nonneoplastic hemopoiesis can be induced in patients with CML.[38,39] The cytogenetic data for CFU-GM from chronic phase CMNL patients following culture with PGE are consistent with data of others which provide little evidence for the persistence of normal committed stem cells in most patients with CML,[40] receiving conventional therapy. Thus, the normalized pattern of Ia-antigen expression and growth responsiveness to normal regulation by PGE induced in CML CFU-GM by suspension preculture represents a phenotypic reversion in the malignant cell population.

The PGE-induced enhancement of CFU-GM Ia-antigen expression, entrance into cell cycle, and restoration of sensitivity to growth regulation observed in suspension preculture contrasts with its inhibitory effect on CFU-GM proliferation observed using agar culture alone. It is possible that in agar one observes a net effect of both positive and negative influences on CFU-GM differentiation; however, investigation of these effects directly in the agar cultures is severely impaired by the semi-solid agar matrix. The addition of PGE to agar cultures 12 to 24 hr after initiation has little effect of CFU-GM proliferation. This result closely occurs as a result of loss of CFU-GM Ia-antigen expression. The addition of small quantities of PGE (10^{-10} *M* to 10^{-12} *M*) to agar cultures at initiation did not restore CFU-GM sensitivity to a larger concentration of PGE (10^{-6} *M*) added 24 hr later. In contrast, these same concentrations of PGE restored Ia-antigen expression and sensitivity to growth inhibition of CFU-GM maintained in suspension culture before culture in soft agar. It appears that the effects of PGE observed in suspension culture may not occur in agar. In this regard, preliminary evidence indicates that the re-expression of CFU-GM Ia-antigen and sensitivity to subsequent growth inhibition by PGE observed following suspension preculture in the presence of PGE requires the interaction of hematopoietic cells and T lymphocytes. Due to the immobilizing properties of soft agar culture such cellular interactions would be prevented.

The ability of PGs of the E series to promote CFU-GM differentiation do not contradict the inhibitory capacity of these compounds. It is apparent that the effects of PGE on hematopoiesis are biphasic. At low as well as high concentrations PGE appears to play a role in CFU-GM differentiation by promoting or modulating CFU-GM cell cycle and coincidently modulating CFU-GM growth regulation as a consequence of appropriate HLA-DR antigen expression. In this capacity, PG appears to maintain adequate numbers of CFU-GM as well as in a state of responsiveness to subsequent regulation as these cells mature and clonally expand. The capacity of PGE to maintain CFU-GM Ia-antigen expression and cell cycle would appear to be a protective role in preventing aberrant myeloid cell proliferation. The demonstration of circulating PGE levels in the range of 10^{-10} *M* to 10^{-12} *M* in human plasma[41] and the insensitivity of human CFU-GM to inhibition at these levels,[9,11,13] at least in primary agar culture, places the CFU-GM differentiating role of PGE well within physiological range. The ultimate degree of CFU-GM expansion to mature granulocytes and monocytes-macrophages is dependent on granulocyte-macrophage colony stimulating factor(s), levels[42,43] as determined by physiologic requirements for adequate cell numbers under homeostatic conditions, or in response to needs for elevated cell production. At high PG concentrations, particularly as a consequence of GM-CSF induced monocyte-macrophage PG production,[8,14,25] clonal expansion of CFU-GM to mature myeloid cells is limited, without compromising the differentiation of earlier stem cells into the CFU-GM compartment. The plateau effect of PGE in promoting CFU-GM cell cycle and differentiation of earlier stem cells into the progenitor cell compartment over the concentration range in which PG also is capable of inhibiting clonal expansion (10^{-6} *M* to 10^{-10} *M*) supports this hypothesis.

REFERENCES

1. Fausser, A. A. and Messner, H. A., Identification of megakaryocytes, macrophages, and eosinophils in colonies of human bone marrow containing neutrophilic granulocytes and erythroblasts, *Blood*, 53, 1023, 1979.
2. Johnson, G., Colony formation in agar by adult bone marrow multipotential hemopoietic cells, *J. Cell. Physiol.*, 103, 371, 1980.

3. Nakahata, T. and Ogawa, M., Hemopoietic colony-forming cells in umbilical cord blood with extensive capability to generate mono- and multipotential hemopoietic progenitors, *J. Clin. Invest.*, 70, 1324, 1982.

4. Fausser, A. A. and Messner, H. A., Granuloerythropoietic colonies in human bone marrow, peripheral blood, and cord blood, *Blood*, 52, 1243, 1978.

5. Chervenick, P. A. and Boggs, D. R., Bone marrow colonies: stimulation *in vitro* by supernatant from incubated human blood cells, *Science*, 169, 691, 1970.

6. Bradley, T. R. and Metcalf, D., The growth of mouse bone marrow cells *in vitro*, *Aust. J. Exp. Biol. Med. Sci.*, 44, 287, 1969.

7. Metcalf, D., *Hemopoietic Colonies*, Springer-Verlag, Berlin, 1977.

8. Kurland, J. I., Broxmeyer, H. E., Pelus, L. M., Bockman, R. S., and Moore, M. A. S., Role for monocyte-macrophage-derived colony-stimulating factor and prostaglandin E in the positive and negative feedback control of myeloid stem cell proliferation, *Blood*, 52, 388, 1978.

9. Pelus, L. M., Broxmeyer, H. E., and Moore, M. A. S., Regulation of human myelopoiesis by prostaglandin E and lactoferrin, *Cell Tissue Kinet.*, 14, 515, 1981.

10. Broxmeyer, H. E., Bognacki, J., Doerner, M. H., and deSousa, M., Identification of leukemia-associated inhibitory activity as acidic isoferritins. A regulatory role for acidic isoferritins in the production of granulocytes and macrophages, *J. Exp. Med.*, 153, 1426, 1981.

11. Pelus, L. M., Broxmeyer, H. E., Clarkson, B. D., and Moore, M. A. S., Abnormal responsiveness of granulocyte-macrophage committed colony-forming cells from patients with chronic myeloid leukemia to inhibition by prostaglandin E, *Cancer Res.*, 40, 2512, 1980.

12. Broxmeyer, H. E., Grossbard, E., Jacobsen, N., and Moore, M. A. S., Persistence of inhibitory activity against normal bone marrow cells during remission of acute leukemia, *N. Engl. J. Med.*, 301, 346, 1979.

13. Pelus, L. M., Saletan, S., Silver, R. T., and Moore, M. A. S., Expression of Ia-antigens on normal and chronic myeloid leukemic human granulocyte-macrophage colony-forming cells (CFU-GM) is associated with the regulation of cell proliferation by prostaglandin E, *Blood*, 59, 284, 1982.

14. Pelus, L. M., Broxmeyer, H. E., Kurland, J. I., and Moore, M. A. S., Regulation of macrophage and granulocyte proliferation: specificities of prostaglandin E and lactoferrin, *J. Exp. Med.*, 150, 277, 1979.

15. Williams, N., Preferential inhibition of murine macrophage colony formation by prostaglandin E, *Blood*, 53, 1089, 1979.

16. Taetle, R. and Koessler, A., Effects of cyclic nucleotides and prostaglandins on normal and abnormal human myeloid progenitor cell proliferation, *Cancer Res.*, 40, 1223, 1980.

17. Aglietta, M., Piacibello, W., and Gavosto, F., Insensitivity of chronic myeloid leukemic cells to inhibition of growth by prostaglandin E, *Cancer Res.*, 40, 2507, 1980.

18. Pelus, L. M., Implications of HLA-DR antigens in the control of human granulocyte and macrophage production, in *Proc. 8th Int. Convocation on Immunol.*, Olgra, P. and Mohen, K., Eds., S. Karger, Basel, in press.

19. Gold, E., Conjalka, M., Pelus, L. M., Broxmeyer, H. E., Jhanwar, S. C., Chaganti, R., Clarkson, B. D., and Moore, M. A. S., Marrow cytogenetic and cell culture analyses of the myelodysplastic syndromes: insights to pathophysiology and prognosis, *J. Clin. Oncol.*, submitted.

20. Pelus, L. M., Association between colony forming units — granulocyte macrophage expression of Ia-like (HLA-DR) antigen and control of granulocyte and macrophage production, *J. Clin. Invest.*, 70, 568, 1982.

21. Broxmeyer, H. E., Relationship of the expression of Ia-like antigenic determinants on normal and leukemic human granulocyte-macrophage progenitor cells in DNA synthesis to the regulatory action of acidic isoferritins, *J. Clin. Invest.*, 69, 632, 1982.

22. Feher, I. and Gidali, J., Prostaglandin E_2 as a stimulator of hemopoietic stem cell proliferation, *Nature (London)*, 247, 550, 1974.

23. Verma, D. S., Spitzer, G., Zander, A. R., McCredie, K. B., and Dicke, K. A., Prostaglandin E_1-mediated augmentation of human granulocyte-macrophage progenitor cell growth *in vitro*, *Leuk. Res.*, 5, 65, 1974.

24. Pelus, L. M., CFU-GM expression of Ia-like, HLA-DR antigen: an association with the humoral control of human granulocyte and macrophage production, *Exp. Hematol.*, 10, 219, 1982.

25. Kurland, J. I., Pelus, L. M., Ralph, P., Bockman, R. S., and Moore, M. A. S., Induction of prostaglandin E synthesis in normal and neoplastic macrophages: role for colony-stimulating factor(s) distinct from effects on myeloid progenitor cell proliferation, *Proc. Natl. Acad. Sci. U.S.A.*, 76, 2326, 1979.

26. Pelus, L. M., Gold, E., Saletan, S., and Coleman, M., Restoration of responsiveness of chronic myeloid leukemia granulocyte-macrophage colony-forming cells to growth regulation *in vitro* following preincubation with prostaglandin E, *Blood*, in press.

27. Fitchen, J. H., Ferrone, S., Quaranta, V., Molinaro, G. A., and Cline, M. J., Monoclonal antibodies to HLA-A, B and Ia-like antigens inhibit colony formation by human myeloid progenitor cells, *J. Immunol.,* 125, 2004, 1980.

28. Moore, M. A. S., Broxmeyer, H. E., Sheridan, A. P. C., Meyers, P. A., Jacobsen, W., and Winchester, R. J., Continuous human bone marrow culture: Ia-antigen characterization of probable pluripotential stem cells, *Blood,* 55, 682, 1980.

29. Janossy, G., Francis, G. E., Capellaro, D., Goldstone, A. H., and Greaves, M. F., Cell sorter analysis of leukemia-associated antigens on human myeloid precursors, *Nature (London),* 276, 176, 1978.

30. Greenberg, P., Grossman, M., Charron, D., and Levy, R., Characterization of antigenic determinants on human myeloid colony forming cells with monoclonal antibodies, *Exp. Hematol.,* 9, 781, 1981.

31. Lanier, L. L. and Warner, N. L., Cell cycle related heterogeneity of Ia-antigen expression on a murine B lymphoma cell line: analysis by flow cytometry, *J. Immunol.,* 126, 626, 1981.

32. Sarkar, S., Glassy, M. C., Ferrone, S., and Jones, O. W., Cell cycle and the differential expression of HLA-A, B and HLA-DR antigens on human B lymphoid cells, *Proc. Natl. Acad. Sci., U.S.A.,* 77, 7297, 1980.

33. Lampson, L. A. and Levy, R., Two populations of Ia-like molecules on a human B cell line, *J. Immunol.,* 125, 293, 1980.

34. Grumet, F. C., Charron, D. J., Fendly, B. M., Levy, R., and Ness, D. B., HLA-DR epitope region definition by use of monoclonal antibody probes, *J. Immunol.,* 125, 2785, 1980.

35. Quaronta, V., Pelligrino, M. A., and Ferrone, S., Serological and immunochemical characterization of the specificity of four monoclonal antibodies to distinct antigenic determinants expressed on subpopulations of human Ia-like antigens, *J. Immunol.,* 126, 548, 1981.

36. Carrel, S., Tosi, R., Gross, N., Tanigaki, N., Carmagnola, A. L., and Accola, R. S., Subsets of human Ia-like molecules defined by monoclonal antibodies, *Mol. Immunol.,* 18, 409, 1981.

37. Newman, R. A. and Greaves, M. F., Characterization of HLA-DR antigens on leukemic cells, *Clin. Exp. Immunol.,* 50, 41, 1982.

38. Singer, J. W., Arlin, Z. A., Najfeld, V., Adamson, J. W., Kempin, S. J., Clarkson, B. D., and Fialkow, P. J., Restoration of nonclonal hematopoiesis in chronic myelogenous leukemia (CML) following a chemotherapy-induced loss of the Ph chromosome, *Blood,* 59, 284, 1982.

39. Goto, T., Nishikori, M., Arlin, Z., Gee, T., Kempin, S., Burchenal, J., Strife, A., Wisniewski, D., Lamber, C., Little, C., Jhanwar, S., Chaganti, R., and Clarkson, B., Growth characteristics of leukemic and normal hematopoietic cells in Ph+ chronic myelogenous leukemia and effects of intensive treatment, *Blood,* 589, 793, 1982.

40. Singer, J. W., Fialkow, P. J., Steinmann, L., Najfeld, V., Stein, S. J., and Robinson, W. A., Chronic myelocytic leukemia (CML): failure to detect residual normal committed stem cells *in vitro,* *Blood,* 53, 264, 1979.

41. Jaffe, B. M., Behrman, H. R., and Parker, C. W., Radioimmunoassay measurement of prostaglandins E, A, and F in human plasma, *J. Clin. Invest.,* 52, 398, 1973.

42. Metcalf, D., Regulation of granulocyte and monocyte-macrophage proliferation by colony-stimulating factor (CSF). A review, *Exp. Hematol.,* 1, 185, 1973.

43. Quesenberry, P. and Levitt, L., Hematopoietic stem cells, *N. Engl. J. Med.,* 301, 819, 1979.

44. Pelus, L. M., unpublished data.

Chapter 5

PROSTAGLANDIN E, LIPOLYSIS, AND DIABETIC KETOACIDOSIS

R. Paul Robertson

TABLE OF CONTENTS

I. INTRODUCTION

Clinical information is now emerging suggesting that prostaglandin (PG) E_2 accumulates in vivo during diabetic ketoacidosis. This finding is relevant to clinical investigators interested in potential biological protective effects of PGs because of the ability of PGE_2 to inhibit hormone-induced lipolysis. This chapter will review the biochemical and physiologic evidence that PGE_2 is an antilipolytic substance and will describe recent results from measurements of PGE_2 during diabetic ketoacidosis.

II. THE FAT CELL HAS RECEPTORS FOR AND SYNTHESIZES PROSTAGLANDINS OF THE E SERIES

A fat cell preparation was used in the first experiments that demonstrated binding of PGE to tissue. These studies were published by Kuehl and Humes[1] who used homogenized fat cells from male Holtzman rats. They observed binding of ^{3}H-PGE_1 to their preparation which could be competed for more avidly by unlabeled PGE_1 and PGE_2 than by other PGs, fatty acids, or hormones. Shortly thereafter, Gorman and Miller[2] reported experiments using adipocyte plasma membrane sacs from male albino rats. They also observed a discrete binding site for PGE_1 and were able to recover in an unmetabolized form the PGE_1 that had been bound to fat cell membranes. Sometime later Schillinger et al.[3] used fat cells from female Wistar rats and also observed binding of ^{3}H-PGE_2.

Studies of the PGE receptor in fat cells from our laboratory for the most part have been in agreement with the results of previous workers. Our experiments utilized intact adipocytes and broken cell preparations from male Sprague-Dawley rats. Despite the differences in animal strains and cellular preparations, our data and that described in the three previously published reports are in close agreement with one exception. The report of Gorman and Miller[2] describes two classes of PGE binding sites. Although the reason for this difference in Holtzman rats is not clear, it may be due to species variation. However, the binding constant of the single class of sites we find agrees reasonably well with that of the high affinity site reported by Gorman and Miller[2] and the single site reported by Kuehl and Humes[1] and Schillinger et al.[3] Since none of the three earlier publications explored studies of down-regulation or post-receptor consequences on lipolysis, this chapter will focus on these aspects of recent studies performed in our laboratory.

Using isolated fat cells, we have performed experiments examining competition by other PGs for binding with ^{3}H-PGE_1 that revealed only a small amount of nonspecific binding (Figure 1). Binding affinities for PGE_1, PGE_2, and the 16,16-dimethyl-PGE_2 analogue were identical, whereas the affinities for the other PGs were 50 to 100 times less. Using competition experiments involving ^{3}H-PGE_1 and unlabeled PGE_1, data were analyzed according to the Scatchard method. The resulting plot (Figure 2) yielded a straight line which indicates a single class of binding sites. A set of experiments was performed wherein five rats were treated with the PGE_2-analogue while litter-mate controls were treated with the diluent in which the analogue was dissolved. The data from the analogue-treated and the control animals yielded linear Scatchard plots with different X-intercepts, i.e., down-regulation of the PGE binding sites was observed. Receptor densities calculated from these intercepts revealed 43% fewer sites in the cells from the analogue-treated rats. Down-regulation was demonstrated using both intact fat cells and triglyceride-free particulate fractions of broken fat cells.

We next examined the post-receptor consequences of down-regulation of the PGE receptor. PGE_1, PGE_2, and 16-16-dimethyl-PGE_2 were all shown to be antilipolytic.

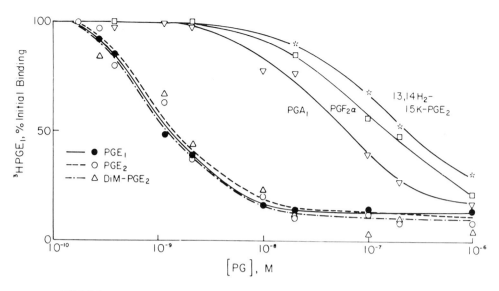

FIGURE 1. Competition by various PGs for ^{3}H-PGE$_1$ binding to isolated fat cells.

We observed that PGE$_2$ was less potent as an antilipolytic substance in cells whose PGE receptors had been diminished in number (Figure 3). This densensitization effect was not observed when insulin was examined. Consequently, we concluded that down-regulation of PGE receptors in the fat cell causes homologous rather than heterologous densensitization.

Although production of arachidonic acid metabolites by fat cells has not been very extensively studied, Shaw and Ramwell[4] reported that extracts of rat epididymal fat pads contained substances that co-chromatographed with PGE$_1$, PGE$_2$, and PGF$_{2\alpha}$. More recently, Axelrod and Levine[5] have observed that isolated adipocytes from Sprague-Dawley rats exposed to norepinephrine synthesize PGE$_2$. Further efforts are needed to intensively examine the kinetics of PGE$_1$ and PGE$_2$ production by isolated adipocytes and to verify such production with inhibitors of PGE synthesis using methodologies such as high performance liquid chromatography (HPLC) and gas chromatography/mass spectroscopy (GC/MS).

III. PROSTAGLANDINS OF THE E SERIES HAVE ANTILIPOLYTIC EFFECTS IN VITRO AND IN VIVO

The initial observation that PGE$_1$ has antilipolytic effects was published by Steinberg et al.[6] They used epididymal fat pads to examine glycerol release, which reflects the rate of lipolysis in this tissue. They observed that PGE$_1$ had an inhibitory effect on basal lipolysis and when lipolysis was stimulated with epinephrine, norepinephrine, ACTH, glucagon, or TSH. Subsequently, many investigators have verified this effect in publications too numerous to completely review in this chapter. Separate lines of evidence indicate that the antilipolytic effect of PGE$_1$ is independent of insulin, the only known antilipolytic hormone. Langslow[7] examined the antilipolytic action of PGE$_1$ on isolated chicken fat cells. PGE$_1$ was found to be potently antilipolytic for glucagon-stimulated lipolysis, whereas insulin had no effect. Loten and Sneyd[8] postulated separate sites of action for insulin and PGE$_1$ based upon experiments demonstrating that only insulin and not PGE$_1$ was able to inhibit lipolysis stimulated by exogenous cyclic AMP (cAMP) in isolated fat cells. Data such as these suggest that interference with cAMP generation may be a mechanism of action for the antilipolytic effects of

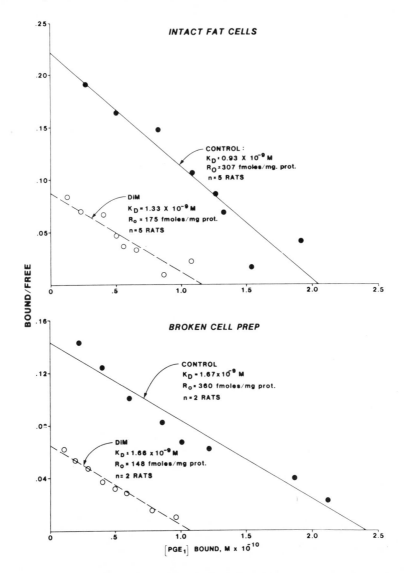

FIGURE 2.   Scatchard plots of specific binding data for control and experimental animals treated with a PGE_2-analogue to induce down-regulation. The data in the upper panel are from intact fat cells whereas those in the bottom panel are from particulate fractions of homogenized fat cells.

PGE. In this regard, Kather and Simon[9] have reported that adenylate cyclase of human fat cell ghosts demonstrate a biphasic response to PGE_2. Inhibition of this enzyme complex occurs at low concentrations, whereas stimulation occurs at much higher concentrations of PGE_2. Furthermore, the expression of the inhibitory effect of PGE_2 was GTP-dependent.

IV. PGE_2 ACCUMULATION DURING DIABETIC KETOACIDOSIS

Evidence for accumulation of PGE_2 during diabetic ketoacidosis in rats has been published by Axelrod and Levine.[10] These investigators measured plasma levels of 13,14-dihydro-15-keto PGE_2, the major circulating metabolite of PGE_2, in normal rats and in rats in which diabetes mellitus and diabetic ketoacidosis had been induced by

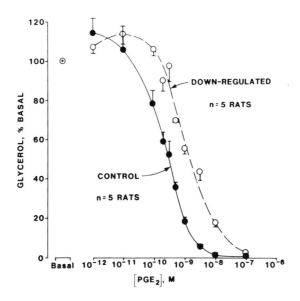

FIGURE 3. Comparison of the antilipolytic effect of PGE_2 on glycerol production by isolated fat cells from control and down-regulated animals.

injections of streptozotocin. They observed that the PGE_2 metabolite levels were six-fold higher in rats with diabetic ketoacidosis than in normal rats. More recently, these investigators have observed elevated circulating levels of the PGE_2 metabolite in human subjects with spontaneous diabetic ketoacidosis.[11]

We have utilized a different approach to the study of arachidonic acid and metabolism in human diabetic ketoacidosis.[12] We have examined plasma PGE metabolite responses in six diabetic human subjects in whom mild ketoacidosis was allowed to develop during a brief period of insulin withdrawal (Figure 4). The amount of time required to reach ketoacidosis was variable, ranging from 12 to 18 hr. The mean data for the group indicated an approximate threefold increase in circulating PGE_2 metabolite just prior to reinstitution of insulin therapy to reverse the ketoacidotic state. The metabolite levels promptly returned to preexperimental values during insulin therapy.

V. HYPOTHESIS

It is now well established that PGEs have binding sites on adipocytes and that they are antilipolytic both in vitro and in vivo. The mechanism of their antilipolytic effect may involve inhibition of adenylate cyclase, the enzyme complex that is required for stimulation of fat cell lipolysis. There is some evidence that fat cells can synthesize PGEs. Data from diabetic ketoacidotic rats indicate that a PGE_2 metabolite accumulates in circulation during acidosis and very preliminary data in humans agree with this observation. This leads to the hypothesis that PGE_2 may be synthesized by fat cells to act locally as a counterregulator of the accelerated lipolysis that is characteristic of diabetic ketoacidosis. In this sense PGE_2 may provide a protective biologic action.

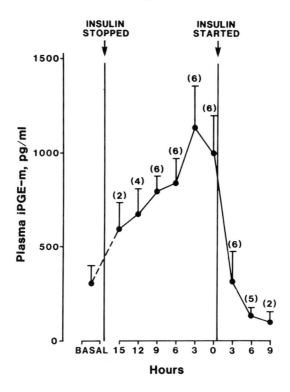

FIGURE 4.   Circulating concentration of 13,14-dihydro-15-keto-PGE$_2$ (PGE-m) levels in 6 diabetic subjects during the evolution of mild ketoacidosis caused by insulin withdrawal for 12 to 18 hr. After insulin therapy, the PGE metabolite levels returned to pre-experimental levels. The numbers in parentheses refer to the number of data points ($\bar{x} \pm$ S.E.) at the designated hour.

REFERENCES

1. Kuehl, F. A., Jr. and Humes, J. L., Direct evidence for a prostaglandin receptor and its application to prostaglandin measurements, *Proc. Natl. Acad. Sci. U.S.A.,* 69, 480, 1972.
2. Gorman, R. R. and Miller, O. V., Specific prostaglandin E$_1$ and A$_1$ binding sites in rat adipocyte plasma membranes, *Biochim. Biophys. Acta,* 323, 560, 1973.
3. Schillinger, E., Prior, G., Speckenbach, A., and Wellershoff, S., Receptor binding in various tissues of PGE$_2$, PGF$_{2\alpha}$ and sulprostone[1], a novel PGE$_2$-derivative, *Prostaglandins,* 18, 293, 1979.
4. Shaw, J. E. and Ramwell, P. W., Release of prostaglandin from rat epididymal fat pad on nervous and hormonal stimulation, *J. Biol. Chem.,* 243, 1498, 1968.
5. Axelrod, L. and Levine, L., Prostacyclin production by isolated adipocytes, *Diabetes,* 30, 163, 1981.
6. Steinberg, D., Vaughan, M., Nestel, P. H., and Bergstrom, S., Effects of prostaglandin E opposing those catecholamines on blood pressure and on triglyceride breakdown in adipose tissue, *Biochem. Pharmacol.,* 12, 764, 1963.
7. Langslow, D. R., The anti-lipolytic action of prostaglandin E$_1$ on isolated chicken fat cells, *Biochim. Biophys. Acta,* 239, 33, 1971.
8. Loten, E. G. and Sneyd, J. G. T., Evidence for separate sites of action for the antilipolytic effects of insulin and prostaglandin E$_1$, *Endocrinology,* 93, 1315, 1973.
9. Kather, H. and Simon, R., Biphasic effects of prostaglandin E$_2$ on the human fat cell adenylate cyclase, *J. Clin. Invest.,* 64, 609, 1979.
10. Axelrod, L. and Levine, L., Plasma prostaglandin levels in rats with diabetes mellitus and diabetic ketoacidosis, *Diabetes,* 31, 994, 1982.

11. Axelrod, L., Shulman, G. I., Blackshear, P. J., Bornstein, W., Roussell, A. M., and Levine, L., Plasma prostaglandin levels in diabetic ketoacidosis, *Diabetes*, 32, 66A, 1983.
12. McRae, J. R., Day, R., and Robertson, R. P., Prostaglandin E (PGE) generation during diabetic ketoacidosis (DKA) in humans, *Diabetes*, 32, 28A, 1983.

Chapter 6

PROSTAGLANDINS AND SHOCK STATES

J. Raymond Fletcher

TABLE OF CONTENTS

I. THE PARTICIPATION OF PROSTAGLANDINS IN SHOCK STATES

A. The Prostaglandin System

The discovery of this group of biologically active fatty acids was made in the 1930s by Kurzrok and Lieb.[1] Two decades later the prostaglandins (PGs) were found to be a family of compounds with unique structures that was elucidated in 1962.[2] Complete synthesis of these substances was achieved by Bergstrom and associates and Van Dorp and colleagues independently in 1964.[3]

Since completion of biosynthesis, a number of changes in this system have been made. Until recently, the PGEs and PGFs were considered the most important. In 1973 several discoveries shifted the focus from these to the PG intermediates (endoperoxides), PGG_2 and PGH_2,[4,5] and to the prostanoids, thromboxane, and PGI_2.[6,7] Another enzymatic pathway was discovered in the late 1970s, thereby establishing two major metabolic degradations of arachidonic acid.[8,9]

Arachidonic acid is released from membrane phospholipids by the action of phospholipases. It is metabolized to oxygenated products by a cyclooxygenase and a lipoxygenase. The cyclooxygenase products consist of the primary or "classical PGs" as well as thromboxane and PGI_2. Thromboxane is formed by platelets, whereas PGI_2 is derived from vascular endothelium. End products from the lipoxygenase enzyme are called leukotrienes.

The arachadonic acid-PG system consists of a class of potent vasoactive polyunsaturated fatty acids which in man are derived mostly from arachidonic acid. PGs are not stored, but are formed immediately prior to release.[10] A variety of physiological, pharmacological, and pathological stimuli trigger their release.[11]

The exact role of the arachidonic acid-PG system in the pathophysiology of shock-like states is unknown despite the many studies performed. These will be reviewed in this chapter.

1. Prostaglandins in Shock

The discovery in 1971 that nonsteroidal anti-inflammatory (NSAI) drugs inhibited the cyclooxygenase enzyme of the arachidonic acid-PG system stimulated more specific scientific investigation in this field. Prior to the use of biological assays and radioimmunoassays, Northover and Subramanian[12] showed that NSAI drugs attenuated the circulatory events in dog endotoxemia. Their initial work has been confirmed by others and extended to various species and different shock-like states.

a. Hemorrhagic (Hypovolemic, Traumatic) Shock

Increases in circulating PGs or PG-like materials are reported in a variety of hemorrhagic shock studies in several species.[13,19] As in all forms of shock, the relationship between circulating PGs and cardiovascular events is complex. PG (cyclooxygenase) inhibitors have been beneficial in the therapy of hemorrhagic shock. They improve survival and this correlates with PG inhibitor-induced improvements in circulatory function.[20-23] PG inhibitors increase blood pressure by altering systemic vascular resistance.[24,25] The mechanism by which this occurs is unknown; however, some data are available.

PGs, like many other circulating vasoactive substances, participate in the homeostatic process of peripheral vascular smooth muscle tone.[20] The vasodilating PGs perhaps inhibit vasoconstriction when present in shock-like states. This inhibition decreases PG synthesis and shifts the balance, allowing more peripheral vasoconstriction.[25]

Observations by others indicate that PGs are involved with pulmonary artery hypertension, and the increase in pulmonary airway pressures.[13,23] PG inhibitors attenuate cellular metabolic derangements (lactic acidosis), protect against vascular endothelial injury, prevent shock irreversibility, and improve survival in hemorrhagic shock.[24,26,28]

While most studies indicate that the PGs may be deleterious, certain observations suggest that some of the PGs may provide beneficial effects in hypovolemic shock.[29-32]

b. Endotoxemia, Sepsis, and Septic Shock

Endotoxemia, endotoxin shock, and sepsis has been the most extensively studied area in the PG field as it relates to shock-like states. Improved survival with analgesic and antipyretic drugs in dog endotoxemia was reported in 1962.[12] While a number of other studies were done between 1962 and 1971 (the year that NSAI drugs were reported to inhibit the PG system), it was only following 1971 that the participation of PGs in sepsis was demonstrated. Plasma PG values are increased in many species including the subhuman primates that have been subjected to endotoxemia.[33-39] Early studies were done assaying the PGs at arbitrary timed intervals rather than when circulatory events were changing. The similarity in the stress in different laboratories was uncertain. Following these early studies, the relationship of PGs to the pathophysiology of endotoxin shock was not clear.

Since then, a number of investigations have shown that shortly after the injection of endotoxin (LD_{50} concentrations), plasma PG concentrations increase in mixed venous and arterial blood.[36,39] These studies indicate the association between the mixed venous PG levels and the increase in pulmonary artery pressures.[34,37,39] In contrast to the early studies that demonstrated that the PGEs and PGFs were the important PGs released, the present understanding is that while the PGEs and PGFs are released, thromboxane and PGI_2 constitute the largest percentage of end products of arachidonic acid metabolism, and are more likely to participate in the pathophysiological events in endotoxemia and sepsis.[40-47]

Thromboxane and PGI_2 have recently received the most attention, especially because specific thromboxane synthetase inhibitors are now being utilized. Bult et al.[48] were first to report that PGI_2 was present in endotoxemia. Harris and co-workers[46] showed a similar time course of an early increase in thromboxane and a more prolonged rise in primate endotoxemia. In rat endotoxemia, Cook et al.[43,47] have demonstrated early and late increases in both thromboxane and PGI_2, and reported that a nonspecific thromboxane inhibitor, imidazole, improves survival. Casey et al.,[42] in a subhuman primate endotoxin model, clearly demonstrated for the first time that a specific thromboxane synthetase inhibitor prevents endotoxin-induced pulmonary artery hypertension and effectively inhibits thromboxane production, but fails to improve survival. In Gram-negative sepsis, thromboxane and PGI_2 are increased as in endotoxemia. In these studies imidazole does not improve survival, even though it inhibits thromboxane synthesis.[49] This suggests that while thromboxane and PGI_2 participate in the pathophysiology of endotoxemia and/or sepsis, the specific inhibition of thromboxane does not improve survival in either type of shock. The role of PGI_2 in these entities has yet to be determined. Interestingly, PGI_2 infusions have improved survival in some forms of shock.[50,51]

The obvious question is, does endotoxemia represent sepsis or septicemia? Live *Escherichia coli* infusions in baboons produce significant increases in plasma PG levels.[52] Animals with bacterial peritonitis show increased plasma values of PG about the time blood cultures are positive for *E. coli*.[45] During Gram-negative sepsis in man, plasma PG levels are increased.[53] Plasma PG values are increased and may participate in the pathophysiology of sepsis.[41]

If the PGs are present, what are their effects in endotoxemia, endotoxin, and septic shock? NSAI drugs have been utilized to elucidate the pathophysiological role that the PGs may have in sepsis. Initial studies utilized greater than therapeutic concentrations of NSAI drugs as pretreatment. Unfortunately, there were great differences between studies in doses and frequencies of NSAI drugs administered.[54-57] Pretreatment with NSAI drugs, however, did show a significant increase in survival and improved circulatory function, whereas post-treatment use of NSAI drugs in overwhelmingly lethal models did not improve survival.[55,57] Subsequently, studies were completed in dogs and baboons with endotoxin shock that demonstrated that NSAI drugs, even when administered after shock had been induced, significantly improved survival.[58] Pre-treatment of animals subjected to Gram-negative peritonitis with NSAI drug (without antibiotics) increased survival. When antibiotics were administered in addition to the NSAI drugs, survival was greater than with antibiotics alone.[59] In addition to Gram-negative sepsis, NSAI drugs are reported to improve survival in Group B streptococcal sepsis.[60]

Several PG effects have been implicated in endotoxemia or sepsis. PGs (1) increase pulmonary artery pressure and decrease systemic arterial pressure,[33-39] (2) exaggerate the metabolic derangements,[30,56,57,61,62] (3) enhance pulmonary dysfunction,[39] and (4) participate in the inflammatory response and in vascular permeability.[63,64] The PGs do not appear to alter the kinin system,[30] serotonin or histamine effects,[62,65] or lysosomal enzyme release in endotoxemia.[37] The inhibition of PGs does not alter the coagulation derangements,[37,61] the complement activation,[37] the leukopenia or thrombocytopenia present in endotoxemia, or sepsis.[61] The documented benefits of PG inhibition in sepsis are the stabilization of cell membranes and the attenuation of circulatory dysfunction. The exact mechanisms by which the PGs participate in the pathophysiology of sepsis are still unknown. With the development of specific inhibitors of other enzymes in the arachidonic acid cascade, more sophisticated and specific information will become available. It is likely that the PGs operate in the hormonal and neurohumoral milieu that homeostatically controls vascular smooth muscle responses.

c. Cardiogenic Shock

The discovery of thromboxane and PGI_2 and their interrelationships have generated a greater understanding of cardiovascular physiology. Thromboxane A_2, a potent vasoconstrictor, is released during platelet aggregation and is essential for the platelet release reaction.[6] PGI_2 is a potent vasodilator which is synthesized by the vascular endothelial cell.[7] PGI_2 prevents platelet aggregation and thereby decreases the synthesis of the vasoconstrictor thromboxane. This balance is now the subject of intense investigation. As platelets are stimulated to adhere to the vessel wall, the arachidonic acid system is activated and thromboxane is synthesized and produces vasoconstriction and further platelet aggregation. In the platelet, the endoperoxides PGG_2 and PGH_2 are formed and if they become available to the endothelial cell, will form PGI_2.[66] Thus, the formation of a vasodilator with antiplatelet aggregating activities may be formed. This balance of vasoconstriction/vasodilatation and aggregation/disaggregation has important implications in processes such as atherosclerosis.

If the proaggregation stimulus can be suppressed without preventing the anti-aggregation process, manipulation of this system could be very important in ischemic attacks of the heart and brain, and even potentially attenuate the progress of peripheral arterial disease. Pharmaceutical manufacturers have developed specific inhibitors of thromboxane that are now being widely studied in animals. Analogues of PGI_2 that will have less vasodilating activities and more platelet anti-aggregating properties are being developed.

Of particular interest to critical care medicine and to physicians in general, are the data suggesting that the PGs are involved in tissue ischemia, especially myocardial injury. Inflammatory cells and platelets are observed in ischemic and infarcted myocardium,[67] suggesting that anti-inflammatory and antiplatelet drugs might preserve cardiac function, thereby reducing morbidity and mortality.[68] The discovery that NSAI drugs inhibit PGs and that PG release is increased during myocardial ischemia implies that PGs may be involved.

It has recently been recognized that acute myocardial ischemia is an evolving process, not a static one.[68] Following experimental coronary occlusion, necrosis is present early but appears complete at 6 hr post-occlusion.[69] Interestingly, there are similarities between cellular reactions in myocardial ischemia and inflammation, i.e., release of hydrolases, proteases, lysosomal membrane destruction, PG release, leukocyte and platelet adhesion, and infiltration.[70-72] The presence of leukocytes and inflammatory cells which are known to release toxic enzymes implies that these enzymes can damage noninjured cells in the ischemic area.[71,72] PGs are also released during myocardial ischemia and may be detrimental.[73-75] Platelet trapping and aggregation with development of fibrin thrombi could extend the area of necrosis.[67] Platelet aggregation is associated with release of a number of agents (adenosine diphosphate, 5-hydroxytryptamine, calcium, PGs, thromboxane A_2) that promote additional platelet aggregates with vasoconstriction, thrombosis, and altered vascular permeability that produce more ischemia.[76] A vicious cycle may be established.

In humans the histologic evolution of myocardial infarction has been studied. In the first few hours, edema, hemorrhage, and inflammatory cells (acute) are present. Acute inflammation is present in the first week, chronic inflammation in the second, then proliferation of connective tissue and collagen deposition with fibrin formation and scarring occur while healing is completed. Complete healing takes from 6 weeks to 6 months.[35]

PGs are increased during and following myocardial ischemia in dogs,[73-75] and during ischemia induced by atrial pacing in humans with ischemic heart disease.[74] The major PG synthesized by the heart is PGI_2 and it may be one of the host defense mechanisms in ischemia.[77] The PGs are clearly involved with vasomotor regulation, mediation of the inflammatory response, and are important in platelet aggregation and thrombosis. Consequently, the ability to manipulate this system to protect against myocardial ischemia, as well as the generalized manifestations of ischemic vascular disease, would seem worthwhile. Currently there are clinical trials utilizing PG infusions to improve limb salvage rates in patients with peripheral vascular disease (see Chapters 12 and 13) and utilizing PG inhibitors for protection against myocardial ischemia (see Chapter 14). The results of these studies will help clarify the roles of PGs in cardiovascular disease.

Experimental studies suggest that cellular and metabolic events in ischemic tissue (inflammatory cells, platelets) are likely to be influenced by the PG system. The discovery that there is a reciprocal relationship between PGI_2 (a vasodilator and antiplatelet aggregating substance) and thromboxane (which has the opposite effects) has great impact on potential treatment and prevention in diseases that alter vascular/blood interfaces. While little information is available in man about PG mediation of these events, there is adequate experimental evidence to state that some component of the PG system is associated with each separate phase in the ischemic process — from initial occlusion of the vessel to completion of the healing.

II. SUMMARY

The PGs appear to participate in a wide variety of shock states: trauma, sepsis, ischemia, and hypotension. The arachidonic acid-PG system is a sensitive indicator of cellular injury. The beneficial effects of PG synthetase inhibitors in endotoxemia and in Gram-negative sepsis imply that PGs may be important in mediating, in part, the irreversibility in these states. The precise mechanism of the beneficial effect of the NSAI drugs is unknown. The data suggest they act on circulatory function.

Which, if any, prostanoid is the key has yet to be determined. The present focus is on thromboxane and PGI_2. The leukotrienes are presently being studied intensively.

There is no doubt that the PGs are involved in shock-like states in animals and man. Additional laboratory studies to define the mechanisms of the NSAI drug-induced beneficial effects are needed. The data base for the manipulation of the PG system is broad and provides an excellent foundation for human studies.

REFERENCES

1. Kurzok, R. and Leib, C. C., Biochemical studies of human semen. II. The action of human semen on the human uterus, *Proc. Soc. Exp. Biol. Med.,* 28, 268, 1930.
2. Bergstrom, S. and Samuelsson, B., The prostaglandins, *Endeavour,* 27, 109, 1968.
3. Samuelsson, B., Biosynthesis of prostaglandins, *Endeavour,* 27, 109, 1968.
4. Hamburg, M. and Samuelsson, B., Detection and isolation of an endoperoxide intermediate in prostaglandin biosynthesis, *Proc. Natl. Acad. Sci. U.S.A.,* 70, 809, 1973.
5. Nugteren, D. H. and Hazelhof, E., Isolation and properties of intermediates in prostaglandin biosynthesis, *Biochim. Biophys. Acta,* 326, 448, 1973.
6. Hamburg, M., Svensson, J., and Samuelsson, B., Thromboxane: a new group of biologically active compounds derived from prostaglandin endoperoxides, *Proc. Natl. Acad. Sci. U.S.A.,* 72, 2994, 1975.
7. Moncada, S., Gryglewski, R., Bunting, S., and Vane, J. R., An enzyme isolated from arteries transforms prostaglandin endoperoxides to an unstable substance that inhibits platelet aggregation, *Nature (London),* 263, 663, 1976.
8. Borgeat, P. and Samuelsson, B., Metabolism of arachidonic acid in polymorphonuclear leukocytes. Structural analysis of novel hydroxylated compounds, *J. Biol. Chem.,* 254, 7865, 1979.
9. Corey, E. J., Clark, D. A., Goto, G., Marfat, A., Meoskowski, C., Samuelsson, B., and Hammarstrom, S., Stereospecific total synthesis of a slow reacting substance of anaphylaxis, leukotriene C-1, *J. Am. Chem. Soc.,* 102, 1436, 1980.
10. Bills, T. K., Smith, J. B., and Silver, M. J., Selective release of arachidonic acid from the phospholipids of human platelets in response to thrombin, *J. Clin. Invest.,* 60, 1, 1977.
11. Smith, J. B., Ingerman, C. M., and Silver, M. J., in *Advances in Prostaglandin and Thromboxane Research,* Samuelsson, B. and Paoletti, R., Eds., Raven Press, New York, 1976, 747.
12. Northover, B. J. and Subramanian, G., Analgesia — antipyretic drugs as antagonists of endotoxin shock in dogs, *J. Pathol. Bacteriol.,* 83, 463, 1962.
13. Fletcher, J. R. and Ramwell, P. W., Modulation of prostaglandins E and F by the lung in baboon hemorrhagic shock, *J. Surg. Res.,* 26, 465, 1979.
14. Fletcher, J. R. and Ramwell, P. W., Altered lung metabolism of prostaglandins during hemorrhagic and endotoxin shock, *Surg. Form,* 18, 184, 1977.
15. Flynn, J. T., Appert, H. E., and Howard, J. M., Arterial prostaglandin A_1, E_1, F_{2o} concentrations during hemorrhagic shock in the dog, *Circ. Shock,* 2, 155, 1975.
16. Flynn, J. T., Bundenbaugh, G. A., and Lefer, A. M., Clearance of PGF_{2o} during circulatory shock, *Life Sci.,* 17, 1699, 1975.
17. Flynn, J. T. and Lefer, A. M., Beneficial effects of arachidonic acid during hemorrhagic shock in the dog, *Circ. Res.,* 40, 422, 1977.
18. Jakshick, B. A., Marshall, G. R., Kourik, J. L., and Needleman, P., Profile of circulating vasoactive substances in hemorrhagic shock and their pharmacologic manipulation, *J. Clin. Invest.,* 54, 842, 1974.
19. Johnston, P. A. and Beck, R. R., Effect of hemorrhage and reinfusion on renal output and systemic arterial concentrations of PGE, *Fed. Proc. Fed. Am. Soc. Exp. Biol.,* 33, 348, 1974.
20. Bond, R. F., Bond, C. H., Perssner, L., and Manning, E. S., Prostaglandin modulation of adrenergic vascular control during hemorrhagic shock, *Am. J. Physiol.,* 241, H85, 1981.
21. Leffler, C. W. and Passmore, J. C., Effects of indomethacin on hemodynamics of dogs in refractory hemorrhagic shock, *J. Surg. Res.,* 23, 392, 1977.
22. Leffler, C. W., Tyler, T. L., and Cassin, S., Effects of indomethacin on cardiovascular hemodynamics of goats in hemorrhagic shock, *Circ. Shock,* 5, 299, 1978.

23. Wilkerson, R. D., Possible role for prostaglandins in the production of alterations in pulmonary function during sphanchnic arterial occlusion, *J. Pharmacol. Exp. Ther.*, 201, 753, 1977.

24. Lefer, A. M., Araki, H., and Okamatsu, S., Beneficial actions of a free radical scavenger in traumatic shock and myocardial ischemia, *Circ. Shock*, 8, 273, 1981.

25. Nasjletti, A. and Malik, K. W., Interrelations between prostaglandins and vasoconstrictor hormones: contribution to blood pressure regulation, *Fed. Proc. Fed. Am. Soc. Exp. Biol.*, 41, 2394, 1982.

26. Miller, W. S. and Smith, J. H., Effect of acetysalicylic acid on lysosomes, *Proc. Soc. Exp. Biol. Med.*, 122, 634, 1966.

27. Noble, W. H., Famewo, C. E., and Garvey, M. B., Pulmonary vascular effects of acetylsalicylic acid, chloroquine, dextran and methylprenisolone given after haemorrhagic shock in dogs, *Can. Anaesth. Soc. J.*, 24, 661, 1977.

28. Perbeck, L. and Hedqvist, P., Prostaglandins E_1 and E_2 antagonize indomethacin-induced decrease in survival rate of haemorrhagically shocked rats, *Acta Chir. Scand.*, 500 (Suppl.), 91, 1980.

29. Blasingham, M. C. and Selkurt, E. E., Influence of PGE_1 on renal function in severe hemorrhagic shock, *Circ. Shock*, 6, 31, 1979.

30. Erdos, E. G., Hinshaw, L. B., and Gill, C. C., Effect of indomethacin in endotoxin shock in the dog, *Proc. Soc. Exp. Biol. Med.*, 125, 916, 1967.

31. Machiedo, G. W., Brown, C. S., Lavigne, J. E., and Rush, B. F., Prostaglandin E_1 as a therapeutic agent in hemorrhagic shock, *Surg. Forum*, 24, 12, 1973.

32. Whitten, R. H., Ryan, N. T., and Egdahl, R. H., PGE_2 in treatment of "irreversible" hemorrhagic shock, *Surg. Forum*, 30, 474, 1979.

33. Anderson, F. L., Jubiz, W., Tsagaris, T. J., and Kuida, H., Plasma prostaglandin levels during endotoxin shock in dogs, *Circulation*, 45, 2, 1972.

34. Anderson, F. L., Tsagaris, T. J., Jubiz, T. J., and Kuida, H., Prostaglandin E and F levels during endotoxemia induced pulmonary hypertension in calves, *Am. J. Physiol.*, 228, 1479, 1975.

35. Collier, J. R., Herman, A. G., and Vane, J. R., Appearance of prostaglandins in renal venous blood of dogs in response to acute systemic hypotension produced by bleeding or endotoxin, *J. Physiol. (London)*, 230, 14, 1973.

36. Fletcher, J. R., Ramwell, P. W., and Herman, C. M., Prostaglandins and the hemodynamic course of endotoxin shock, *J. Surg. Res.*, 20, 589, 1976.

37. Fletcher, J. R. and Ramwell, P. W., Modification by aspirin and indomethacin of the haemodynamic and prostaglandin releasing effects of *E. coli* endotoxin in the dog, *Br. J. Pharmacol.*, 51, 175, 1977.

38. Kessler, E., Hughes, R. C., and Bennett, E. N., Evidence for the presence of prostaglandin-like material in the plasma of dogs with endotoxin shock, *J. Clin. Med.*, 81, 85, 1973.

39. Parratt, J. R. and Sturgess, R. M., Evidence that prostaglandin release mediates pulmonary vasoconstriction induced by *E. coli* endotoxin, *J. Physiol. (London)*, 246, 79, 1975.

40. Bult, H., Beetens, J., and Vercriysse, P., Blood levels in 6-keto-$PGF_{1\alpha}$, the stable metabolite during endotoxin induced hypotension, *Arch. Int. Pharmacodyn.*, 236, 285, 1978.

41. Butler, R. R., Wise, W. C., and Haluska, P. V., Elevated plasma levels of thromboxane and prostacyclin in septic shock, *Circ. Shock*, 8, 213, 1981.

42. Casey, L. C., Fletcher, J. R., Zmudka, M. I., and Ramwell, P. W., Prevention of endotoxin-induced pulmonary hypertension in primates by use of a selective thromboxane synthetase inhibitor, OKY 1581, *J. Pharmacol. Exp. Ther.*, 22, 441, 1982.

43. Cook, J., Wise, W., and Haluska, P., Elevated thromboxane levels in the rat during endotoxin shock, *J. Clin. Invest.*, 65, 227, 1980.

44. Demling, R. H., Smith, M., and Gunther, R., Pulmonary injury and prostaglandin production during endotoxemia in conscious sheep, *Am. J. Physiol.*, 240, H348, 1981.

45. Fletcher, J. R., Short, B. L., Casey, L., and Ramwell, P. W., Thromboxane and prostacyclin in gram-negative sepsis, *J. Trauma*, in press.

46. Harris, R. H., Zmudka, M. I., Maddox, Y., Ramwell, P., and Fletcher, J. R., Relationships of TxB_2 and 6-keto-PGF_α to the hemodynamic changes during baboon endotoxin shock, in *Advances in Prostaglandin Thromboxane Research*, Vol. 7, Raven Press, New York, 1980, 843.

47. Wise, W. C., Cook, J. A., and Haleska, P. V., Implications for thromboxane A_2 in the pathogenesis of endotoxin shock, *Adv. Shock Res.*, 6, 83, 1981.

48. Bult, H., Beetens, J., Vercruysse, P., and Herman, A. G., Blood levels of 6-keto-$PGF_{1\alpha}$, the stable metabolite of prostacyclin during endotoxin induced hypotension, *Arch. Int. Pharmacodyn.*, 236, 285, 1978.

49. Fletcher, J. R., Short, B. L., Casey, L. C., Walker, R. I., Gardiner, M., and Ramwell, P. W., Thromboxane inhibition in gram-negative sepsis fails to improve survival, in *Advances in Thromboxane and Prostaglandin Research*, Vol. 12, Samuelsson, B., Paoletti, R., and Ramwell, P., Eds., Raven Press, New York, 1983, 117.

50. Fletcher, J. R. and Ramwell, P. W., The effects of prostacyclin (PGI$_2$) on endotoxin shock and endotoxin-induced platelet aggregation in dogs, *Circ. Shock*, 7, 299, 1980.

51. Lefer, A., Tabas, J., and Smith, E., Salutory effects of prostacyclin in endotoxin shock, *Pharmacology*, 21, 206, 1980.

52. Urist, M. M., Casey, L. C., Ramwell, P. W., and Fletcher, J. R., Prostacyclin and thromboxane metabolism in endotoxemia or sepsis in the baboon (abstract), *Assoc. Acad. Surg.*, 1981.

53. Ramwell, P. W., Fletcher, J. R., and Flamenbaum, W., The arachidonic acid — prostaglandin system in endotoxemia, *6th Int. Congr. Pharmacol.*, Helsinki, 1975, 175.

54. Greenway, C. V. and Murthy, V. S., Mesenteric vasoconstriction after endotoxin administration in cats pre-treated with aspirin, *Br. J. Pharmacol.*, 43, 259, 1971.

55. Hinshaw, L. B., Solomon, L. A., Erdos, E. G., Reins, D. A., and Gunter, B. J., Effects of salicylic acid on the canine response to endotoxin, *J. Pharmacol. Exp. Ther.*, 157, 1967.

56. Parratt, J. R. and Sturgess, R. M., The effect of indomethacin in the cardiovascular and metabolic responses to *E. coli* endotoxin in the cats, *Br. J. Pharmacol.*, 50, 177, 1974.

57. Parratt, J. R. and Sturgess, R. M., *E. coli* endotoxin shock in the cat, treatment with indomethacin, *Br. J. Pharmacol.*, 53, 485, 1975.

58. Fletcher, J. R. and Ramwell, P. W., Indomethacin improves survival after endotoxin in baboons, in *Advances in Prostaglandin Thromboxane Research*, Vol. 7, Raven Press, New York, 1980, 821.

59. Short, B. L., Gardiner, W. M., Walker, R., and Fletcher, J. R., Indomethacin improves survival in gram negative sepsis, *Adv. Shock Res.*, 6, 27, 1981.

60. Short, B. L., Miller, M. R., and Fletcher, J. R., Improved survival in the suckling rat model of group B streptococcal sepsis after treatment with nonsteroidal anti-inflammatory drugs, *Pediatrics*, 70, 343, 1982.

61. Fletcher, J. R. and Ramwell, P. W., Lidocaine or indomethacin improves survival in baboon endotoxin shock, *J. Surg. Res.*, 24, 154, 1978.

62. Parratt, J. R. and Sturgess, R. M., The possible roles of histamine, 5-hydroxy-tryptamine and prostaglandin F$_2$ as mediators of the acute pulmonary effects of endotoxin shock, *J. Surg. Res.*, 24, 154, 1978.

63. Battacherjee, R., Release of prostaglandin-like substance by Shigella endotoxin and its inhibition by non-steroidal anti-inflammatory compounds, *Br. J. Pharmacol.*, 54, 489, 1975.

64. Spector, W. G. and Willoughby, D. A., Salicylate and increased vascular permeability, *Nature (London)*, 196, 1104, 1962.

65. Hall, R. C., Hodge, R. L., and Irvine, R., The effect of aspirin on the response to endotoxin, *Aust. J. Exp. Biol. Med. Sci.*, 50, 589, 1972.

66. Bunting, S., Gryglewski, R., Moncada, S., and Vane, J. R., Arterial walls generate from prostaglandin endoperoxides a substance (prostaglandin X) which relaxes strips of mesenteric and coeliac arteries and inhibits platelet aggregation, *Prostaglandin*, 12, 897, 1976.

67. Sommers, H. M. and Jennings, R. B., Experimental acute myocardial infarction. Histologic and histochemical studies of early myocardial infarcts induced by temporary or permanent occlusion, *Lab. Invest.*, 13, 1491, 1964.

68. Braunwald, E., Introductory remarks in protection of ischemic myocardium, *Circulation,* (Suppl.1), I-53, 1976.

69. Reimer, K. A. and Jennings, R. B., The changing anatomic reference base of evolving myocardial infarction. Underestimation of myocardial blood flow and overestimation of experimental anatomic infarct size due to tissue edema, hemorrhage and acute inflammation, *Circulation*, 60, 866, 1979.

70. Brachfeld, N., Maintenance of cell viability, *Circulation,* 39, (Suppl. 4), 202, 1969.

71. Fox, A. C., Hoffstein, S., and Weissman, G., Lysosomal mechanisms in production of tissue damage during myocardial ischemia and effects of treatment with steroids, *Am. Heart J.,* 91, 394, 1976.

72. Lefer, A. M. and Spath, J. A., Preservation of myocardial integrity by a protease inhibitor during myocardial ischemia, *Arch. Int. Pharmacodyn.,* 211, 225, 1974.

73. Berger, H., Zaret, B., Speroff, L., and Cohen, L. S., Regional cardiac prostaglandin release during myocardial ischemia in anesthetized dogs, *Am. J. Cardiol.,* 39, 481, 1977.

74. Berger, H. J., Zaret, B. L., Speroff, L., Cohen, L. S., and Wolfson, S., Cardiac prostaglandin release during myocardial ischemia induced by atrial pacing in patients with coronary artery disease, *Am. J. Cardiol.,* 39, 481, 1977.

75. Ogletree, M. L., Flynn, J. T., Feota, M., and Lefer, A. M., Early prostaglandin release from ischemic myocardium in the dog, *Surg. Gynecol. Obstet.,* 144, 734, 1977.

76. Packham, M. A. and Mustard, J. F., Clinical pharmacology of platelets, *Blood*, 50, 555, 1977.

77. Isakson, P. G., Raz, A., Denny, S. E., Pure, E., and Needleman, P., A novel prostaglandin is the major product of arachidonic acid metabolism in the rabbit heart, *Proc. Natl. Acad. Sci. U.S.A.,* 74, 101, 1977.

Chapter 7

CANCER

Alan Bennett

TABLE OF CONTENTS

I. INTRODUCTION

Unlike many disease topics, the question of biological protection by prostaglandins (PGs) in cancer involves two separate aspects, the host and the cancer. Furthermore, both can produce the PGs and related substances to which the malignant and host cells may be exposed. When cancer cells form, the host defenses would normally try to eradicate them. The fact that cancer cells survive implies that the host defenses are not capable of working properly and/or are hindered by mechanisms operated by the cancer cells. The defense of the host and of the cancer are discussed separately below, although in many cases the findings are variable and may apply to both aspects.

II. DEFENSE OF THE HOST

A. Cell Differentiation

There is substantial evidence that some PGs can induce cells to differentiate. This applies to the development of normal cells and also to malignant cells that can then become morphologically and functionally normal. The mechanism is thought to involve an increased cellular content of cAMP. PGs causing differentiation can therefore be regarded as antimalignant, protecting the host. Malignant cells that can be induced to differentiate (mainly with PGE and PGA compounds — PGF compounds are usually ineffective) include mouse leukemic cells,[1,4] Friend erythroleukemic cells,[5,6] neuroblastoma,[7-9] and rat mammary malignant cells.[10] In some cases the PG synthesis inhibitor indomethacin inhibited differentiation.[3,5] There are some cells that do not differentiate with PGE compounds, namely human leukemic cells,[1,11,12] unlike their normal counterparts or murine leukemic cells; however, there are no reports that PGs favor the cancer by decreasing differentiation. It is not possible to simply describe the various effects of different PGs on various cell types. More detailed accounts of this and other aspects are given by Bennett,[13] together with many references, including recently published reviews on PGs and cancer.

B. Cell Proliferation

Many papers report an inhibitory effect of PGE and PGA compounds on the proliferation of malignant or transformed cells in culture; however, again the results vary greatly and these PGs have no effect in some cell types and can even cause enhancement in others. there are also variations with other PGs. To make matters even more complicated, the effect on Raji cells from Burkitt lymphoma is concentration-dependent, with stimulation at low concentrations of PGE_1 or PGE_2 and inhibition at high concentrations.[14] Details of these results are presented in more detail in Reference 13. The effects of PG synthesis inhibitors on cell proliferation are also contradictory, with enhancement, no effect, or inhibition of proliferation.[13]

C. Immunity

Cancer immunology is highly complex and controversial, as are the influences of PGs on immunologic pathways. Aspects that may be affected include the differentiation and proliferation of cells of the immune system, antibody expression, lymphokine production, and other aspects of cell activity. Most of the work on the immune system has concerned the lymphocytes. Only a few of the reports indicate that PGs favor the host defense by stimulating the proliferation or activity of T and B lymphocytes from man and laboratory animals. Similarly, in few cases does indomethacin inhibit the immune response. In contrast, most studies report that PGs reduce and indomethacin enhances lymphocyte proliferation or activity. Part of the reason these results are bewildering and complex is because there are so many steps involved in the measured immune responses. Even adding the PGs at different stages of responses may alter the effect obtained. A brief overview, together with lists of reviews are given in Reference 13, and effects of PGs in protecting the cancer are discussed in Section III. C.

Thromboxanes and lipoxygenase products may also be important in affecting the immune system. Thromboxane A_2 may have a role in lymphocyte transformation.[15,16] 5-HETE inhibits transformation, whereas under other circumstances 5,12-dihydroxy-HETE and other polyhydroxy-related eicosatetraenoic acids may promote transformation.[17] Leukotrienes C and D appear to be immunosuppressive.[18] It is important to remember that inhibitors of cyclooxygenase may make more substrate available for conversion by lipoxygenases into leukotrienes, etc. Another aspect is that the extent of an immune response may determine the extent of inflammation, which in turn may affect tumor spread.[19]

III. PROTECTION OF THE CANCER

Results in some of the topics discussed in Section II are variable, either favoring the host or the cancer. Some of the variability is due to differences in the types of cancer and PGs studied. Appropriate aspects are therefore reconsidered in the topics below.

A. Initiation and Promotion of Carcinogenesis

There is some evidence that PGs may be involved in the earliest development of cancers. Some arachidonate products are themselves mutagenic, or may cause other compounds to be metabolized into mutagenic agents. Malondialdehyde, formed by thromboxane synthetase from PG endoperoxides, is carcinogenic in mice.[20] PGs may be required for tetraphorbol acetate to initiate epidermal hyperproliferation and hyperplasia in mouse skin.[21-23]

The conversion of arachidonate to PGH_2 can provide oxygen that converts relatively inert chemicals into carcinogens,[24,25] an effect blocked by cyclooxygenase inhibitors.

With regard to promoters of carcinogenesis which shorten the latent period between the exposure to the chemical carcinogen and the formation of a tumor, PGs or in some cases possibly lipoxygenase products, may be involved. The subject has been discussed in recent reviews.[21,26] Most studies indicate that PGs themselves are not promoters, but may play a role in the process.

B. Cell Proliferation

This topic is relevant to both the host and the cancer, because the results are variable. The work is discussed in Section II. B.

C. Immunity

The host's immune defenses are often depressed in cancer. A substantial amount of evidence indicates that PGs may be involved, and a main source of these inhibitory PGs may be leukocytes.[26-30] The way that malignant cells stimulate leukocyte PG production, and the extent to which malignant cells produce PGs are not clear. One effect of PGE and PGA compounds is to inhibit human and murine natural killer cells.[31,32] Indomethacin frequently increases the immune response (see Reference 13).

D. Platelet Aggregation

This topic may be important with regard to metastatic spread via the bloodstream. The aggregation of platelets around a malignant cell may protect it from attack by host leukocytes and aid its penetration into various tissues. This may explain why aspirin, an inhibitor of platelet aggregation, reduced the metastatic spread of various malignant cell lines injected into mice.[33] Other studies in mice support this view. Thromboxane synthesis inhibitors decreased, and 15-HPETE (which blocks PGI_2 synthesis) increased the metastasis of B-16 amelanotic melanoma to the lungs.[34] In other tumor cell lines, a high ratio of thromboxane:PGI_2 production favored metastatic spread.[35] Thus, thromboxane A_2 may protect the cancer and PGI_2 may protect the host. In addition, various studies both in man and laboratory animals show that tumors can release PGs into the venous blood supply (see Reference 13). Clearly these might have numerous effects, including an alteration of platelet aggregation.

E. Vascular Effects and Blood Supply

It has been hypothesized that PGE_2 and possibly other substances released from tumors may cause local vasodilatation and possibly aid the dispersion of clumps of malignant cells.[36]

Once cancer cells have survived the difficult task of escaping destruction by the host and then penetrating into an appropriate distant site, the formation of a blood supply is necessary to allow continued growth. Angiogenesis is therefore important, and it has been suggested that PGs may be involved in the formation of new blood vessels.[37]

F. Bone

Many human carcinomas commonly spread to the skeleton, such as those of breast, lung, kidney, and prostate. Animal data show that certain PGs such as PGE_2 and PGI_2 are potent bone-resorbing agents, and drugs that inhibit PG synthesis can inhibit bone destruction by malignant cells in vivo.[38-41] Furthermore, in some patients with "solid" tumors, hypercalcemia may occur. This disease responds to treatment with aspirin or indomethacin,[42] although not all investigators have found this.[43] We were initially intrigued with the possibility that malignant breast metastatic cells capable of producing large amounts of PGs were those that most easily formed bone metastases. Our early work showed a higher median production of PG-like material from breast carcinomas in patients with isotopic scan evidence of bone metastasis near the time of breast surgery.[44,45] Work by others[46] showed that those tumors that most actively resorbed bone in vitro were most commonly assoicated with spread to the skeleton in vivo. It now appears, however, that the difference in median values was not due to a higher PG production in the tumors that spread to bone; instead, there was a low PG production by the primary tumor in patients with no evidence of bone metastases.[47,48] Thus, while PGs may have a role in bone metastasis, their contribution does not seem to be of great importance.*

IV. GENERAL CONSIDERATIONS OF PROSTAGLANDINS AND THEIR SYNTHESIS INHIBITORS IN CANCER

Since there are so many interacting variables in so many types of cancer, we cannot expect a clear and simple analysis. At best, we could hope for knowledge of how a given type of cancer at a particular stage in its development responds to PGs or drugs that modify their formation or catabolism. It remains to be determined in all cases of human disease whether PGs or their synthesis inhibitors can be used to improve treatment. Whatever the outcome, the results will increase our understanding of tumor biology.

PGs administered in vivo appear to be beneficial in some cases[49-51] The mechanisms are diverse, and in the latter study[51] $PGF_{2\alpha}$ acted by lowering blood progesterone levels in rats with a hormone-dependent mammary adenocarcinoma. In contrast PGE_2 or

---

* Editor's note: See the following chapter for a different view.

$PGF_{2\alpha}$ enhanced murine carcinogenesis,[52,53] whereas patients with breast cancer or leukemia given PGA_1, PGA_2, or PGE_2 in a pilot study showed no evidence of disease regression.[54]

The practical importance in cancer of using drugs that inhibit PG synthesis may be substantial. Such drugs are widely used by patients with cancer, often to treat unrelated conditions, but sometimes to treat the side effects of conventional therapy such as radiation-induced mucositis[55] or diarrhea.[56] Furthermore, corticosteroids that inhibit the release of PG precursors[57] commonly form part of regimes using cytotoxic drugs.

Fortunately, almost all the data from animal studies indicate that inhibitors of PG synthesis are beneficial, or at least have no harmful effects in cancer (see Reference 13). For example, mice with a methylcholanthrene-induced tumor survived longer when treated with indomethacin,[58] and mice with a transplanted mammary adenocarcinoma lived longer when PG synthesis inhibitors were given together with cytotoxic chemotherapy.[59] It remains to be seen what happens in man, although a few results are available. For example, flurbiprofen increased the response of patients previously insensitive to cytotoxic therapy,[60] but benorylate did not affect the formation of bone metastasis or survival in patients with breast cancer.[61] Our double-blind controlled trial with flurbiprofen in breast cancer is nearing an end and will soon be available for analysis.

It also remains to be seen how cancer is affected by drugs that alter particular parts of the PG cascade. Drugs are now available that selectively inhibit thromboxane formation, and drugs acting selectively at other sites may well emerge in the future.

The word "cytoprotection" which has been used in relation to GI mucosa[62] may be due to various factors such as blood flow, mucus production, and bicarbonate secretion. But do PGs protect at the cellular level? Our indirect evidence indicates that they do not in the two cell lines studied, hepatoma cells (HTC, Flow Laboratories) and human normal embryological cells of intestinal epithelium (407, Flow Laboratories). The inclusion of indomethacin 0.1 or 1 $\mu g/m\ell$ in the culture medium reduced the viability of the tumor cells, but not of the normal epithelial cells. X-irradiation dose relatedly inhibited cell proliferation, but this was not altered by indomethacin in the normal cells; it was additive with the inhibitory effect of indomethacin on the tumor cells.[63] The fact that indomethacin did not increase the response of irradiation argues against a "cytoprotective" effect of endogenous PGs. These cell culture results suggest that PG synthesis inhibitors would not adversely affect the tumor response to radiotherapy, although they do not assess the effect of any PGs that might reach cancer cells in vivo from other cells. However, studies in vivo suggest that combination of a PG synthesis inhibitor with X-irradiation is beneficial.[64-66]

REFERENCES

1. Collins, S. J., Bodner, A., Ting, R., and Gallo, R. C., Induction of morphological and functional differentiation of human promyeloctyic leukemia cells (HL-60) by compounds which induce differentiation of murine leukemia cells, *Int. J. Cancer,* 25, 213, 1980.
2. Honma, Y., Kasukabe, T., Hozumi, M., and Koshihara, Y., Regulation of prostaglandin synthesis during differentiation of cultured mouse myeloid leukemia cells, *J. Cell. Physiol.,* 104, 349, 1980.
3. Honma, Y., Kasukabe, T., and Hozumi, M., Inhibition of differentiation of cultured mouse myeloid leukemia cells by nonsteroidal antiinflammatory agents and counteraction of the inhibition by prostaglandin E, *Cancer Res.,* 39, 2190, 1979.
4. Takenaga, K., Honma, Y., and Hozumi, M., Inhibition of differentiation of mouse myeloid leukemia cells by phenolic antioxidants and alpha-tocopherol, *Gann,* 72, 104, 1981.

5. Santoro, M. G. and Jaffe, B. M., Role of prostaglandins on the growth and differentiation of Friend erythroleukemia cells, in *Prostaglandins and Cancer: First International Conference,* Powles, T. J., Bockman, R. S., Honn, K. V., and Ramwell, P., Eds., Alan R. Liss, New York, 1982, 425.

6. Santoro, M. G., Bennedetto, A., and Jaffe, B. M., Prostaglandin A_1 induces differentiation in Friend erythroleukemia cells, *Prostaglandins,* 17, 719, 1979.

7. Prasad, K. N., Role of prostaglandins in differentiation of neuroblastoma cells in culture, in *Prostaglandins and Cancer: First International Conference,* Powles,T. J., Bockman, R. S., Honn, K. V., and Ramwell, P., Eds., Alan R. Liss, New York, 1982, 437.

8. Adolphe, M., Giroud, J. P., Timsit, J., Fontagne, J., and Leckat, P., Action de la prostaglandine A_2 sur la proliferation et la differenciation morphologique d'une lignee cellulaire de neuroblastome murin, *C. R. Seances Soc. Biol., Paris,* 6-7, 694, 1974.

9. Lazo, J. S. and Ruddon, R. W., Neurite extension and malignancy of neuroblastoma cells after treatment with prostaglandin E_1 and papaverine, *J. Natl. Cancer Inst.,* 59, 137, 1977.

10. Rudland, P. S. and Warburton, M. J., Prostaglandins induce differentiation and reduce the neoplastic potential of a rat mammary tumour stem cell line, in *Prostaglandins and Cancer: First International Conference,* Powles, T. J., Bockman, R. S., Honn, K. V., and Ramwell, P., Eds., Alan R. Liss, New York, 1982, 465.

11. Taetle, R., Guittard, J. P., and Mendelsohn, J. M., Abnormal modulation of granulocyte/macrophage progenitor proliferation by prostaglandin E in chronic myeloproliferative disorders, *Exp. Hematol.,* 8, 1190, 1980.

12. Moore, M. A., Mertelsmann, R., and Pelus, L. M., Phenotypic evaluation of chronic myeloid leukemia, *Blood Cells,* 7, 217, 1981.

13. Bennett, A., in *Handbook of Prostaglandins and Related Lipids,* Willis, A. L., Ed., CRC Press, Boca Raton, Florida, in press.

14. Karmali, R. A., Horrobin, D. F., Menezes, J., and Patel, P., The relationship between concentrations of prostaglandin A_1, E_1, E_2 and E_2 α and rates of cell proliferation, *Pharmacol. Res. Commun.,* 11, 69, 1979.

15. Parker, C. W., Stenson, W. F., Huber, M. G., and Kelly, J. P., Formation of thromboxane B_2 and hydroxyarachidonic acids in purified human lymphocytes in the presence and absence of PHA, *J. Immunol.,* 122, 1572, 1979.

16. Kelly, J. P., Johnson, M. C., and Parker, C. W., Effect of inhibitors of arachidonic acid metabolism on mitogenesis in human lympocytes: possible role of thromboxanes and products of the lypoxygenase pathway, *J. Immunol.,* 122, 1563, 1979.

17. Parker, C. W., Arachidonate metabolites and immunity, in *Prostaglandins and Cancer: First International Conference,* Powles, T. J., Bockman, R. S., Honn, K. V., and Ramwell, P., Eds., Alan R. Liss, New York, 1982, 595.

18. Thomson, D. M. P., Phelan, K., and Bach, M. K., Leukotrienes released by human monocytes mediate tumor antigen induced leukocyte adherence inhibition (L. A. I.), in *Prostaglandins and Cancer: First International Conference,* Powles, T. J., Bockman, R. S., Honn, K. V., and Ramwell, P., Eds., Alan R. Liss, New York, 1982, 667.

19. Van den Brenk, H. A. S., Stone, M., Kelly, H., Orton, C., and Sharpington, C., Promotion of growth of tumor cells in acutely inflammed tissues, *Br. J. Cancer,* 30, 246, 1974.

20. Shamberger, R. J., Adreone, T. L., and Willis, C. E., Antioxidants and cancer. IV. Initiating activity of malonaldehyde as a carcinogen, *J. Natl. Cancer Inst.,* 53, 1771, 1974.

21. Levine, L., Arachidonic acid transformation and tumor production, *Adv. Cancer Res.,* 35, 49, 1981.

22. Furstenberger, G. and Marks, F., Early prostaglandin E synthesis is an obligatory event in the induction of cell proliferation in mouse epidermis in vivo by the phorbol ester TPA, *Biochem. Biophys. Res. Commun.,* 92, 749, 1980.

23. Furstenberger, G., Gross, M., and Marks, F., On the role of prostaglandins in the induction of epidermal proliferation, hyperplasia and tumor promotion in mouse skin, in *Prostaglandins and Cancer: First International Conference,* Powles, T. J., Bockman, R. S., Honn, K. V., and Ramwell, P., Eds., Alan R. Liss, New York, 1982, 239.

24. Miller, J. A., Carcinogenesis by chemicals: an overview, *Cancer Res.,* 70, 559, 1970.

25. Miller, J. A. and Miller, E. C., The initiation stage of chemical carcinogenesis: an introductory overview, in *Prostaglandins and Cancer: First International Conference,* Powles, T. J., Bockman, R. S., Honn, K. V., and Ramwell, P., Eds., Alan R. Liss, New York, 1982, 81.

26. Honn, K. V., Bockman, R. S., and Marnett, L. J., Prostaglandins and cancer: a review of tumor initiation through tumor metastasis, *Prostaglandins,* 21, 833, 1981.

27. Salmon, S. E., Interrelationship of endogenous macrophages, prostaglandin synthesis and tumor cell clonogenicity in human tumor biopsies, in *Prostaglandins and Cancer: First International Conference,* Powles, T. J., Bockman, R. S., Honn, K. V., and Ramwell, P., Eds., Alan R. Liss, New York, 1982, 633.

28. Goodwin, J. S. and Webb, D. R., Regulation of the immune response by prostaglandins, *Clin. Immunol. Immunopathol.*, 15, 106, 1980.

29. Goldyne, M. E. and Stobo, J. D., Immunoregulatory role of prostaglandins and related lipids, *CRC Crit. Rev. Immunol.*, 2, 189, 1981.

30. Goodwin, J. S. and Webb, D. R., Regulation of the immune response by prostaglandins, in *Suppressor Cells in Human Disease,* Goodwin, J. S., Ed., Marcel Dekker, New York, 1981, 99.

31. Brunda, M. J., Herberman, R. B., and Holden, H. T., Inhibition of murine natural killer cell activity by prostaglandins, *J. Immunol.*, 124, 2682, 1980.

32. Bankhurst, A. D., The modulation of human natural killer cell activity by prostaglandins, *J. Lab. Clin. Immunol.*, 7, 85, 1982.

33. Gasic, G. J., Gasic, T. B., Galanti, N., Johnson, T., and Murphy, S., Platelet-tumor-cell interactions in mice. The role of platelets in the spread of malignant disease, *Int. J. Cancer,* 11, 704, 1973.

34. Honn, K. V., Prostacyclin/thromboxane ratios in tumor growth metastasis, in *Prostaglandins and Cancer: First International Conference,* Powles, T. J., Bockman, R. S., Honn, K. V., and Ramwell, P., Eds., Alan R. Liss, New York, 1982, 733.

35. Donati, M. B., Borowska, A., Bottazzi, B., Dejana, E., Giavazzi, R., Rotilio, D., and Manotvani, A., in *Proc. 5th Int. Conf. Prostaglandins,* Fordazlone Giovanni Lorenzini, Milan, 1982, 136.

36. Bennett, A., Prostaglandins: relationships to breast cancer and its spread, in *New Aspects of Breast Cancer,* Vol. 5, *Endocrine Relationships in Breast Cancer,* Stoll, B. A., Ed., Heinemann, London, 1982, 156.

37. Form, D. M., Sidky, Y. A., Kubai, L., and Auerbach, R., PGE_2-induced angiogenesis, in *Prostaglandins and Cancer: First International Conference,* Powles, T. J., Bockman, R. S., Honn, K. V., and Ramwell, P., Eds., Alan R. Liss, New York, 1982, 685.

38. Powles, T. J., Clark, S. A., Easty, D. M., Easty, G. C., and Neville, A. M., The inhibition by aspirin and indomethacin of osteolytic tumor deposits and hypercalcaemia in rats with Walker tumor, and its possible application to human breast cancer, *Br. J. Cancer,* 28, 316, 1973.

39. Strausser, H. R. and Humes, J. L., Prostaglandin synthesis inhibition: effect on bone changes and sarcoma tumor induction in balb/c mice, *Int. J. Cancer,* 15, 724, 1975.

40. Galasko, C. S. B. and Bennett, A., Relationship of bone destruction in skeletal metastasis to osteoclast activation and prostaglandins, *Nature (London),* 263, 508, 1976.

41. Galasko, C. S. B., Rawlins, R., and Bennett, A., Timing of indomethacin in the control of prostaglandins, osteoclasts and bone destruction produced by VX_2 carcinoma in rabbits, *Br. J. Cancer,* 40, 360, 1979.

42. Seyberth, H. W., Segre, G. V., Morgan, J. L., Sweetman, B. J., Potts, J. T., and Oates, J. A., Prostaglandins as mediators of hypercalcemia associated with certain types of cancer, *N. Engl. J. Med.,* 293, 1278, 1975.

43. Coombes, R. C., Neville, A. M., Bondy, P. K., and Powles, T. J., Failure of indomethacin to reduce hypercalcemia in patients with breast cancer, *Prostaglandins,* 12, 1027, 1976.

44. Bennett, A., McDonald, A. M., Simpson, J. S., and Stamford, I. F., Breast cancer, prostaglandins and bone metastases, *Lancet,* 1, 148, 1975.

45. Bennett, A., Charlier, E. M., McDonald, A. M., Simpson, J. S., Stamford, I. F., and Zebro, T., Prostaglandins and breast cancer, *Lancet,* 2, 124, 1977.

46. Powles, T. J., Dowsett, M., Easty, D. M., Easty, G. C., and Neville, A. M., Breast-cancer osteolysis, bone metastases, and anti-osteolytic effect of aspirin, *Lancet,* 1, 608, 1976.

47. Bennett, A., Prostaglandins and inhibitors of their synthesis in cancer growth and spread, in *Endocrinology of Cancer,* Vol. 3, Rose, D. P., Ed., CRC Press, Boca Raton, Fla., 1982, 113.

48. Bennett, A., Berstock, D. A., Carroll, M. A., Stamford, I. F., and Wilson, A. J., Breast cancer, its recurrence, and patient survival in relation to tumor prostaglandins, *Adv. Prostaglandin, Thromboxane, Leukotriene Res.,* 12, 299, 1983.

49. Santoro, M. G., Philpott, G. W., and Jaffe, B. M., Inhibition of tumour growth in vivo and in vitro by prostaglandin E, *Nature (London),* 263, 777, 1976.

50. Josse, R. G., Wilson, D. R., Heersche, J. N., Mills, J. R., and Murray, T. M., Hypercalcemia with ovarian carcinoma, *Cancer,* 48, 1233, 1981.

51. Jacobson, H., Oncolytic action of prostaglandin, *Cancer Chemother. Rep.,* 58, 503, 1974.

52. Lupulescu, A., Enhancement of carcinogenesis by prostaglandins, *Nature (London),* 272, 634, 1978.

53. Lupulescu, A., Hormonal regulation of epidermal tumor development, *J. Invest. Dermatol.,* 77, 186, 1981.

54. Powles, T. J., Coombes, R. C., Depledge, M., Muindi, J., and Powles, R., Prostaglandin administration to patients with cancer, in *Prostaglandins and Cancer: First International Conference,* Powles, T. J., Bockman, R. S., Honn, K. V., and Ramwell, P., Eds., Alan R. Liss, New York, 1982, 825.

55. Tanner, N. S. B., Stamford, I. F., and Bennett, A., Plasma prostaglandins in mucositis due to radiotherapy and chemotherapy for head and neck cancer, *Br. J. Cancer,* 43, 767, 1981.

56. Mennie, S. A. T., Dalley, V., Dinneen, L. C., and Collier, H. O. J., Treatment of radiation-induced gastrointestal distress with acetylsalicylate, *Lancet*, 2, 942, 1975.

57. Gryglewski, R. J., Panczenko, B., Korbut, R., Grodzinska, L., and Ocetkiewicz, A., Corticosteroids inhibit prostaglandin release from perfused mesenteric blood vessels of rabbit and from perfused lungs of sensitized guinea pig, *Prostaglandins*, 10, 343, 1975.

58. Lynch, N. R., Castes, M., Astoin, M., and Solomon, J. C., Mechanism of inhibition of tumor growth by aspirin and indomethacin, *Br. J. Cancer*, 38, 503, 1978.

59. Bennett, A., Berstock, D. A., and Carroll, M. A., Increased survival of cancer-bearing mice treated with inhibitors of prostaglandin synthesis alone or with chemotherapy, *Br. J. Cancer*, 45, 762, 1982.

60. Powles, T. J., Alexander, P., and Millar, J. L., Enhancement of anti-cancer activity of cytotoxic chemotherapy with protection of normal tissues by inhibition of PG synthesis, *Biochem. Pharmacol.*, 27, 1389, 1978.

61. Powles, T. J., Dady, P. J., Williams, J., Easty, G. C., and Coombes, R. C., Use of inhibitors of prostaglandin synthesis in patients with breast cancer, *Adv. Prostaglandin Thromboxane Res.*, 6, 511, 1980.

62. Robert, A., Effect of prostaglandins on gastrointestinal functions, in *Prostaglandins and Thromboxanes*, Berti, F. and Velo, G. P., Eds., Plenum Press, New York, 1977, 287.

63. Gaffen, J. G., Northway, M. G., and Bennett, A., unpublished data.

64. Bennett, A., Houghton, J., Leaper, D. J., and Stamford, I. F., Cancer growth, response to treatment and survival time in mice: beneficial effect of the prostaglandin synthesis inhibitor flurbiprofen, *Prostaglandins*, 17, 179, 1979.

65. Northway, M.G., Bennett, A., Carroll, M. A., Feldman, M. S., Mamel, J. J., Libshitz, H. I., Swarc, I. A., and Eastwood, G., Comparative effects of anti-inflammatory agents and radiotherapy on normal esophagus and tumors in animals, *Gastroenterology*, 78, 1229, 1980.

66. Hellmann, K. and Pym, B. A., Antitumour activity of flurbiprofen in vivo and in vitro, in *Prostaglandins and Cancer: First International Conference*, Powles, T. J., Bockman, R. S., Honn, K. V. and Ramwell, P., Eds., Alan R. Liss, New York, 1982, 767.

Chapter 8

BREAST CANCER

G. N. Hortobagyi

TABLE OF CONTENTS

I. INTRODUCTION

Prostaglandins (PGs) constitute a family of arachidonic acid metabolites found in virtually every type of mammalian tissue. They act mostly near the sites of synthesis and, therefore, are considered local and regional mediators that participate in a variety of biologic processes.[1] The effects are protean, and different PGs may have opposing actions within the same tissue or different doses may elicit various end-organ responses.[2] These metabolites have been implicated in processes of cell differentiation,[3,4] growth,[5] and function. In neoplastic diseases they are known to participate in the processes of carcinogenesis,[6,7] promotion,[7] tumor growth, replication,[5,8] and modulation of the metastatic process.[7,9] Most somatic cells, including transformed cells, have the ability to produce and are often under the influence of various PGs.[1] More recently, PGs have been studied in the area of oncology because of their presumed involvement in hypercalcemia of malignancy,[10] neovascularization,[11] modulation of the immune system,[12,13] and the metastatic process.[14] Many of these studies have been performed in experimental mammary tumors, and some information is available about the basic biology of PGs in human breast cancer as well as preliminary data from in vivo therapeutic studies with PGs and inhibitors of PG synthetase.

In this chapter I will briefly review basic experimental information about PGs in cancer (see also Chapter 7) and will emphasize those aspects that are pertinent to breast carcinoma. I will also discuss the available information with respect to the role of PGs in human breast cancer, particularly their influence in therapeutic interventions up to the present time.

II. CELL GROWTH AND REPLICATION

That PGs bind to specific membrane receptors is well established.[1] Both nonspecific and specific binding can be measured and quantitated in benign and malignant tissues. In this regard, PGs are like steroid[15] or polypeptide hormones.[16] Little is known, however, about the correlation of the concentration of specific binding sites with the biological activity of each PG. Cyclic nucleotides are mediators for various cell functions, including cell growth. PGs, not unlike polypeptide hormones, modulate cyclic nucleotide activity.[17] Stimulation of cyclic AMP (cAMP) synthesis inhibits cell replication. Consequently, PGs are known to influence the growth of both tumor cells and normal host cells, a function that is particularly important in the case of cells responsible for immune reaction. PGs also may simultaneously stimulate tumor growth and inhibit host cell activation, thus tilting the host-tumor interaction in favor of the tumor.[18]

PG synthetase has also been implicated in the process of carcinogenesis.[19] Of specific importance in the area of breast cancer is the interaction between PG synthetase and steroid hormone (estrogens) binding to DNA.[6] Estrogens and other steroid hormones are known to induce tumors in various hormone-dependent tissues in experimental animals,[20,21] and probably in humans.[22] The hypothesis has been made that specific target organ enzymes (peroxidase) may catalyze the oxidation of hormones (i.e., diethylstilbestrol) to intermediates that bind nucleic acids and other cellular macromolecules.[19] PG synthetase in these same organs also may catalyze this reaction.[6] Estradiol induces PG synthetase-catalyzed binding to DNA. The interaction of estrogens and PG synthetase may potentiate this interaction on estrogen-dependent tissues. In addition, estrogens and other steroid hormones have been implicated as promoters and may serve as both initiators and promoters of carcinogenesis in hormone-dependent tissues such as breast, endometrium,[23] and prostate.

PGs of the A series are known to inhibit tumor cell proliferation and induce differentiation.[24] In vitro incubation of B16$_a$ cell suspensions with PGA$_1$ and PGA$_2$ will produce dose-dependent inhibition of DNA synthesis. Similar results are obtained with Lewis lung carcinoma cells.[7] Other studies have shown that PGAs induce differentiation in murine erythroleukemia cells,[3] in mouse neuroblastoma,[4] and in Lewis lung carcinoma (3LL) cell lines.[24] While inhibition of DNA synthesis has been observed with PGE_2 analogues, the effects on differentiation occur predominantly with PGA compounds. The induction of differentiation, as opposed to cytotoxic therapy, is an attractive avenue of investigation for the control of human neoplasms. In this area, along with vitamins, dimethylsulfoxide (DMSO), and other substances, PGs are effective in inducing differentiation.

III. IMMUNOLOGICAL EFFECTS

Published reports implicate PGs, mostly of the E type, in exerting a wide variety of regulatory effects on host defenses.[25] As a broad generalization, PGs are believed to inhibit immunologic reactivity; however, in some specific situations enhancement rather than inhibition has been observed. While all immune cells are able to produce PGs, macrophages and monocytes seem to be the major source of endogenous PGs.[18,26] PGs of the E and F classes induce proliferation and differentiation of thymocytes in vitro, but the significance of this effect in vivo is unclear. Several reports have suggested that PGE, PGF, and PGA may inhibit ^3H thymidine incorporation in PHA-stimulated peripheral blood lymphocytes. Conversely, there is evidence that indomethacin enhances ^3H thymidine uptake by T cells. Similarly, other investigators have reported that PGE_2 inhibits PHA and ConA stimulated mitogenesis but has no effect on PWM-induced mitogenesis. This observation suggests that the inhibitory effect of PGE_2 on T cells is stronger than that on B cells. While PGs inhibit the formation of plaque-forming cells from mouse spleen lymphocytes in culture, spleen cell cultures incubated with indomethacin and antigen produce more plaque-forming colonies than the controls.

The effect of PGs on humoral immunity has been inadequately studied. More detailed studies of the effect of PGs on T cells suggest that PGs may activate suppressor T cells, thus depressing the immune response.[27] This hypothesis was indirectly confirmed following the administration of PG synthetase inhibitors, such as indomethacin, which resulted in restoration of T cell function.[28] PGs also may promote lymphokine production (PGE_1). The killing of target cells by cytotoxic T cells is a cyclic nucleotide-mediated phenomenon that can be influenced by various substances including PGs. Interferon is known to activate natural killer (NK) cells and at the same time to stimulate cellular PG biosynthesis.[29] Both E and A type PGs inhibit NK cell activity in vitro, while PG synthetase inhibitors potentiate NK cell activity, suggesting that PGs participate in the feedback mechanism to regulate NK cell activity in vivo.

Honn and co-workers[7] have shown that prostacyclin (PGI_2) is a potent vasodilator that inhibits platelet aggregation and, therefore, interferes with the process of metastasis by inhibiting tumor cell platelet thrombus formation. Thromboxane has exactly the opposite effect — that of vasoconstriction and increasing platelet aggregation. By modulating the PGI_2/thromboxane ratio in experimental tumor systems, tumor growth could be enhanced or inhibited. In line with this research, a new compound, nafazatrom, which is a potent stimulator of PGI_2 biosynthesis, has been shown to substantially decrease the metastatic potential of several tumor systems.

The major problem in assessing the physiologic and therapeutic effects of PGs and PG synthetase inhibitors on the immune system is the paucity of in vivo information, especially in humans.

IV. HYPERCALCEMIA

Many publications during the last 15 years have reflected the interrelation of hypercalcemia, bone resorption, and PGs. Klein and Raisz[31] in 1970 reported their results showing that PGs stimulate bone resorption in vitro. PGEs were the most potent stimulators of bone resorption, although other PGs did so to a lesser extent.[32,33] Numerous investigators have described that the stimulation of bone resorption by PGs is different and separate from that related to parathyroid hormone. Coombes et al.[34] reported that tumor cells, monocytes, and macrophages also release PGs. Co-cultures of fresh tumor cells and chunks of healthy bone result in bone resorption within 24 to 72 hr. Bennett et al.[35] found that breast cancer cells, especially from patients known to have bone metastasis, synthesize large quantities of PGs in vitro, mostly of the E series. Powles and co-workers[36] stated that 60% of human breast carcinomas produce osteolysis in culture. The bone resorption mechanisms of PGs and of parathyroid hormone are similar, although independent, and proceed through the activation of adenyl cyclase and accumulation of cAMP. A close interaction of host and tumor cells appears necessary for this effect to occur. Macrophages or monocytes in the tumor area are thought to release PGs, which in turn act on the local and regional lymphocytes and stimulate release of the osteoclase-activating factor (OAF) by these cells.[10] Thus, PGs do not directly produce bone resorption, but stimulate the lymphocyte-mediated bone resorption through OAF.

Galasko and co-workers[37] have shown that bone metastasis and hypercalcemia can be prevented in rabbits with mammary carcinoma in vivo by administering aspirin and indomethacin during the early osteoclastic phase of bone resorption. In later stages of the disease, however, these same drugs were unable to alter either the metastatic process or bone resorption. PGs of the E series are responsible in some animal models for the development of hypercalcemia.[38] One must remember that PGs are local or regional mediators and, therefore, they do not circulate in sufficient quantities to explain the development of generalized metastases or hypercalcemia or to determine the appropriate therapeutic intervention. There are many factors involved in these processes. Attempts to induce hypercalcemia or bone resorption by the administration of PGs usually have failed.[39,40] Similarly, the use of PG synthetase inhibitors has helped to control hypercalcemia in only a few instances.[10,41] It is an accepted fact today that the hypercalcemic effect of PGs or the bone resorption stimulating effect of PGs is a local or regional one.

V. PROSTAGLANDIN PRODUCTION BY TUMORS

Many transformed cell lines (animal and human) synthesize and release considerable amounts of PGs into the growth media.[42-44] In vitro PG synthesis can be modulated by modifying the composition of culture media. Thus, by increasing the concentration of precursor fatty acids, PG production is markedly increased.[42] Conversely, the addition of corticosteroids to the media completely inhibits PG biosynthesis.

Our experience with many long-term breast cancer cell lines shows that most produce and release considerable quantities of PGs into the culture media.[43] All these cell lines are pure and do not contain other host cells. Most cell lines originate from pleural effusions, all of which contain high concentrations of PGE_2. Attempts to analyze in vitro PG production and the clinical characteristics of the patients from whom the cell lines originated showed that older patients with slower-growing tumors (long disease-free interval, long survival with metastases) were more likely to have PGE_2-producing tumors than patients with the opposite characteristics. There was no detectable correlation between osseous metastases, hypercalcemia, and in vitro PG production.

Evaluation of PG synthesis and release in fresh tumors or short-term cultures showed that macrophages and monocytes within the tumor, and not the tumor cells, were responsible for PG production.[18] There are indications that macrophage-produced PGs are necessary for tumor colony formation, reflecting the intimate and complete interaction of tumor and host cells.

PG synthesis in normal and malignant mammary tissue varies with the stage of estrus cycle, which indicates a close interrelation with systemic hormonal levels,[45] or that the macrophage content of the tumor changes with tumor growth or regression secondary to hormonal intervention.

The PG content of malignant breast tumors has also been measured and found to be elevated,[46,47] although this finding has not been correlated with any meaningful biological or clinical factor. The plasma (or serum) concentration of PGE_2 was measured in patients with breast carcinoma. While elevated levels were found in a large proportion of patients, they did not correlate with tissue concentrations of PGs or with the clinically important parameters.[47,48]

Studies in human breast tumors show that they contain a high intratumoral concentration of PGE_2 and PGF_2. This is true in most but not all tumors. The intratumoral concentration does not correlate with plasma or serum levels of these same PGs. Whether the ability to produce high concentrations of PGs correlates with disease-free interval or survival in these patients has not been determined at this point.

VI. THERAPEUTIC ATTEMPTS

A. Preclinical

PGs inhibit in vitro cell replication and DNA synthesis in many cell systems.[7,14,24] In addition, the systemic administration of PGs of the A and E series to tumor-bearing mice delays the growth of B16 melanoma and results in prolonged survival of the animals. The administration of 16-16 dimethyl PGF_2 produced similar inhibition of growth in a human colorectal cancer xenograft in mice.[49]

PG synthetase inhibitors have been employed in a greater number of experiments and clinical trials with antitumor purposes.[50,51] Early experiments with aspirin and indomethacin gave, at best, conflicting results.[52] Newer nonsteroidal anti-inflammatory (NSAI) agents with a more potent PG synthetase inhibitor activity have demonstrated antitumor activity more consistently. Hellman and Pym[53] reported in 1981 that flurbiprofen was ineffective in inhibiting the appearance of distant metastasis of Lewis lung carcinoma and B16 melanoma in rodents. They also reported that when flurbiprofen was given simultaneously with local radiation therapy, the inhibitory effect of this combination was greater than that of radiation therapy alone. Whether this was due to a radiomimetic effect of flurbiprofen or a direct antitumor effect of flurbiprofen could not be established from their experiment. That flurbiprofen failed to inhibit the appearance of metastases in the B16 model is somewhat surprising since this drug had a direct, dose-related, growth-inhibiting effect in vitro against B16 melanoma cells.

In a series of experiments with mouse mammary tumor virus treated with irradiation and flurbiprofen, tumor weights decreased in response to increased doses of radiation.[54] Tumor weight and volume were smaller in the animals treated with flurbiprofen, and fewer and less severe radiotherapy effects occurred.

Other experiments with mouse mammary tumors have suggested that flurbiprofen could enhance the effect of radiotherapy or chemotherapy;[51] however, these experiments have not been uniformly reproduced.

PG synthetase inhibitors were added in vitro to mammary tumor cells and chunks of bone. The most effective antiosteolytic combination was found to be a PG synthetase inhibitor and a diphosphonate.[50] The experiment suggested the flurbiprofen is also effective in inhibiting osteolysis.

B. Clinical Trials

Three major clinical trials have been undertaken in an attempt to evaluate the antitumor and antiosteolytic effects of PG synthetase inhibitors in human breast cancer. All three trials were conducted in England by a group of investigators who have demonstrated interest and experience in the field of PG research.

Powles and associates, in 1975, initiated a clinical trial in patients with primary breast cancer and high risk of relapse or metastasis after mastectomy. One hundred and sixty (160) patients were entered into this study over a period of 2½ years, and after appropriate stratification were randomized to receive benorylate, a selective inhibitor of cyclooxygenase, 4 g, twice per day, or placebo over a period of 18 months. Two reports have been published so far from this study, both of which indicate that benorylate was not effective in reducing overall recurrence or metastasis, specifically bone metastasis.[55,56] This was true even though benorylate produced marked reduction in plasma thromboxane B_2 levels.

The purpose of the second trial was to evaluate the effect of nonsteroidal or anti-inflammatory drugs on the appearance or progression of osteolytic bone metastasis.[56] This was an open trial and included 26 patients with breast cancer. Eight of them were treated with a combination of soluble aspirin (2.7 g/day) and indomethacin (75 mg/day), 2 patients were treated with indomethacin (300 mg/day), 9 patients were given flurbiprofen (300 mg/day), and 7 received benoxyprofen (300 mg/day). All patients were evaluated clinically and a variety of biochemical tests were conducted to monitor bone metabolism. Pain and analgesic requirements were assessed regularly. Although 20% of patients treated with the various anti-inflammatory agents received relief from pain and hypercalcemia decreased in 2 of 4 patients treated with flurbiprofen and 1 of 2 patients treated with benoxyprofen, no objective evidence of change or improvement in the osteolytic process was observed in any of these patients.

The third trial was to evaluate the combination of chemotherapy and flurbiprofen. One hundred and one (101) patients with metastatic breast carcinoma not previously treated with chemotherapy were given a combination of Adriamycin and vindesine (or vincristine) at standard doses once a month.[57] These patients were randomized to receive either flurbiprofen 100 mg 3 times a day or placebo for 2 weeks of each cycle. There was no difference in objective response rate or rate of stabilization between the groups treated with flurbiprofen or placebo; furthermore, there was no difference in responsiveness of osseous metastasis between these two groups of patients. The median duration of response and the median survival of patients treated with flurbiprofen or placebo were identical. Of some interest, however, was the fact that in the patients treated with flurbiprofen the incidence of severe leukopenia and peripheral neuropathy related to the vinca alkaloids was lower than in the control group. This is especially important since the doses of chemotherapy received by both groups of patients were similar.

Powles et al.[57] reported a small series of patients with breast carcinoma treated with exogenous PGs. Four patients who had been treated with local and systemic therapy for recurrent disease and in whom progressive disease of soft tissue was observed were given PGE by means of intravenous infusion over a 48-hr period, followed by oral administration of the same PG 6 times a day. No objective response occurred, although tolerance was acceptable. Seven additional patients with metastatic or locally recurrent breast cancer in whom disease progression was confirmed following chemotherapy or endocrine therapy were treated with pure crystalline PGA_1 and liquid PGA_2 dissolved in ethanol. The drugs were given intravenously in a 6-hr infusion once a week. No objective response was observed in any of these patients, but all of them tolerated this treatment without severe complications or toxicity. While in vitro and in vivo studies in experimental animal systems show tumor inhibition by various PGs, evidence in humans is not sufficient to assess the antitumor activity of these substances.

VII. COMMENTS

That PGs of the various types are intimately involved in the biologic processes of tumor growth, differentiation, modulation, metastasis, and possibly treatment has been amply documented. While in vitro experiments show that PGs can both stimulate and inhibit tumor growth, insufficient information exists about their effect on the various experimental and human tumors in vivo. The failure of earlier clinical trials with PGs as inhibitors to produce any sort of conclusive evidence may be due to the lack of pertinent information. PGs are just one of many factors that modulate these important biologic processes, and to expect major, clinically detectable changes in established tumors by adjusting only PG synthesis may be unrealistic. These efforts may be more successful in the early stages of tumor development, although much more information may be needed regarding the specific type of PG or the specific PG synthesis inhibitor and the histologic characteristics of the tumor before a successful clinical result can be achieved.

Similar questions must be answered about the interaction of PGs and immune reactivity. Substantial and often contradictory information exists about the effect of PGs and inhibitors of PG synthesis in vitro. In vivo information, both in experimental tumor systems and in humans, will be necessary in order to better understand these interactions and before any modulation of this PG-induced immunosuppression for therapeutic purposes can be attempted.

Most successful therapeutic experiments have been performed on models not relevant to the clinical situation. For instance, therapeutic intervention before tumor implantation or before metastatic spread occurs is not applicable to the medical situation in which cancer is diagnosed in patients after two thirds of the natural history of the tumor has elapsed and often when metastases are firmly established. The inhibitory effect of PG synthetase inhibitors occurs only in the early stages of osteolysis. For this reason, therapeutic attempts should be undertaken only in early stages of tumor growth and before the development of demonstrable metastatic disease.

Finally, one should recognize that the PG system represents a local or, at best, regional mediator system and that the systemic administration of PGs or their inhibitors may be totally ineffective. Conversely, they may produce different and sometimes opposing effects in the various organ systems. Research in regional or targeted therapeutic intervention might be more successful by adjusting the processes of immunosuppression, osteolysis, and metastasis in favor of the host.

REFERENCES

1. McCarthy, J. A., Prostaglandins; an overview, in *Advances in Pediatrics,* Vol. 25, Barness, L. A., Bongiovanni, A. M., Morrow, G., Oski, F., and Rudolph, A. M., Eds., Yearbook Medical Publishers, Chicago, 1978, 121.
2. Manku, M. S., Horrobin, D. F., Karmazyn, M., and Cunnane, C. C., Prolactin and zinc effects on rat vascular reactivity: possible relationship to dihomo-λ-linolenic acid and to prostaglandin synthesis, *Endocrinology,* 104, 774, 1979.
3. Santoro, M. G. and Jaffe, B. M., Role of prostaglandins on the growth and differentiation of Friend erythroleukemia cells, in *Prostaglandins and Cancer: First International Conference,* Vol. 2, Powles, T. J., Bockman, R. S., Honn, K. V., and Ramwell, P., Eds., Alan R. Liss, New York, 1982, 425.
4. Prasad, K. N., Role of prostaglandins in differentiation of neuroblastoma cells in culture, in *Prostaglandins and Cancer: First International Conference,* Vol. 2, Powles, T. J., Bockman, R. S., Honn, K. V., and Ramwell, P., Eds., Alan R. Liss, New York, 1982, 437.
5. Goodwin, J. S., Husby, G., and Williams, R. C., Jr., Prostaglandin E and cancer growth, *Cancer Immunol. Chemother.,* 8, 3, 1980.

6. Bennett, S., Marshall, W., and O'Brien, P. J., Metabolic activation of diethylstilbestrol by prostaglandin synthetase as a mechanism for its carcinogenicity, in *Prostaglandins and Cancer: First International Conference,* Vol. 2, Powles, T. J., Bockman, R. S., Honn, K. V., and Ramwell, P., Eds., Alan R. Liss, New York, 1982, 143.

7. Honn, K. V., Bockman, R. S., and Marnett, L. J., Prostaglandins and cancer: a review of tumor initiation through tumor metastasis, *Prostaglandins,* 21, 833, 1981.

8. Jubiz, W., Frailey, J., and Smith, J. B., Inhibitory effect of prostaglandin E_{2a} on the growth of a hormone-dependent rat mammary tumor, *Cancer Res.,* 39, 998, 1979.

9. Honn, K. V., Dunn, J. R., and Meyer, J., Thromboxanes and prostacyclin: positive and negative modulators of tumor cell proliferation, in *Prostaglandins and Cancer: First International Conference,* Vol. 2, Powles, T. J., Bockman, R. S., Honn, K. V., and Ramwell, P., Eds., Alan R. Liss, New York, 1982, 375.

10. Mundy, G. R., Involvement of prostaglandin synthesis in mechanisms of malignant hypercalcemia, in *Prostaglandins and Cancer: First International Conference,* Vol. 2, Powles, T. J., Bockman, R. S., Honn, K. V., and Ramwell, P., Eds., Alan R. Liss, New York, 1982, 501.

11. Form, D. M., Sidky, Y. A., Kubai, L., and Auerbach, R., PGE_2-induced angiogenesis, in *Prostaglandins and Cancer: First International Conference,* Vol. 2, Powles, T. J., Bockman, R. S., Honn, K. V., and Ramwell, P., Eds., Alan R. Liss, New York, 1982, 685.

12. Alexander, P., Prostaglandins in relation to tumour-host ineractions, in *Prostaglandins and Cancer: First International Conference,* Vol. 2, Powles, T. J., Bockman, R. S., Honn, K. V., and Ramwell, P., Eds., Alan R. Liss, New York, 1982, 581.

13. Parker, C. W., Arachidonate metabolites and immunity, in *Prostaglandins and Cancer: First International Conference,* Vol. 2, Powles, T. J., Bockman, R. S., Honn, K. V., and Ramwell, P., Eds., Alan R. Liss, New York, 1982, 595.

14. Honn, K. V., Cicone, B., and Skoff, A., Prostacyclin: a potent antimetastatic agent, *Science,* 212, 1270, 1981.

15. Chan, L. and O'Malley, B. W., Mechanism of action of the sex steroid hormones, *N. Engl. J. Med.,* 294, 1322, 1976.

16. Murad, F. and Haynes, R. C., Jr., Hormones and hormone antagonists, in *The Pharmacological Basis Therapeutics,* Goodman, L. S., Gilman, A. G., and Gilman, A., Eds., Macmillan, New York, 1980, 1367.

17. Teller, N., Malachi, T., and Halbrecht, I., Prostaglandin E_2 and cyclic AMP levels in human breast tumors, *J. Cancer Res. Clin. Oncol.,* 93, 275, 1979.

18. Salmon, S. E., Interrelationship of endogenous macrophages, prostaglandin synthesis and tumor cell clongenicity in human tumor biopsies, in *Prostaglandins and Cancer: First International Conference,* Vol. 2, Powles, T. J., Bockman, R. S., Honn, K. V., and Ramwell, P., Eds., Alan R. Liss, New York, 1982, 633.

19. Marnett, L. J., Bienkowski, M. J., Leithauser, M., Pagels, W. R., Panthananickal, A., and Reed, G. A., Prostaglandin synthetase-dependent cooxygenation, in *Prostaglandins and Cancer: First International Conference,* Vol. 2, Powles, T. J., Bockman, R. S., Honn, K. V., and Ramwell, P., Eds., Alan R. Liss, New York, 1982, 97.

20. Bradley, C. J., Kledzik, G. S., and Meites, J., Prolactin and estrogen dependency of rat mammary cancers at early and late stages of development, *Cancer Res.,* 36, 319, 1976.

21. Rudali, G., Jullien, P., Vives, C., and Apiou, F., Dose-effect studies on estrogen induced mammary cancers in mice, *Biomedicine,* 29, 45, 1978.

22. Bibbo, M., Haenszel, W. M., Wied, G. L., Hubby, M., and Herbst, A. L., A twenty-five-year follow-up study of women exposed to diethylstilbestrol during pregnancy, *N. Engl. J. Med.,* 298, 763, 1978.

23. Mack, T. M., Pike, M. C., Henderson, B. E., Pfeffer, R. I., Gerkins, V. R., Arthur, M., and Brown, S. E., Estrogen and endometrial cancer in a retirement community, *N. Engl. J. Med.,* 294, 1262, 1976.

24. Turner, W. A., Taylor, J. D., and Honn, K. V., Effects of prostaglandin "A" series on tumor cells in vitro, in *Prostaglandins and Cancer: First International Conference,* Vol. 2, Powles, T. J., Bockman, R. S., Honn, K. V., and Ramwell, P., Eds., Alan R. Liss, New York, 1982, 369.

25. Parker, C. W., Arachidonate metabolites and immunity, in *Prostaglandins and Cancer: First International Conference,* Vol. 2, Powles, T. J., Bockman, R. S., Honn, K. V., and Ramwell, P., Eds., Alan R. Liss, New York, 1982, 595.

26. Fulton, A., Rios, A., Loveless, S., and Heppner, G., Prostaglandins in tumor-associated cells, in *Prostaglandins and Cancer: First International Conference,* Vol. 2, Powles, T. J., Bockman, R. S., Honn, K. V., and Ramwell, P., Eds., Alan R. Liss, New York, 1982, 701.

27. Fulton, A. M. and Levy, J. G., The possible role of prostaglandins in mediating immune suppression by nonspecific T suppressor cells, *Cell. Immunol.,* 52, 29, 1980.

28. Mavligit, G. M., Raphael, L. S., Calvo, D. B., III, and Wong, W. L., Indomethacin-induced, monocyte-dependent restoration of local graft-versus-host reaction among cells from cancer patients, *J. Natl. Cancer Inst.*, 65, 317, 1980.

29. Fitzpatrick, F. A. and Stringfellow, D. A., Host defense: trilateral relationships among virus, interferon induction and cellular prostaglandin biosynthesis, in *Prostaglandins and Cancer: First International Conference*, Vol. 2, Powles, T. J., Bockman, R. S., Honn, K. V., and Ramwell, P., Eds., Alan R. Liss, New York, 1982, 333.

30. Eling, T. E., Honn, K. V., Busse, W. D., Seuter, F., and Marnett, L. J., Stimulation of PGI$_2$ biosynthesis by nafazatrom (BAY G 6575), in *Prostaglandins and Cancer: First International Conference*, Vol. 2, Powles, T. J., Bockman, R. S., Honn, K. V., and Ramwell, P., Eds., Alan R. Liss, New York, 1982, 783.

31. Klein, D. C. and Raisz, L. G., Prostaglandins: stimulation of bone resorption in tissue culture, *Endocrinology*, 86, 1436, 1970.

32. Martin, T. J. and Partridge, N. S., Prostaglandins and cellular bone resorption, in *Prostaglandins and Cancer: First International Conference*, Vol. 2, Powles, T. J., Bockman, R. S., Honn, K. V., and Ramwell, P., Eds., Alan R. Liss, New York, 1982, 525.

33. Bennett, A., McDonald, A. M., Simpson, J. S., and Stamford, I. F., Breast cancer, prostaglandins and bone metastases, *Lancet*, 1, 1218, 1975.

34. Coombes, R. C., Neville, A. M., Gazet, J. C., Fort, H. T., Nash, A. G., Baker, J. W., and Powles, T. J., Agents affecting osteolysis in patients with breast cancer, *Cancer Chemother. Pharmacol.*, 3, 41, 1979.

35. Bennett, A., Charlier, E. M., McDonald, A. M., Simpson, J. S., Stamford, I. F., and Zebro, T., Prostaglandins and breast cancer, *Lancet*, 2, 624, 1977.

36. Powles, T. J., Clark, S. A., Easty, D. M., Easty, G. C., and Neville, A. M., The inhibition by aspirin and indomethacin of osteolytic tumour deposits and hypercalcemia in rats with Walker tumour, and its possible application to human breast cancer, *Br. J. Cancer*, 28, 316, 1973.

37. Galasko, C. S. B., Rawlins, R., and Bennett, A., Prostaglandins, osteoclasts and bone destruction produced by VX2 carcinoma in rabbits: effects of administering indomethacin at different doses and times, *Br. J. Cancer*, 40, 360, 1979.

38. Seyberth, H. R., Segre, G. V., Morgan, J. L., Sweetman, B. J., Potts, J. T., Jr., and Oates, J. A., Prostaglandins as mediators of hypercalcemia associated with certain types of cancer, *N. Engl. J. Med.*, 293, 1278, 1975.

39. Franklin, R. B. and Tashjian, A. H., Jr., Intravenous infusions of prostaglandin E$_2$ raises plasma concentrations in the rat, *Endocrinology*, 97, 240, 1975.

40. Beliel, O. M., Singer, F. R., and Coburn, J. W., Prostaglandins: effect on plasma calcium concentration, *Prostaglandins*, 3, 327, 1973.

41. Caro, J. F., Besarab, A., and Flynn, J. T., Prostaglandin E and hypercalcemia in breast carcinoma: only a tumor marker? A need for perspective, *Am. J. Med.*, 66, 337, 1979.

42. Hammarstrom, S., Endogenous prostaglandin production and cell replication in vitro, in *Prostaglandins and Cancer: First International Conference*, Vol. 2, Powles, T. J., Bockman, R. S., Honn, K. V., and Ramwell, P., Eds., Alan R. Liss, New York, 1982, 297.

43. Hortobagyi, G. N., Schultz, P., Cailleau, R., Samaan, N., and Blumenschein, G., In vitro prostaglandin production by metastatic breast cancer, in *Prostaglandins and Cancer: First International Conference*, Vol. 2, Powles, T. J., Bockman, R. S., Honn, K. V., and Ramwell, P., Eds., Alan R. Liss, New York, 1982, 567.

44. Owen, K., Gomolka, D., and Droller, M. J., Prostaglandin E$_2$ by tumor cells in vitro, *Cancer Res.*, 40, 3167, 1980.

45. Foecking, M. K., Panganamala, R. V., Abou-Issa, H., and Minton, J. P., Modulation of prostaglandins in hormone dependent mammary carcinoma, in *Prostaglandins and Cancer: First International Conference*, Vol. 2, Powles, T. J., Bockman, R. S., Honn, K. V., and Ramwell, P., Eds., Alan R. Liss, New York, 1982, 657.

46. Gunasegaram, R., Loganath, A., Peh, K. L., Chiang, S. C., and Ratman, S. S., Identification of prostaglandins in infiltrating duct carcinoma of the human breast, *IRCS Med. Sci.*, 8, 747, 1980.

47. Malachi, T., Chaimoff, Ch., Feller, N., and Halbrecht, I., Prostaglandin E$_2$ and cyclic AMP in tumor and plasma of breast cancer patients, *J. Cancer Res. Clin. Oncol.*, 102, 71, 1981.

48. Powles, T. J., Coombes, R. C., Neville, A. M., Ford, H. T., and Gazet, J. C., 15-keto-13,14-dihydroprostaglandin E concentrations in serum of patients with breast cancer, *Lancet*, 2, 138, 1967.

49. Tutton, P. J. and Barkla, D. H., Influence of prostaglandin analogues on epithelial cell proliferation and xenograft growth, *Br. J. Cancer*, 41, 47, 1980.

50. Galasko, C. S. B., Samuel, A. W., Rushton, S., and Lacey, E., The effect of prostaglandin synthesis inhibitors and diphosphonates on tumour-mediated osteolysis, *Br. J. Surg.*, 67, 493, 1980.

51. Leaper, D. J., French, B. T., and Bennett, A., Breast cancer and prostaglandins: a new approach to treatment, *Br. J. Surg.*, 66, 683, 1979.

52. Dowsett, M., Easty, D. M., Easty, G. C., and Neville, A. M., Breast-cancer osteolysis, bone metastases, and anti-osteolytic effect of aspirin, *Lancet,* 1, 608, 1976.

53. Hellman, K. and Pym, B. A., Antitumor activity of flurbiprofen *in vivo* and *in vitro,* in *Prostaglandins and Cancer: First International Conference,* Vol. 2, Powles, T. J., Bockman, R. S., Honn, K. V., and Ramwell, P., Eds., Alan R. Liss, New York, 1982, 767.

54. Northway, M. G., Bennett, A., Carroll, M. A., Eastwood, G. L., Feldman, M. S., Libshitz, H. I., Mamel, J. J., and Szwarc, I. A., Effects of anti-inflammatory agents and radiotherapy on esophageal mucosa and tumors in animals, in *Prostaglandins and Cancer: First International Conference,* Vol. 2, Powles, T. J., Bockman, R. S., Honn, K. V., and Ramwell, P., Eds., Alan R. Liss, New York, 1982, 799.

55. Powles, T. J., Dady, P. J., Williams, J., Easty, G. C., and Coombes, R. C., Use of inhibitors of prostaglandin synthesis in patients with breast cancer, in *Advances in Prostaglandin and Thromboxane Research,* Vol. 6, Samuelsson, B., Ramwell, P. W., and Paoletti, R., Eds., Raven Press, New York, 1980, 511.

56. Powles, T. J., Muindi, J., and Coombes, R. C., Mechanisms for development of bone metastases and effects of anti-inflammatory drugs, in *Prostaglandins and Cancer: First International Conference,* Vol. 2, Powles, T. J., Bockman, R. S., Honn, K. V., and Ramwell, P., Eds., Alan R. Liss, New York, 1982, 541.

57. Powles, T. J., Coombes, R. C., Depledge, M., Muindi, J., and Powles, R., Prostaglandin administration to patients with cancer, in *Prostaglandins and Cancer: First International Conference,* Vol. 2, Powles, T. J., Bockman, R. S., Honn, K. V., and Ramwell, P., Eds., Alan R. Liss, New York, 1982, 825.

Chapter 9

PROSTACYCLIN IN THE CONTROL OF TUMOR METASTASIS

Kenneth V. Honn, James M. Onoda, David G. Menter, John D. Taylor, and
Bonnie F. Sloane

TABLE OF CONTENTS

I. METASTATIC CASCADE

Advances in surgery and radiation therapy of primary tumors have left metastasis as a principal obstacle to cancer cure. Metastasis, simply defined, is the loss of contiguity between cells or clumps of cells and the primary tumor followed by their dissemination to distant organs (Figure 1). After transformation (i.e., chemical, radiation, or viral) a neoplastic cell can undergo proliferation until limited by its blood supply and its invasive properties. To establish a metastatic focus the tumor cells must first dissociate from the primary tumor and intravasate or invade into the circulatory system. During transport in the circulatory system the tumor cells may interact with host platelets to induce platelet aggregation. This in turn may enhance attachment of tumor cells to the blood vessel wall. Tumor cell extravasation through the vessel wall is thought to be facilitated by proteolytic enzymes released from the tumor cell. At the metastatic site the processes of proliferation, angiogenesis, invasion and metastasis (from a metastasis) can recur (Figure 1).

An estimated 0.001% of cells that detach from the primary tumor survive to form a metastatic lesion, indicating that metastasis is a very inefficient process.[1-3] Pathophysiological properties of the tumor cells (i.e., "pre-existing metastatic phenotype"[4]) as well as properties of the host (i.e., tumor cell/platelet interaction[5]) may affect survival. Survival might simply be a random event[3] or a combination of random and nonrandom events.

Successful arrest and/or adhesion of the tumor cells to the vessel wall and the factors (e.g., platelets, endothelial cell surface determinants, tumor cell surface determinants, etc.) that activate and/or enhance this process may be the most important events in metastasis since the presence of viable circulating tumor cells does not correlate with patient survival.[6] Although carcinomas were once believed to metastasize via the lymphatics and mesenchymal tumors via the vascular system, there is now substantial evidence that malignant cells can pass freely between the lymphatics and the vasculature.[7-11] This indicates that at some point in the metastatic cascade tumor cells are transported via the vasculature.

Abnormalities in platelet function and blood coagulability often occur in animals bearing transplantable tumors and in patients with malignant neoplasms.[12-15] These abnormalities include hyperaggregability of platelets[16] with resultant thrombocytopenia[17] and a reduction in fibrinogen concomitant with an increase in fibrin-fibrinogen degradation products.[12,15,18] Tumor cells have been reported to possess both a platelet activating material[19-22] and a procoagulant activity responsible for alterations in the fibrin-fibrinogen system.[23-25] The role of platelets and blood coagulation in tumor metastasis has been the subject of debate for many years.[26] Morphologists from the beginning of the century have described tumor cells enmeshed within a thrombus and adherent to the capillary wall.[27-31] In a classic study Wood[32] visualized (via continuous cinemicrography of rabbit ear chambers) the fate of intra-arterially injected V_2 squamous carcinoma cells. He observed that small clumps (6 to 10) of tumor cells arrested in the capillaries and became enmeshed in a clot of fibrin and platelets. Wood[32] concluded that the initial site of arrest was not determined by vessel diameter or rate of blood flow, an idea also supported by the observations of Zeidman.[33] Additional morphological evidence to support a role of platelets in tumor arrest has been provided by the studies of Warren and Guldner[34] and Sindelar et al.[35]

Gasic et al.[36] were the first to provide direct experimental evidence for a role of platelets in tumor cell metastasis. They had noted that pretreatment of mice with neuraminidase resulted in formation of fewer lung colonies following injection of TA3 ascites tumor cells. These results were found to be attributable to induction of thrombocytopenia and were also observed when thrombocytopenia was induced with anti-

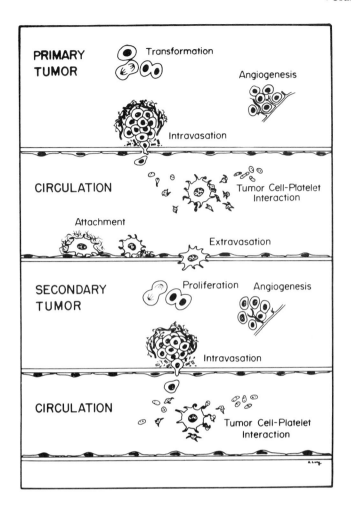

FIGURE 1. Overiew of the metastatic cascade. (From Honn, K. V. et al., in *Cancer Invasion and Metastasis: Biologic and Therapeutic Aspects,* Nicholson, G. L. and Milas, L., Eds., Raven Press, New York, in press. With permission.)

platelet antiserum. In addition, the antimetastatic effects of neuraminidase could be reversed by platelet infusion.

In subsequent papers, Gasic et al.[19,37,38] demonstrated that numerous human and animal tumor cells and plasma membrane vesicles shed from tumor cells were capable of aggregating platelets in vitro with a concomitant stimulation of the release reaction (measured as [14C]-serotonin released from prelabeled platelets). Other laboratories have confirmed the in vitro aggregation of platelets by both animal and human tumor cells and the induction of thrombocytopenia following i. v. injection of several tumor lines.[21,39-47] Recent work from Pearlstein and co-workers[21] provides more direct evidence that a direct relationship exists between platelets, tumor cells, and metastasis. Using ten cell lines derived from the polyoma virus-induced PW20 Wistar-Furth rat renal sarcoma, they found a significant correlation between the ability of the tumor cells to metastasize spontaneously and their platelet aggregating activity in vitro. Recent reviews of this area can be found in the work of Jamieson[48] and Honn and Sloane;[49] however, most of the studies to date still only provide circumstantial evidence that host platelets facilitate hematogenous metastasis.

The mechanisms by which platelets might enhance metastasis have not been established. It is generally accepted that tumor cells are damaged during transport from the site of intravasation to the site of extravasation. This circulatory trauma may be due to humoral factors (i.e., macrophages, natural killer cells, antibodies) and physical factors (i.e., shear forces, mechanical trauma due to passage through the microvasculature). Tumor cells shielded within platelet thrombi may be protected from some or all of the above. In addition, platelets may enhance tumor cell adhesion to endothelial or de-endothelized surfaces via platelet bridges. Recently Turner et al.[50] have demonstrated that during Walker 256 carcinosarcoma (W256) tumor cell-induced platelet aggregation (TCIPA), fibronectin released from the platelet α-granules becomes associated with the surface of the W256 cells. Prior to TCIPA the tumor cell surface was devoid of fibronectin. Thus, platelet-derived fibronectin could facilitate tumor cell adhesion. Nicolson and co-workers[51] have demonstrated that fibronectin may function as a tumor cell attachment protein. However, Liotta and co-workers[52,53] found that the more metastatic tumor cells seem to use laminin as an attachment protein.

The contribution of each of the above-suggested mechanisms to platelet enhancement of tumor cell metastasis is not known; however, it is generally accepted that platelets enhance metastasis by facilitating processes which occur during tumor cell arrest and/or adhesion. Therefore, in an effort to reduce metastasis, cancer therapy aimed at interrupting the metastatic cascade has been attempted with antiplatelet and/or anticoagulant agents such as heparin,[54] warfarin,[55] and dipyridamole.[56] The results to date have been inconsistent with the exception of those with warfarin.[57]

II. PROSTACYCLIN, THROMBOXANES, PLATELETS, AND METASTASIS

Compounds derived from arachidonic acid (prostacyclin [PGI$_2$] and thromboxane A$_2$ [TXA$_2$], Figure 2) have been demonstrated to have a profound, but possibly not exclusive,[58] role in platelet aggregation and normal hemostasis. Hamberg et al.[59] demonstrated the formation of TXA$_2$ from the endoperoxide intermediate PGH$_2$ (Figure 2). Subsequently, platelet TXA$_2$ biosynthesis was found to be stimulated by numerous aggregating agents and was believed to be an absolute requirement for platelet aggregation.[60] This view has recently been challenged by the observation that in some cases the endoperoxide PGH$_2$ initiates platelet aggregation independent of its conversion to TXA$_2$.[61]

One year following the discovery of TXA$_2$, Vane and co-workers[62] discovered prostacyclin (PGI$_2$) as a transformation product of PG endoperoxides (Figure 2). PGI$_2$ is the most potent endogenous inhibitor of platelet aggregation; it was discovered to be 30 to 40 times more potent that PGE$_1$[63] and 1000 times more potent than adenosine.[64] It has been suggested that PGI$_2$ and TXA$_2$ play an antagonistic and pivotal role in the control of thrombosis centered upon their bidirectional (PGI$_2$ increases, TXA$_2$ decreases) effect on platelet cAMP levels; however, proaggregatory agents (i.e., 1-0-alkyl-2-0-acetyl-2sn-glyceryl3-phosphorylcholine [PAF-acether]) in addition to TXA$_2$ should also be considered in this pivotal role.

Our working hypothesis has been that the normal intravascular balance between PGI$_2$ and platelet arachidonic acid metabolites (i.e., TXA$_2$) can be altered in favor of thrombosis and metastasis by the presence of a primary tumor, circulating tumor cells, and/or their shed membrane vesicles.[5] This hypothesis can be tested experimentally, and the evidence supporting a role for exogenous and endogenous PGI$_2$ as an antimetastatic agent is presented below.

A. Prostacyclin Effects In Vivo and In Vitro
1. Prostacyclin Effects on TCIPA
In vitro, the addition of elutriated[65] W256 cells to human platelet-rich plasma (PRP)

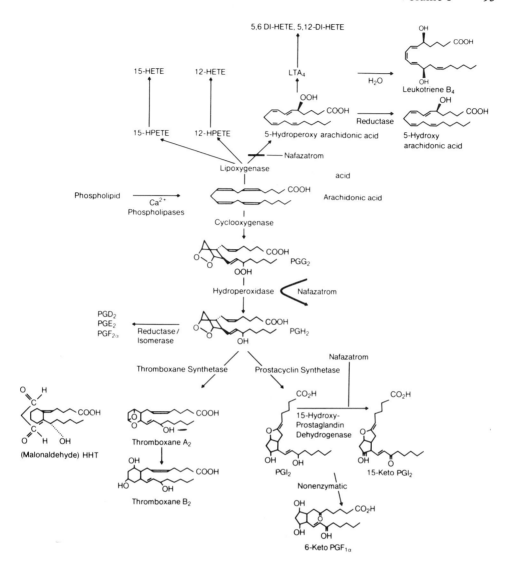

FIGURE 2. Arachidonic acid metabolism via the lipoxygenase pathway resulting in hydroperoxy fatty acids and leukotrienes and via the PG endoperoxide synthetase (cyclooxygenase + hydroperoxidase) pathway resulting in PGs (including prostacyclin) and thromboxanes. Possible sites of action of nafazatrom include: (1) inhibition of lipoxygenase activity, (2) reducing co-factor for the hydroperoxidase of PG endoperoxide synthetase, and (3) inhibition of PGI₂ degradation by 15-hydroxy-PG dehydrogenase. (From Honn, K. V., et al., *Biochem. Pharmacol.*, 32, 1, 1983. With permission.)

resulted in irreversible platelet aggregation after a short lag period of 0.5 to 1 min.[66,67] This aggregation was inhibited by PGI₂ in a dose-dependent manner with maximal inhibition observed at PGI₂ dose of 10 ng/mℓ.[66] PGI₂ was tested against a variety of tumor types. Complete inhibition of TCIPA with PGI₂ (10 ng/mℓ) was observed in the B16 amelanotic melanoma (B16a),[67] 15091A mammary adenocarcinoma, and Lewis lung carcinoma (3LL).[66] Two additional PGs (PGE₁ and PGD₂) known to inhibit platelet aggregation[68] were 100 times less potent than PGI₂ in inhibiting W256-induced platelet aggregation.[66] The stable metabolite of PGI₂, 6-keto-PGF₁ₐ, was only effective at supraphysiological doses.[66]

It is well-known that circulating tumor cells may exist as single cells or multicellular clumps and that aggregates of tumor cells are more efficient in generating lung colonies than single cells.[9,69-71] Liotta et al.[71] demonstrated that the intravenous injection of 10^3 T241 fibrosarcoma cells in clumps of 6 to 7 cells produced 10 times as many pulmonary tumors as 10^3 single cells. In these experiments, doubling the size of the homotypic emboli doubled the number of tumors. In in vitro studies in our laboratory, W256 cells underwent spontaneous homotypic adhesion into clumps of 5 to 10 cells, which could be visualized by scanning electron microscopy (Figure 4A). PGI$_2$ at a dose of 100 ng/ mℓ completely prevented homotypic aggregation of W256 cells.[72] The relevance of these observations to PGI$_2$ effects in vivo are unknown at present. However, it is clear that PGI$_2$ can prevent various cell-cell interactions involving tumor cells.

2. Prostacyclin Effects on Tumor Cell-Induced Platelet Release Reaction (TCIPR)

During the release reaction materials stored in platelet granules (dense granules, α-granules, and lysosomes) are released into the environment. The dense granules contain high concentrations of amines (serotonin), adenine nucleotides, and divalent cations. The α-granules contain a variety of proteins, among which are heparin neutralizing protein (PF4), β-thromboglobulin, fibrinogen, fibronectin, platelet-derived growth factors, etc.[73] Lysosomes contain acid hydrolases including acid phosphatase, β-N-acetylglucosaminidase, β-glucuronidase, cathepsin D, collagenase, and others.[74,75] Several of these platelet factors could conceivably aid in tumor metastasis. Dense granule serotonin is a potent vasoconstrictor and can further stimulate platelet aggregation.[73] α-Granule-derived β-thromboglobulin inhibits production of PGI$_2$, which has demonstrated antimetastatic activity, by the vascular endothelium.[76] Platelet-derived fibronectin could coat tumor cells and increase adhesiveness as discussed above and in addition α-granule fibrinogen could contribute to tumor cell-associated fibrin.[38]

A variety of human and animal tumor cells have been found to evoke the release of platelet dense granules.[38] We have demonstrated that PGI$_2$ inhibits the release of dense granules during TCIPA (measured as release of ^{14}C-serotonin from prelabeled platelets).[67] In addition, PGI$_2$ caused a dose-dependent decrease in platelet α-granule release (measured as β-thromboglobulin release) induced during W256 TCIPA.[67]

PGI$_2$ inhibition of W256 TCIPA, including inhibition of release of platelet α- and dense granules, was confirmed morphologically by transmission electron microscopy (TEM). Tumor cells and platelets were coincubated in an aggregometer cuvette and fixed prior to the first phase of aggregation, between the first and second phases of aggregation, and after complete aggregation. Even prior to the first phase of aggregation (Figure 3A) platelet pseudopod formation had initiated and granules had been released. At the end of the first phase (Figure 3B) a platelet aggregate had formed and platelet and tumor cell membranes had become closely apposed. Fibrin had polymerized and was found in association with the platelet-tumor cell aggregate by the end of the second phase (Figure 3C). In the presence of 10 ng/mℓ PGI$_2$, the platelets did not undergo aggregation or release of α- and dense granules in response to W256 cells (Figure 3D).

In virtually all of the experiments examined thus far, there does not appear to be an engulfing of the tumor cell by platelets. When attachment occurred it seemed to be between a limited number of platelets and tumor cells. Generally this was followed by activation of surrounding platelets to form aggregates. This does not preclude, of course, that preformed platelet aggregates may also attach to tumor cells. If the attachment of a limited number of platelets to the tumor cells is a selective process, this suggests that heterogenous platelet populations may exist. Indeed there are some recent studies which indicate that functionally heterogenous platelet populations do exist.[77-79]

These TEM studies suggested a change in the surface topology of the tumor cell in response to platelets. Therefore, we more fully examined the interaction between platelets and W256 tumor cells using scanning electron microscopy (SEM) under conditions in which platelet aggregation did occur. The surface topology of control tumor cells (incubated without platelets) was characterized by pseudopods and fine microvilli which resulted in the tumor cells having a fuzzy image by SEM (Figure 4A). After 2 min of coincubation with the tumor cells a few platelets that had not undergone shape change could be seen attached to the tumor cell (Figure 4B). At 12 min of coincubation the tumor cell surface was covered with platelets that had formed pseudopods (Figure 4C). In turn the tumor cell membrane seemed to have lost its fine surface microvilli and many of its pseudopods. These SEM images suggest that there may be bidirectional interactions between tumor cells and platelets that could result in modifications of the tumor cell membrane and alter the adhesive properties of the tumor cell.

3. Prostacyclin Effects on Platelet-Induced Tumor Cell Adhesion In Vitro

Fantone et al.[80] have recently demonstrated that the adherence of W256 cells to plastic plates or nylon fibers can be stimulated by the tumor promoter phorbol myris tate acetate and the chemotactic peptide f-Met-Leu-Phe. PGI_2 directly inhibited this increased adhesion, however, PGI_2 had no effect on basal (unstimulated) W256 cell adhesion.[80] Hara et al.[42] reported that tumor cells will not aggregate washed platelets; however, the addition of a small amount (2% v/v) of platelet poor plasma (PPP) restored a full aggregation response, suggesting an absolute requirement for a plasma factor during TCIPA.[42,81]

The adhesion of W256 cells to plastic plates was increased in the presence of washed rat platelets.[72] The addition of PGI_2 (30 $\mu g/m\ell$) completely prevented the increased adhesion under both aggregatory and nonaggregatory conditions. The PGI_2 effect was dose-dependent both in the presence and absence of PPP with a 40% decrease observed at 1 μg $PGI_2/m\ell$. PGI_2 had no effect on basal (unstimulated) W256 cell attachment.[72] Rat platelets also enhanced the attachment of W256 cells to cultured rat endothelial cells, a response which can be blocked with PGI_2.[82] These in vitro results suggest that platelets may increase tumor cell adhesion to endothelium in vivo and PGI_2 may limit the formation of a stable tumor cell-endothelial cell interaction.

4. Prostacyclin Effects On Metastasis In Vivo

We have previously reported that bolus i.v. injection of PGI_2 into mice reduced lung colony formation from tail vein-injected B16a cells by greater than 70% and in combination with a phosphodiesterase inhibitor (theophylline) by more than 93%.[83] PGE_2, $PGF_{2\alpha}$, and the stable hydrolysis product of PGI_2, 6-keto-$PGF_{1\alpha}$, were ineffective.[83] PGD_2 is also antimetastatic as reported by Stringfellow and Fitzpatrick;[84] however, we found PGD_2 to be less than one third as effective as PGI_2.[83] These results correlate well with the effects of these various eicosanoids on TCIPA.[5,66,67] Pretreatment of animals with some antiplatelet agents has resulted in increased extrapulmonary tumors;[85] however, using [^{125}I] deoxyuridine labeled B16a cells we demonstrated that PGI_2 does not cause extrapulmonary redistribution of cells.[83]

The results with exogenous PGI_2 demonstrate its efficacy as an antimetastatic agent. We have also proposed that the production of PGI_2 by the vascular endothelium may be a natural deterrent to metastasis.[83] To test this hypothesis we perfused mice with a lipoxygenase product of arachidonic acid, 15-hydroperoxyeicosatetraenoic acid (15-HPETE), prior to tail-vein injection of B16a tumor cells. Hydroperoxy fatty acids in general are potent ($K_i \sim 10^{-7}$ M) inhibitors of PGI_2 synthase.[86] Little structural specificity is evident in the inhibition, since a number of isomeric hydroperoxides are equally effective.[86] If mice were pretreated (approximately 20 min) with 15-HPETE (100 to 200 μg per animal) prior to tail-vein injection of B16a cells, 300 to 500% more pulmonary tumor colonies were observed 26 days later.[72] Increased macroscopic tu-

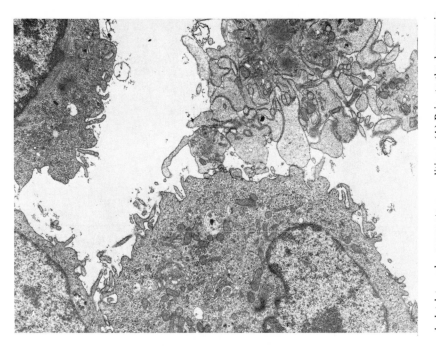

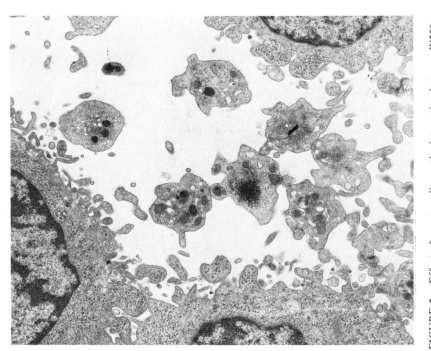

FIGURE 3.   Effect of prostacyclin on the interaction between W256 tumor cells and platelets under aggregatory conditions. (A) Prior to the decrease in light transmittance indicating platelet aggregation, the platelets had already begun to form pseudopods and to release their granules. (Magnification × 9900.) (B) Platelet aggregates had formed by the end of the first phase of aggregation and close membrane appositions were present between platelets and tumor cells. Most of the platelets had released their granules. (Magnification × 10,700.) (C) By the end of the second phase of aggregation fibrin was seen in association with the tumor cells and platelet aggregates and the tumor cell membrane seemed to have lost its microvilli. (Magnification × 10,500.) (D) In the presence of 10 ng/mℓ prostacyclin, platelets did not undergo aggregation in response to tumor cells. (Magnification × 6300.)

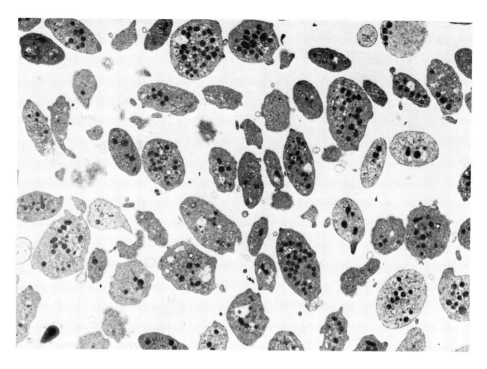

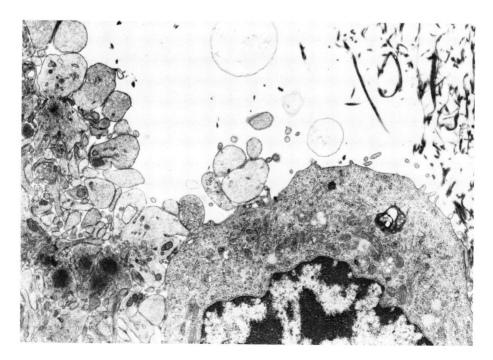

FIGURE 3 (continued)

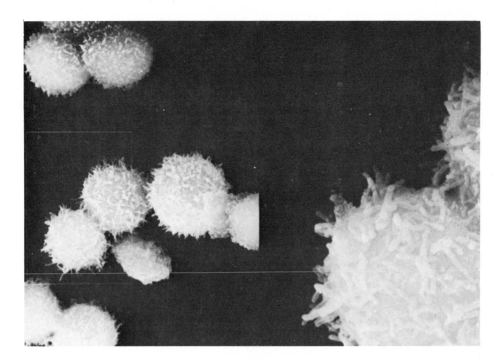

A

FIGURE 4.   Interaction between W256 tumor cells and platelets under non-aggregatory conditions. (A) Control tumor cells have fine surface microvilli which give them a fuzzy appearance. (Magnification × 1600, left; × 5300, right.) (B) After 2 min of coincubation a few platelets can be seen adherent to the tumor cells. The tumor cells seem to have lost their surface microvilli but still have pseudopods. (Magnification × 18,200.) (C) After 12 min of coincubation many platelets were adherent to the tumor cells and these platelets had undergone shape changes and formed pseudopods. The tumor cell surface topology appears to have become mostly smooth with no microvilli and few pseudopods. (Magnification × 6900, left; × 15,900, right.)

mors were also found in the liver and spleen of 15-HPETE treated animals.[72] Collectively these results suggest that endogenous PGI_2 production may function as a natural deterrent to metastasis, possibly by limiting tumor cell-platelet-vessel wall interactions.

B. Effect of Agents that Stimulate or Synergize with Endogenous PGI_2 Production
1. Agents that Alter PGI_2 Metabolism
One such compound which may represent the prototype of a new class of pharmacologically active agents is nafazatrom (Bay g 6575; 2,4-dihydro-5-methyl-2[2-(2napthyloxy)ethyl]-3H-pyrazol-3-one). Nafazatrom has been reported to possess significant antithrombotic activity in several models of experimental thrombosis.[87] The antithrombotic activity of nafazatrom may be due in part to its effects on vascular wall PGI_2 production. Vermylen et al.[88] first presented evidence for increased PGI_2 production. Plasma obtained from human volunteers after ingestion of a single dose (1.2 g) of nafazatrom stimulated PGI_2 release from slices of rat aorta. Others also have reported increased PGI_2 production.[89,90]

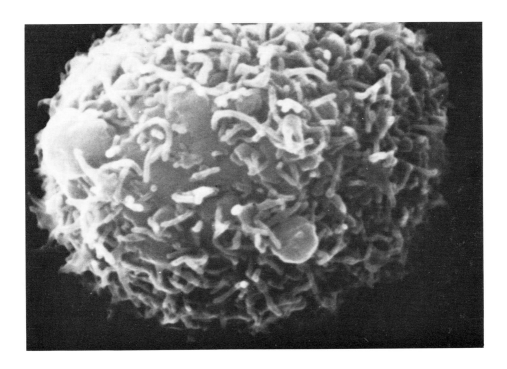

FIGURE 4B.

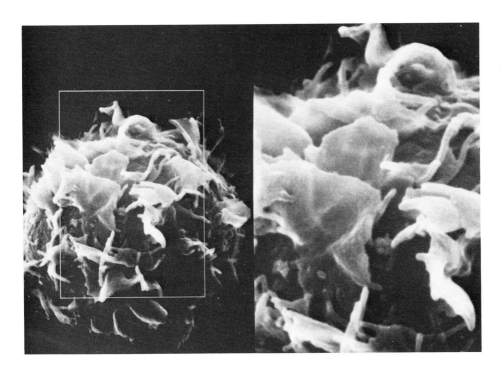

FIGURE 4C.

Three biochemical mechanisms have been proposed to explain the PGI_2 stimulating effects of nafazatrom (Figure 2). First, nafazatrom has been found to inhibit the cytosolic lipoxygenase (generation of HPETE) of B16a cells[91] as well as that of human and rabbit neutrophils.[92] Since vascular endothelial cells have been found to produce 12-HPETE by lipoxygenation of arachidonic acid[93] and hydroperoxy fatty acid has been proposed as an endogenous regulator of PGI_2 biosynthesis, nafazatrom may interfere with PGI_2 synthase inhibition. Second, nafazatrom may act as a reducing cofactor for the hydroperoxidase activity of PG endoperoxide synthase.[94,95] Third, nafazatrom has been reported to inhibit the enzymatic degradation of PGI_2 to 15-keto-PGI_2 by 15 hydroxy-PG dehydrogenase.[96] This is the major route of PGI_2 catabolism in the cat[97] and man.[98] Any or all of the above mechanisms would result in increased endogenous PGI_2 levels.

Nafazatrom has been evaluated for its antimetastatic activity against tail-vein injected elutriated B16a and 3LL tumor cells and found to inhibit lung colony formation by more than 70%.[5,99,100] In addition, this compound significantly reduces spontaneous pulmonary metastasis from subcutaneous B16a and 3LL tumors.[99] Ambrus et al.[101] have also reported antimetastatic activity of nafazatrom in three of four experimental tumor lines tested. Nafazatrom is currently in Phase I clinical study.[102] Collectively, these results point to significant antimetastatic properties of this PGI_2 enhancing agent.

2. Thromboxane Synthase Inhibitors

As stated above, we had initially proposed that the intravascular balance between PGI_2 and TXA_2 was disrupted by metastasizing tumor cells. This led us to suggest several therapeutic strategies including the use of thromboxane synthase inhibitors as antimetastatic agents. We initially investigated a series of endoperoxide analogues that were thromboxane synthase inhibitors.[103,104] One endoperoxide analogue, thromboxane synthase inhibitor U54701 (9,11-iminoepoxy-prosta-5,13-dienoic acid[105]) completely inhibited TXA_2 production by human platelets in response to elutriated 3LL cells concomitant with an inhibition of platelet aggregation;[67] however, W256 TCIPA was only inhibited 25% by a comparable dose of U54701 even though TXA_2 biosynthesis was almost completely inhibited.[67] Furthermore, TX synthase inhibitors which are imidazole derivatives (i.e., OKY-1553; 1-[7-carboxyheptyl]imidazole) did not inhibit in vitro TCIPA even in the presence of inhibited platelet TXA_2 production. These aberrant results suggest that tumor cells can initiate platelet aggregation by a mechanism independent of, or in addition to, TXA_2 biosynthesis.[5] For example, in vitro the endoperoxide PGH_2 can initiate platelet aggregation via the TXA_2 receptor.[106] Generation of PGH_2 would not be altered by selective TX synthase inhibitors. Nevertheless, TX synthase inhibitors have demonstrated antimetastatic activity in vivo. For example, U54701 (200 μg per animal) inhibits lung colony formation (experimental metastasis) by 95%.[107] The imidazole derivative, OKY-1553, also inhibits experimental metastasis.[107] In addition, OKY-1553 inhibits spontaneous metastasis from subcutaneous B16a and 3LL tumors.[107] These in vivo results appear to be at variance with the effects of these compounds on in vitro TCIPA.

TX synthase inhibitors result in decreased platelet adhesion to injured vascular wall[108] and increased platelet sensitivity to PGI_2 inhibition,[109] presumably because the lower the platelet TXA_2 biosynthetic capability, the lower the dose of PGI_2 required for inhibition of aggregation.[110] In addition, TX synthase inhibitors have been reported to reorient platelet endoperoxide (PGH_2, Figure 2) metabolism toward PGI_2 biosynthesis by the vessel wall.[111] This hypothesis, originally termed the "steal hypothesis", was first proposed by Gryglewski et al.[112] The hypothesis states that under conditions in which aggregating platelets are juxtaposed to the endothelium in a narrow vessel lumen, platelet PGH_2 may be utilized by vessel wall PGI_2 synthase to augment basal

PGI_2 production. These results are consistent with the work of Needleman et al.,[113] which suggested that normally the "steal" of precursor by the vessel wall may not be an important pathway fo PGI_2 biosynthesis; however, under conditions of a strong stimulus for platelet aggregation (i.e., circulating tumor cells), the selective blockage of TXA_2 synthase could drive platelet PGH_2 metabolism into PGI_2 biosynthesis by the vessel wall. In vivo evidence for the "steal hypothesis" has been recently provided by the experiments of Aiken et al.[110]

We propose that the discrepancy between lack of consistent inhibition of TCIPA by TX synthase inhibitors in vitro and their antimetastatic activity in vivo is due to the operation of the "steal hypothesis" in vivo. In vitro TCIPA may proceed by pathways independent of TXA_2 biosynthesis. Thus, the antimetastatic activity of TX synthase inhibitors in vivo may ultimately be due to augmented endogenous PGI_2 biosynthesis.

3. Calcium Channel Blocker Compounds (CCBC)

A number of vascular and myocardial disorders can be alleviated by inducing vaso-dilation with calcium channel blockers including vasospastic angina, acute myocardial infarction, arrhythmias, pulmonary hypertension, etc. (for recent reviews see Braunwald,[114] Henry,[115] and Godfraind[116]). Recent attention has been focused on the effects of CCBC on platelet aggregation. Verapamil has been reported to reduce ADP-induced rat platelet aggregation in vitro and in vivo;[117] however, verapamil has been reported to be ineffective in reducing ADP-induced platelet aggregation of human[118] and cat[119] platelets. Two dihydropyridine class CCBCs (nimodipine and nifedipine) have also produced mixed results when tested for inhibition of ADP-induced platelet aggregation.[82] We reinvestigated the effect of nimodipine and nifedipine on ADP and thrombin-induced aggregation of human platelet-rich plasma and found both compounds to be effective inhibitors.[82]

Therefore, we evaluated the effects of two CCBCs (nimodipine and nifedipine) on TCIPA and spontaneous pulmonary metastasis of B16a. Both CCBC compounds effected a dose-dependent inhibition of B16a TCIPA over a dose range of 4 to 400 μg/ $m\ell$.[82] In addition, the platelet stimulated adhesion of [^{125}I]-Udr labeled W256 cells to cultured rat endothelial cells was inhibited 60% with 40 μg/$m\ell$ nimodipine.[82] In vivo the daily administration of nimodipine (80 mg/kg) to C57BL/6J mice bearing subcutaneous B16a tumors inhibited spontaneous pulmonary metastasis by more than 81%.[82] Similar qualitative results were obtained with nifedipine. We next examined the possibility of a synergism between CCBC and PGI_2 in inhibition of TCIPA in vitro. PGI_2 at a dose of 100 fg/$m\ell$ does not significantly affect TCIPA induced by W256 cells (Figure 5). Similarly nimodipine (15 μg/$m\ell$) produces only a 15% inhibition of TCIPA (Figure 5); however, the combination of PGI_2 (100 fg/$m\ell$) plus nimodipine (15 μg/$m\ell$) results in a greater than 50% inhibition of W256 TCIPA (Figure 5). Although preliminary, these in vitro results suggest a possible synergism between CCBC and PGI_2 in inhibition of tumor cell metastasis in vivo.

III. CONCLUSIONS

It is intuitive that for hematogenous metastasis to occur the tumor cell must arrest in the microvasculature and attach to the vessel wall prior to extravasation and growth into a metastatic focus. Indirect evidence supports the concept that tumor cells interact with platelets during this process as discussed above. We propose that the metabolism of arachidonic acid in the tumor cell, the platelet, and the vessel wall plays an essential role in the sum total of these interactions (Figure 6). For example, the production of PGI_2 by the vessel wall and of TXA_2 by the platelet is thought to play a key, although possibly not an exclusive, role in thrombosis.

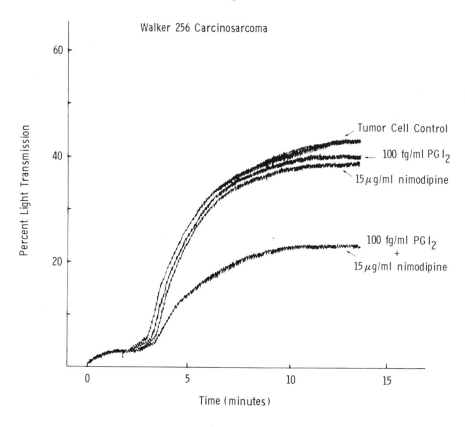

FIGURE 5.   Synergism between PGI₂ and the calcium channel blocker nimodipine on inhibition of platelet aggregation induced by W256 cells. (From Honn, K. V. et al., in *Cancer Invasion and Metastasis: Biologic and Therapeutic Agents,* Nicholson, G. L. and Milas, L., Eds., Raven Press, New York, in press. With permission.)

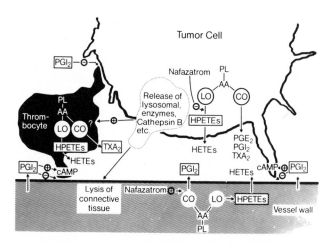

FIGURE 6.   Interactions among tumor cells, platelets (thrombocytes), and the blood vessel wall. Direct interactions are possible between the platelet and the vessel wall, the tumor cell and vessel wall, and the platelet(s) and tumor cell(s). Any one or all of the above may enhance tumor cell arrest and metastasis. PGI₂ may prevent attachment of tumor cell(s) to platelet(s) or to vessel wall. Abbreviations: PL, phospholipids; AA, arachidonic acid; CO, cyclooxygenase; LO, lipoxygenase; HPETE, hydroperoxyeicosatetraenoic acid; HETE, hydroxyeicosatetraenoic acid; PGI₂, prostacyclin; and TXA₂, thromboxane A₂. (From Honn, K. V., et al., *Biochem. Pharmacol.,* 32, 1, 1983. With permission.)

Exogenous PGI_2 may function as an antimetastatic agent by inhibiting the association of the tumor cell with the vessel wall (Figure 6). The interactions between the vessel wall and tumor cells or platelets may be inhibited by stimulation of platelet cAMP or tumor cell cAMP by exogenous PGI_2. Similarly, vessel wall PGI_2 may serve as a natural deterrent to metastasis by inhibiting these interactions (Figure 6). A new class of antimetastatic agents may be compounds that have the ability to stimulate endogenous PGI_2 production and/or prolong the half-life of PGI_2 (e.g., nafazatrom). In addition, PGI_2 and/or TXA_2 production by the tumor cell may be important in tumor cell platelet vessel wall interactions. Donati and co-workers[120] have recently examined arachidonic acid metabolites produced by several sublines that developed from the murine FS6 sarcoma. These cell lines were reported to produce PGI_2, TXA_2, PGD_2, PGE_2, and $PGF_{2\alpha}$.[120] These lines differed widely in their abilities to metastasize. A comparison between arachidonic acid metabolism and metastatic potential revealed an inverse correlation between tumor cell PGI_2 production and metastatic potential and a positive correlation with TXA_2 production. These authors suggested that the balance between PGI_2 and TXA_2 was shifted towards a proaggregatory condition in the highly metastatic cells.[120] A new proposal to explain the in vivo antimetastatic effects of TX synthase inhibitors ("steal hypothesis") may result from enhanced endogenous PGI_2 production, synthesized from endoperoxide PGH_2 generated during TCIPA. Finally, a heretofore unsuspected class of pharmacologic agents (calcium channel blockers) are reported by us to have potent antimetastatic activity, which in part may result from a synergism with PGI_2.

ACKNOWLEDGMENTS

This investigation was supported by grant numbers CA29405 and CA29997 awarded by the National Cancer Institute, Department of Health and Human Services, and by American Cancer Society Grant BC-356, Miles Institute for Preclinical Pharmacology, and Bayer AG. The excellent technical assistance of Marjorie Carufel, Deborah Moilanen, Gregory Neagos, and Kim Pampalona is appreciated. The expert typing of Susan Lyman is gratefully acknowledged.

REFERENCES

1. Weiss, L., Cancer cell traffic from the lungs to the liver: an example of metastatic inefficiency, *Int. J. Cancer,* 25, 385, 1980.
2. Weiss, L., Metastatic inefficiency, in *Tumor Invasion and Metastasis,* Liotta, L. A. and Hart, I. R., Eds., Martinus Nijhoff, The Hague, 1982, 81.
3. Weiss, L., Overview of the metastatic cascade, in *Hemostatic Mechanisms and Metastasis,* Honn, K. V. and Sloane, B. F., Eds., Martinus Nijhoff, The Hague, in press.
4. Poste, G. and Fidler, I. J., The pathogenesis of cancer metastasis, *Nature (London),* 283, 139, 1980.
5. Honn, K. V., Busse, W. D., and Sloane, B. F., Commentary: prostacyclin and thromboxanes. Implications for their role in tumor cell metastasis, *Biochem. Pharmacol.,* 32, 1, 1983.
6. Salsbury, A. J., The significance of the circulating cancer cell, *Cancer Treat. Rev.,* 2, 55, 1975.
7. Fisher, E. R. and Fisher, B., Recent observations on concepts of metastasis, *Arch. Pathol.,* 83, 321, 1967.
8. Hilgard, P., Beyerle, L., Hohage, R., Hiemeyer, V., and Kubler, M., The effect of heparin on the initial phase of metastasis formation, *Eur. J. Cancer,* 8, 347, 1972.
9. Fidler, I. J., The relationship of embolic homogeneity, number, size and viability to the incidence of experimental metastasis, *Eur. J. Cancer,* 9, 223, 1973.
10. del Regato, J. A., Pathways of metastatic spread of malignant tumors, *Semin. Oncol.,* 4, 33, 1977.
11. Weiss, L., A pathobiologic overview of metastasis, *Semin. Oncol.,* 4, 5, 1977.
12. Goodnight, S. H., Bleeding and intravascular clotting in malignancy: a review, *Ann. N. Y. Acad. Sci.,* 230, 271, 1974.
13. Zacharski, L. R., Henderson, W. G., Rickles, F. R., Forman, W. B., Cornell, C. J., Forcier, R. J., Harower, H. W., and Johnson, R. O., Rationale and experimental design for the VA cooperative study of anticoagulation (Warfarin) in the treatment of cancer, *Cancer,* 44, 732, 1979.
14. Donati, M. B. and Poggi, A., Malignancy and haemostasis, *Br. J. Haematol.,* 44, 173, 1980.
15. Edwards, R. L., Rickles, F. R., and Cronlund, M., Abnormalities of blood coagulation in patients with cancer. Mononuclear cell tissue factor generation, *J. Lab. Clin. Med.,* 98, 917, 1981.
16. Yahara, Y., Okawa, S., Onozawa, Y., Motomiya, T., Tanoue, K., and Yamazaki, H., Activation of platelets in cancer, especially with reference to genesis of disseminated intravascular coagulation, *Thromb. Res.,* 29, 27, 1983.
17. Brain, M. C., Azzopardi, J. G., Baker, L. R. I., Pineo, G. F., Roberts, P. D., and Dacie, J. V., Microangiopathic haemolytic anemia: the possible role of vascular lesions on pathogenesis, *Br. J. Haematol.,* 18, 183, 1970.
18. Harker, L. A. and Slichter, S. J., Platelet and fibrinogen consumption in man, *N. Engl. J. Med.,* 287, 999, 1972.
19. Gasic, G. J., Boettiger, D., Catalfamo, J. L., Gasic, T. B., and Stewart, G. J., Aggregation of platelets and cell membrane vesiculation by rat cells transformed *in vitro* by Rous sarcoma virus, *Cancer Res.,* 38, 2950, 1978.
20. Pearlstein, E., Cooper, L. B., and Karpatkin, S., Extraction and characterization of a platelet-aggregating material from SV 40-transformed mouse 3T3 fibroblasts, *J. Lab. Clin. Med.,* 93, 332, 1979.
21. Pearlstein, E., Salk, P. L., Yogeeswaran, G., and Karpatkin, S., Correlation between spontaneous metastatic potential, platelet-aggregating activity of cell surface extracts, and cell surface sialylation in 10 metastatic variant derivatives of rat renal sarcoma cell line, *Proc. Natl. Acad. Sci. U.S.A.,* 77, 4336, 1980.
22. Karpatkin, S., Smerling, A., and Pearlstein, E., Plasma requirement for the aggregation of rabbit platelets by an aggregating material derived from SV 40-transformed 3T3 fibroblasts, *J. Lab. Clin. Med.,* 96, 994, 1980.
23. Gordon, S. G., Franks, J. J., and Lewis, B., Cancer procoagulant A: a factor X activating procoagulant from malignant tissue, *Thromb. Res.,* 6, 127, 1975.
24. Curatolo, L., Colucci, M., Cambini, A. L., Poggi, A., Morasca, L., Donati, M. B., and Semeraro, N., Evidence that cells from experimental tumours can activate coagulation factor X, *Br. J. Cancer,* 40, 228, 1979.
25. Gordon, S. G. and Cross, B. A., A factor X activating cysteine protease from malignant tissue, *J. Clin. Invest.,* 67, 1665, 1981.
26. Karpatkin, S. and Pearlstein, E., Role of platelets in tumor cell metastases, *Ann. Intern. Med.,* 95, 636, 1981.
27. Iwasaki, T., Histological and experimental observations on the destruction of tumor cells in blood vessels, *J. Pathol. Bacteriol.,* 20, 85, 1915.
28. Willis, R. A., *The Spread of Tumours in the Human Body,* J. & A. Churchill, London, 1934.
29. Saphir, O., The fate of carcinoma emboli in the lung, *Am. J. Pathol.,* 23, 245, 1947.
30. Durham, J. R., Ashley, P. F., and Dorencamp, D., Cor pulmonale due to tumor emboli: review of literature and report of a case, *JAMA,* 175, 757, 1961.

31. Morgan, A. D., The pathology of subacute cor pulmonale in diffuse carcinomatosis of the lungs, *J. Pathol. Bacteriol.*, 61, 75, 1949.
32. Wood, S., Jr., Mechanisms of establishment of tumor metastases, *Pathobiol. Annu.*, 281, 1971.
33. Zeidman, I., The fate of circulating tumor cells. I. Passage of cells through capillaries, *Cancer Res.*, 21, 38, 1961.
34. Warren, B. A. and Guldner, F.-H., Ultrastucture of the adhesion of HeLa cells to human vein wall, *Angiologica*, 6, 32, 1969.
35. Sindelar, W. F., Tralka, T. S., and Ketcham, A. S., Electron microscopic observations on formation of pulmonary metastases, *J. Surg. Res.*, 18, 137, 1975.
36. Gasic, G. J., Gasic, T. B., and Stewart, C. C., Antimetastatic effects associated with platelet reduction, *Proc. Natl. Acad. Sci. U.S.A.*, 61, 46, 1968.
37. Gasic, G. J., Gasic, T. B., Galanti, N., Johnson, T., and Murphy, J., Platelet tumor-cell interactions in mice. The role of platelets in the spread of malignant disease, *Int. J. Cancer*, 11, 704, 1973.
38. Gasic, G. J., Koch, P. A. G., Hsu, B., Gasic, T. B., and Niewiarowski, S., Thrombogenic activity of mouse and human tumors: effects on platelets, coagulation and fibrinolysis, and possible significance for metastasis, *Z. Krebsforsch.*, 86, 263, 1976.
39. Hilgard, P., The role of blood platelets in experimental metastases, *Br. J. Cancer*, 28, 429, 1973.
40. Gastpar, H., Ambrus, J., and Thurber, L. E., Study of platelet aggregation *in vivo*. II. Effect of benecylane on circulating metastatic tumor cells, *J. Med.*, 8, 53, 1977.
41. Paschen, W., Patscheke, H., and Worner, P., Aggregation of activated platelets with Walker 256 carcinoma cells, *Blut*, 38, 17, 1979.
42. Hara, Y., Steiner, M., and Baldini, M. G., Characterization of the platelet aggregating activity of tumor cells, *Cancer Res.*, 40, 1217, 1980.
43. Skolnik, G., Alpsten, M., and Ivarsson, L., Studies on mechanisms involved in metastasis formation from circulating tumor cells, *J. Cancer Res. Clin. Oncol.*, 97, 249, 1980.
44. Bastida, E., Ordinas, A., and Jamieson, G. A., Idiosyncratic platelet responses to human tumor cells, *Nature (London)*, 291, 661, 1981.
45. Pearlstein, E., Abrogio, C., Gasic, G., and Karpatkin, S., Inhibition of the platelet-aggregating activity of two human adenocarcinomas of the colon and an anaplastic murine tumor with a specific thrombin inhibitor, dansyl-arginine N-(3-ethyl-1,5-pentanediyl)amide, *Cancer Res.*, 41, 4535, 1981.
46. Bastida, E., Ordinas, A., Giardina, S. L., and Jamieson, G. A., Differentiation of platelet-aggregating effects of human tumor cell lines based on inhibition studies with apyrase, hirudin and phospholipase, *Cancer Res.*, 42, 4348, 1982.
47. Tanaka, N., Ashida, S.-I, Tohgo, A., and Ogawa, H., Platelet-aggregating activities of metastasizing tumor cells, *Invasion Metastasis*, 2, 289, 1982.
48. Jamieson, G. A., Ed., *Interaction of Platelets and Tumor Cells*, Alan R. Liss, New York, 1982.
49. Honn, K. V. and Sloane, B. F., Eds., *Hemostatic Mechanisms and Metastasis*, Martinus Nijhoff, The Hague, in press.
50. Turner, W. A., Menter, D. G., Honn, K. V., and Taylor, J. D., Tumor cell induced platelet fibronectin release, *Proc. Am. Assoc. Cancer Res.*, 24 (Abstr.), 25, 1983.
51. Nicolson, G. L., Irimura, T., Gonzalez, R., and Ruoslahti, E., The role of fibronectin in adhesion of metastatic melanoma cells to endothelial cells and their basal lamina, *Exp. Cell Res.*, 135, 461, 1981.
52. Murray, J. C., Liotta, L., Rennard, S. I., and Martin, G. R., Adhesion characteristics of murine metastatic and nonmetastatic tumor cells *in vitro*, *Cancer Res.*, 40, 347, 1980.
53. Terranova, V. P., Liotta, L. A., Russo, R. G., and Martin, G. R., Role of laminin in the attachment and metastasis of murine tumor cells, *Cancer Res.*, 42, 2265, 1982.
54. Elias, E. G., Sepulveda, F., and Mink, I. B., Increasing the efficiency of cancer chemotherapy with heparin: clinical study, *J. Surg. Oncol.*, 5, 189, 1973.
55. Lione, A. and Bosmann, H. B., The inhibitory effect of heparin and warfarin treatments on the intravascular survival of B16 melanoma cells in syngeneic C57 mice, *Cell Biol. Int. Rep.*, 2, 81, 1978.
56. Gastpar, H., Platelet cancer cell interaction in metastasis formation: a possible therapeutic approach to metastasis prophylaxis, *J. Med.*, 8, 103, 1977.
57. Maat, B. and Hilgard, P., Anticolagulant and experimental metastases — evaluation of antimetastatic effects in different model systems, *J. Cancer Res. Clin. Oncol.*, 101, 275, 1981.
58. Vargaftig, B. B., Chignard, M., and Benveniste, J., Present concepts on the mechanism of platelet aggregation, *Biochem. Pharmacol.*, 30, 263, 1981.
59. Hamberg, M., Svensson, J., and Samuelsson, B., Thromboxanes: a new group of biologically active compounds derived from prostaglandin endoperoxides, *Proc. Natl. Acad. Sci. U.S.A.*, 72, 2994, 1975.
60. Gorman, R. R., Modulation of human platelet function by prostacyclin and thromboxane A_2, *Fed. Proc. Fed. Am. Soc. Exp. Biol.*, 38, 83, 1979.

61. Heptinstall, S., Bevan, J., Cockbill, S. R., Hanley, S. P., and Parry, M. J., Effects of a selective inhibitor of thromboxane synthetase on human blood platelet behaviour, *Thromb. Res.,* 20, 219, 1980.

62. Moncada, S., Gryglewski, R. J., Bunting, S., and Vane, J. R., An enzyme isolated from arteries transforms prostaglandin endoperoxides to an unstable substance that inhibits platelet aggregation, *Nature (London),* 263, 663, 1976.

63. Moncada, S. and Vane, J. R., The discovery of prostacyclin (PGX); a fresh insight into arachidonic acid metabolism, in *Biochemical Aspects of Prostaglandins and Thromboxanes,* Kharasch, N. and Fried, J., Eds., Academic Press, New York, 1977, 155.

64. Mullane, K. M., Dusting, G. J., Salmon, J. A., Moncada, S., and Vane, J. R., Biotransformation and cardiovascular effects of arachidonic acid in the dog, *Eur. J. Pharmacol.,* 54, 217, 1979.

65. Sloane, B. F., Dunn, J. R., and Honn, K. V., Lysosomal cathepsin B: correlation with metastatic potential, *Science,* 212, 1151, 1981.

66. Honn, K. V. and Sloane, B. F., Prostaglandins in tumor cell metastasis, in *Basic Mechanisms and Clinical Treatments of Tumor Metastasis,* Torisu, M. and Yoshida, Y., Eds., Academic Press, New York, in press.

67. Honn, K. V., Menter, D., Moilanen, D., Cavanaugh, P. G., Taylor, J. D., and Sloane, B. F., Role of prostacyclin and thromboxanes in tumor cell-platelet-vessel wall interactions, in *Protective Agents in Human Experimental Cancer,* Slater, T. F., Ed., Academic Press, New York, in press.

68. Vane, J. R., Bunting, S., and Mocada, S., Prostacyclin in physiology and pathophysiology, in *International Review of Experimental Pathology,* Vol. 23, Richter, G. W. and Epstein, M. A., Eds., Academic Press, New York, 1982, 161.

69. Watanabe, S., Metastasizability of tumor cells, *Cancer,* 7, 215, 1954.

70. Liotta, L. A., Kleinerman, J., and Saidel, G. M., Quantitative relationships of intravascular tumor cells, tumor vessels, and pulmonary metastases following tumor implantation, *Cancer Res.,* 34, 997, 1974.

71. Liotta, L. A., Kleinerman, J., and Saidel, G. M., The significance of hematogenous tumor cell clumps in the metastatic process, *Cancer Res.,* 36, 889, 1976.

72. Honn, K. V., Menter, D. G., Onoda, J. M., Taylor, J. D., and Sloane, B. F., Role of prostacyclin as a natural deterrent to hematogenous tumor metastasis, in *Cancer Invasion and Metastasis: Biologic and Therapeutic Aspects,* Nicolson, G. L. and Milas, L., Eds., Raven Press, New York, in press.

73. Kaplan, K. L., Platelet granule proteins: localization and secretion, in *Platelets in Biology and Pathology,* Vol. 2, Gordon, J. L., Ed., Elsevier/North Holland, Amsterdam, 1981, 77.

74. Gordon, J. L., Blood platelet lysosomes and their contribution to the pathophysiological role of platelets, in *Lysosomes in Biology and Pathology,* Vol. 4, Dingle, J. T. and Dean, R. T., Eds., Elsevier/North Holland, Amsterdam, 1975, 3.

75. Holmsen, H. and Weiss, H. J., Secretable storage pools in platelets, *Annu. Rev. Med.,* 30, 119, 1979.

76. Hope, W., Martin, T. J., Chesterman, C. N., and Morgan, F. J., Human β-thromboglobulin inhibits PGI$_2$ production and binds to a specific site in bovine aortic endothelial cells, *Nature (London),* 282, 210, 1979.

77. George, J. N., Thoi, L. L., and Morgan, R. K., Quantitative analysis of platelet membrane glycoproteins: effect of platelet washing procedures and isolation of platelet density subpopulations, *Thromb. Res.,* 23, 69, 1981.

78. Santoro, S. A. and Cunningham, L. W., The interaction of platelets with collagen, in *Platelets in Biology and Pathology,* Gordon, J. L., Ed., Elsevier/North Holland, Amsterdam, 1981, 249.

79. Thompson, C. B., Eaton, K., Princiotta, S. M., Rushin, C. A., and Valleri, C. R., Size dependent platelet subpopulations: relationship of platelet volume to ultrastructure, enzymatic activity and function, *Br. J. Haematol.,* 50, 509, 1982.

80. Fantone, J., Kunkel, S., and Varani, J., Inhibition of tumor cell adherence by prostaglandins, in *Prostaglandins and Cancer,* Powles, T. J., Bockman, R. S., Honn, K. V., and Ramwell, P., Eds., Alan R. Liss, New York, 1982, 673.

81. Cavanaugh, P. G., Sloane, B. F., Bajkowski, A., Gasic, G. J., Gasic, T. B., and Honn, K. V., Involvement of a cathepsin B-like cysteine proteinase in platelet aggregation induced by tumor cells and their shed membrane vesicles, submitted.

82. Honn, K. V., Menter, D. G., Onoda, J. M., Taylor, J. D., and Sloane, B. F., Unpublished data, 1983.

83. Honn, K. V., Cicone, B., and Skoff, A., Prostacyclin: a potent antimetastatic agent, *Science,* 212, 1270, 1981.

84. Stringfellow, D. A. and Fitzpatrick, F. A., Prostaglandin D$_2$ controls pulmonary metastasis of malignant melanoma cells, *Nature (London),* 282, 76, 1979.

85. Willmott, N., Malcolm, A., McLeod, T., Gracie, A., and Calman, K. C., Changes in anatomical distribution of tumor lesions induced by platelet-active drugs, *Invasion Metastasis,* 3, 32, 1983.

86. Salmon, J. A., Smith, D. R., Flower, R. S., Moncada, S., and Vane, J. R., Further studies on the enzymatic conversion of prostaglandin endoperoxide into prostacyclin by porcine aortic microsomes, *Biochem. Biophys. Acta,* 523, 250, 1978.

87. Seuter, F., Busse, W. D., Meng, K., Hoffmeister, F., Moller, E., and Horstmann, H., The antithrombotic activity of Bay g 7575, *Arzneim. Forsch.,* 29, 54, 1979.

88. Vermylen, J., Chamone, D. A. F., and Verstraete, M., Stimulation of prostacyclin release from vessel wall by Bay g 6575, an antithrombotic compound, *Lancet,* 1, 518, 1979.

89. Carreras, L. O., Chamone, D. A. F., Klerckx, P., and Vermylen, J., Decreased vascular prostacyclin (PGI$_2$) in diabetic rats. Stimulation of PGI$_2$ release in normal and diabetic rats by the antithrombotic compound Bay g 6575, *Thromb. Res.,* 19, 663, 1980.

90. Chamone, D. A. F., van Damme, B., Carreras, L. O., and Vermylen, J., Increased release of vascular prostacyclin-like activity after long-term treatment of diabetic rats with Bay g 6575, *Haemostasis,* 10, 297, 1981.

91. Honn, K. V. and Dunn, J. R., Nafazatrom (Bay g 6575) inhibition of tumor cell lipoxygenase activity and cellular proliferation, *FEBS Lett.,* 139, 65, 1982.

92. Busse, W. D., Mardin, M., Grutzmann, R., Dunn, J. R., Theodoreau, M., Sloane, B. F., and Honn, K. V., Nafazatrom (Bay g 6575): an inhibitor of cellular lipoxygenase, *Fed. Proc. Fed. Am. Soc. Exp. Biol.,* 41 (Abstr.), 1717, 1982.

93. Herman, A. G., Claeys, M., Moncada, S., and Vane, J. R., Biosynthesis of prostacyclin (PGI$_2$) and 12L-hydroxy-5,8,10,14-eicosatetraenoic acid (HETE) by pericardium, pleura, peritoneum and aorta of the rabbit, *Prostaglandins,* 18, 439, 1979.

94. Eling, T. E., Honn, K. V., Busse, W. D., Seuter, F., and Marnett, L. J., Stimulation of PGI$_2$ biosynthesis by nafazatrom (Bay g 6575), in *Prostaglandins and Cancer,* Powles, T. J., Bockman, R. S., Honn, K. V., and Ramwell, P., Eds., Alan R. Liss, New York, 1982, 783.

95. Marnett, L. J., Eling. T. E., and Honn, K. V., Unpublished data, 1983.

96. Wong, P. Y.-K, Chao, P. H.-W., and McGiff, J. C., Nafazatrom (Bay g 6575), an antithrombotic and antimetastatic agent, inhibits 15-hydroxyprostaglandin dehydrogenase, *J. Pharmacol. Exp. Ther.,* 223, 757, 1982.

97. Machleidt, C., Forstermann, U., Anhut, H., and Hertting, G., Formation and elimination of prostacyclin metabolites in the cat in vivo as determined by radioimmunoassay of unextracted plasma, *Eur. J. Pharmacol.,* 74, 19, 1981.

98. Rosenkranz, B., Fischer, C., Weimer, K. E., and Frolich, J. C., Metabolism of prostacyclin and 6-keto-prostaglandin F$_{1\alpha}$ in man, *J. Biol. Chem.,* 255, 10194, 1980.

99. Honn, K. V., Meyer, J., Neagos, G., Henderson, T., Westley, C., and Ratanatharathorn, V., Control of tumor growth and metastasis with prostacyclin and thromboxane synthetase inhibitors: evidence for a new antitumor and antimetastatic agent (Bay g 6575), in *Interaction of Platelets and Tumor Cells,* Jamieson, G. A., Ed., Alan R. Liss, New York, 1982, 295.

100. Honn, K. V. and Sloane, B. F., Prostacyclin, thromboxanes, and hematogenous metastasis, in *Advances in Prostaglandin, Thromboxane, and Leukotriene Research,* Vol. 12, Samuelsson, B., Paoletti, R., and Ramwell, P., Eds., Raven Press, New York, 1983, 313.

101. Ambrus, J. L., Ambrus, C. M., Gastpar, H., and Williams, P., Study of platelet aggregation in vivo. IX. Effect of nafazatrom on in vivo platelet aggregation and spontaneous tumor metastasis, *J. Med.,* 13, 35, 1982.

102. Baker, L., Haas, C., Young, J., Evans, L., Kyle, G., and Honn, K., Human in-vivo and in-vitro evaluation of nafazatrom (NFZ), *Proc. Am. Assoc. Cancer Res.,* 24 (Abstr.), 135, 1983.

103. Honn, K. V., Menter, D., Cavanaugh, P. G., Neagos, G., Moilanen, D., Taylor, J. D., and Sloane, B. F., A review of prostaglandins and the treatment of tumor metastasis, *Acta Clin. Belg.,* 38, 53, 1983.

104. Mentor, D., Neagos, G., Dunn, J., Palazzo, R., Tchen, T. T., Taylor, J. D., and Honn, K. V., Tumor cell induced platelet aggregation: inhibition by prostacyclin, thromboxane A$_2$ and phosphdiesterase inhibitors, in *Prostaglandins and Cancer,* Powles, T. J., Bockman, R. S., Honn, K. V., and Ramwell, P., Eds., Alan R. Liss, New York, 1982, 809.

105. Fitzpatrick, F., Bundy, G., Gorman, R., Honohan, T., McGuire, J., and Sun, F., 9,11-Iminoepoxyprosta-5,13-dienoic acid is a selective thromboxane A$_2$ synthetase inhibitor, *Biochim. Biophys. Acta,* 573, 238, 1979.

106. Hornby, E. J. and Skidmore, I. F., Evidence that prostaglandin endoperoxides can induce platelet aggregation in the absence of thromboxane A$_2$ production, *Biochem. Pharmacol.,* 31, 1158, 1982.

107. Honn, K. V., Inhibition of tumor cell metastasis by modulation of the vascular prostacyclin/thromboxane A$_2$ system, *Clin. Exp. Metastasis,* 1, 103, 1983.

108. Hall, E. R., Chen, Y. C., Ho, T., and Wu, K. K., The reduction of platelet thrombi on damaged vessel wall by a thromboxane synthetase inhibitor in platelets, *Thromb. Res.,* 27, 501, 1982.

109. Bertele, V., Falanga, A., Roncaglioni, M. C., Cerletti, C., and deGaetano, G., Thromboxane synthetase inhibition results in increased sensitivity to prostacyclin, *Thromb. Haemostasis,* 47, 294, 1982.

110. Aiken, J. W., Shebuski, R. J., Miller, O. V., and Gorman, R. R., Endogenous prostacyclin contributes to the efficacy of a thromboxane synthetase inhibitor for preventing coronary artery thrombosis, *J. Pharm. Exp. Ther.*, 219, 299, 1981.

111. Defreyn, G., Deckmyn, H., and Vermylen, J., A thromboxane synthetase inhibitor reorients endoperoxide metabolism in whole blood towards prostacyclin and prostaglandin E_2, *Thromb. Res.*, 26, 389, 1982.

112. Gryglewski, R. J., Bunting, S., Moncada, S., Flower, R. J., and Vane, J. R., Arterial walls are protected against deposition of platelet thrombi by a substance (prostaglandin X) which they make from prostaglandin endoperoxides, *Prostaglandins*, 12, 685, 1976.

113. Needleman, P., Wyche, A., and Raz, A., Platelet and blood vessel arachidonate metabolism and interactions, *J. Clin. Invest.*, 63, 345, 1979.

114. Braunwald, E., Mechanism of action of calcium-channel-blocking agents, *N. Engl. J. Med.*, 307, 1618, 1982.

115. Henry, P. D., Comparative pharmacology of calcium antagonists, nifedipine, verapamil, and diltiazem, *Am. J. Cardiol.*, 46, 1047, 1980.

116. Godfraind, T., Mechanism of action of calcium entry blockers, *Fed. Proc. Fed. Am. Soc. Exp. Biol.*, 40, 2866, 1981.

117. Ribeiro, L. G. T., Brandon, T. A., Horak, J. K., Solis, R. T., and Miller, R. R., Inhibition of platelet aggregation by verapamil: further rationale for the use of calcium antagonists in coronary artery disease, *Circulation*, 62 (Abstr.), 293, 1980.

118. Addonizio, V. P., Fisher, C. A., and Edmunds, L. H., Effects of verapamil and nifedipine on platelet activation, *Circulation*, 62 (Abstr.), 326, 1980.

119. Schmunk, G. A. and Lefer, A. M., Anti-aggregatory actions of calcium channel blockers in cat platelets, *Res. Commun. Chem. Pathol. Pharmacol.*, 35, 179, 1982.

120. Donati, M. B., Borowska, A., Bottazzi, B., Dejana, E., Giavazzi, R., Rotilio, D., and Montovani, A., Metastatic potential correlates with changes in the thromboxane-prostacyclin balance, in *Proc. 5th Int. Conf. Prostaglandins*, (Abstract), 136, 1982.

Chapter 10

ROLE OF PROSTAGLANDINS IN TRANSPLANTATION

J. R. L. Shaw

TABLE OF CONTENTS

I. INTRODUCTION

Transplantation of organs from one individual to another is now an established part of routine clinical practice. The mechanical problems encountered in transplantation of kidneys, heart, lung, and liver have been largely overcome and it is likely that the surgical problems encountered in segmental pancreatic allografting will also be solved in the near future. There remains, however, several important difficulties in the maintenance of satisfactory graft function. The greatest of these challenges is the control of graft rejection. In this chapter the potential uses of prostaglandin (PG) modulation in clinical transplantation of solid organs will be reviewed, and this will include modification of platelet activity by PGs.

II. CURRENT PROBLEMS IN CLINICAL TRANSPLANTATION

A. Organ Procurement

Donor availability is still a major hurdle to be overcome in most parts of the world, but with steady improvements in graft and recipient survival, it is hoped that clinicians caring for brain-dead patients will be more aware of the great benefit that may derive from their involvement in the supply of organs for transplantation.

Damage to organs for transplantation may be caused during the premorbid condition of the donor, particularly if hypotension is associated with poor circulation of blood through an organ. Prior to transplantation, organs are usually preserved by cooling. Most of the damage to an organ during procurement is inflicted by ischemia while the organ is warm, and attempts are made to reduce the warm ischemia time as much as possible during removal and insertion of organs. Ideally, good perfusion during removal should be followed by rapid cooling after removal and rapid re-warming after insertion into the recipient. In many clinical situations this ideal is not achieved. The circulation in the donor patient may be impaired by the injury or disease-state that led to brain death. Organ microperfusion may be impaired by hypotension, distribution of blood away from that organ, vasospasm within the organ, or occlusion of capillaries by platelet aggregates. After removal of the organ, with the persistence of vasoconstrictive agents and of platelet aggregates within the organ, vasospasm may impair rapid perfusion with cold preservative solution. Later rewarming after transplantation could also be impaired. Factors released by platelets are capable of initiating the clotting cascade, causing further capillary occlusion. These factors, by prolonging the warm ischemia time, could therefore impair graft function.

In the kidney, a prolonged warm ischemia time results in acute tubular necrosis which leads to post-transplantation anuria. The patient can be maintained on dialysis while graft function is awaited. Liver, heart, and lung transplants must function immediately for staisfactory results, and reduction of graft damage is therefore particularly important. The lungs are very susceptible to contusion and to damage by circulatory particles such as platelet aggregates. Damage is manifested by reduced compliance and reduced gas transfer capability. Ventilation inflation pressure increases and hypoxia develops. Platelet and white cell aggregates are found in the capillaries together with local release of serotonin, histamine, and other products that damage capillaries and alveoli, increasing their permeability to protein, thus increasing the risk of pulmonary edema. In the heart, platelet aggregates may be associated with coronary spasm and reduced myocardial oxygenation.

B. Organ Preservation

Kidneys can be preserved very satisfactorily for at least 24 hr by storing in an ice-cooled container after flushing with a cold preservative medium. Graft function should be immediate, but during any temporary impairment of function dialysis will support the patient until graft function returns. With liver and heart transplants immediate function is essential and present methods of preservation do not allow storage of organs for more than a few hours, certainly less than 24 hr. This means that expensive air-travel is often necessary to transport organs from donor to recipient, and the time available for cross-matching and histocompatibility matching is correspondingly shortened.

C. Early Organ Function

Satisfactory function should be immediate in heart, lung, and liver grafts. In kidney and pancreas grafts a temporary delay in function is not so critical, but delayed function often makes diagnosis of rejection very difficult. In a functioning kidney, a rising serum creatinine and falling urinary output will suggest rejection, but in a kidney with acute tubular necrosis these features are not present and severe rejection may be overlooked until graft salvage is no longer possible. There is, therefore, a need for improvements in graft protection during procurement and storage, and some evidence will be presented to suggest that PGs may be useful.

D. Hyperacute Rejection

Rejection of organs occurring within minutes or hours of transplantation is usually due to preformed antibodies against the graft; this is not at present treatable. If the transplanted organ is essential for life support, for example the heart or liver, this event is fatal.[1] It is possible that PGs may inhibit the events that result from antibody reactions with graft antigen. If so, patients with antibodies against grafts could possibly receive a transplanted organ, and xenografts could be considered in the future.

E. Acute Rejection

Acute rejection is still the main cause of graft failure after transplantation, and the major hurdle to be overcome in clinical transplantation. Conventional immunosuppression with steroids and azathioprine has enabled clinical transplantation to be developed over the last 20 years. Associated morbidity is high, because the immunosuppression is not selective and death due to opportunistic infections is common. Side effects of steroids are severe, and many episodes of acute rejection are not controllable. Cyclosporin A is a very powerful immunosuppressant that is replacing conventional drugs in many centers.[2] Steroids can often be avoided or kept at very low doses. A serious problem with the use of Cyclosporin A is its nephrotoxicity, which seems to be dose related, and which often leads to severe renal impairment requiring dialysis.[3-5] It is often difficult to tell whether renal impairment is due to rejection of a transplanted kidney or to nephrotoxicity. The former would require an increased dose of Cyclosporin A, the latter a reduction in dosage. Renal biopsy may be helpful,[6] but carries appreciable morbidity. It is possible that modulation of PG metabolism in combination with other immunosuppression would result in better control of rejection with lower doses of such drugs as Cyclosporin A (perhaps avoiding nephrotoxicity). Changes in endogenous PG metabolism during rejection may be a noninvasive clinical tool for separating graft impairment due to rejection from that due to nephrotoxicity.

F. Chronic Rejection

Chronic rejection is a difficult clinical problem, and its exact cause is undetermined. It is often associated with accelerated graft arteriosclerosis,[7] which may be related to increased platelet deposition, and may be controllable by drugs influencing platelet activity. The long-term results of Cyclosporin A immunosuppression upon graft function have yet to be determined.

G. Neoplasia

Immunosuppression is associated with an increased incidence of benign and malignant tumors. Presumably this relates to a reduced ability to overcome infections with oncogenic viruses or a disturbance of immunological surveillance. Early studies with Cyclosporin A used together with steroids resulted in a high incidence of neoplasms,[2] particularly lymphomas, and this also occurs during immunosuppression following cardiac transplants.

Therefore, in clinical transplantation there is a need for improvement in organ preservation and storage and the control of rejection. Evidence will be presented to suggest that in the future PG modulation may be a useful adjunct to present schedules.

III. ROLE OF PLATELETS IN TRANSPLANTATION

Because of the close interaction between platelet activity and PG metabolism, it may be useful to study the involvement of platelets in transplantation. If they were important, PGs could be used to change their activity.

A. Organ Procurement and Preservation

Accumulation of platelets may occur during hypoperfusion of organs being removed for transplantation, and as already described, this may impair preservation and later perfusion by blood after transplantation, prolonging warm ischemia. It is interesting that in human kidney allografts renal blood flow at the time of transplantation is lower in kidneys that later have severe rejection episodes.[8]

B. Hyperacute Rejection

Platelets accumulate early in hyperacute rejection or xenograft rejection. In hyperacute rejection of dog kidneys there is a rapid uptake of platelets by the graft[9,10] with a concomitant reduction in blood flow through that organ until the degree of ischemia leads to graft necrosis. Platelet accumulation also occurs early in hyperacute cardiac allograft rejection in the rat,[11] and this is followed by widespread endothelial damage. Similar platelet accumulation occurs when pig kidneys are transplanted to dogs.[12]

C. Acute Rejection

Platelet accumulation is seen early in acute renal allograft rejection as shown by histology in human kidneys.[13-16] Indium-labeled platelets accumulate early in graft rejection,[17] and immunoreactive thromboxane (TX)B_2 release in rejection of kidneys[18] and hearts[19] may be in part due to platelet activation. Serotonin levels are reduced in platelets during rejection of kidneys.[20] Platelet accumulation in the graft is probably secondary to an immune attack, but may be an important factor in determining the extent of damage to the graft caused by the immune attack.

Platelet aggregation and degranulation in a kidney undergoing rejection may contribute to renal damage in at least two ways. First, the epithelium may be damaged by products of degranulation[21] or complement fixation,[11] facilitating cellular infiltration of the organ and helper cell activation. If helper cell activation can be suppressed, specific tolerance is more likely to be induced.[22] Second, blockage of arterioles and capillaries by platelet aggregates and vasoconstriction from products of platelet degranulation and release of lysosomal cationic inflammatory mediators[21] may reduce renal blood flow[23] causing ischemic necrosis, and possibly reducing the effect of high zone tolerance. If platelet accumulation is prevented, perhaps graft damage during acute rejection could be reduced.

D. Chronic Rejection

Platelet uptake does occur in chronic rejection as shown by indium-labeled platelet imaging[24] and this may be responsible for the intimal thickening.[14] There may be a component resulting from previous graft ischemia and vascular damage during acute rejection, and if so a reduction in graft damage during the early stages of transplantation could reduce the extent of chronic rejection.

There are therefore several theoretical reasons why drugs modifying platelet behavior might be of use in transplantation.

IV. ROLE OF ENDOGENOUS PROSTAGLANDINS IN TRANSPLANTATION IMMUNOLOGY

PGs appear to be involved in the regulation of cellular and humoral immunity,[25-28] and changes in lymphocyte activity are related to intracellular cyclic AMP (cAMP) concentration[29] which may be affected by macrophage-derived PGs.[30] It is therefore likely that interference with this communication between cells involved in immune phenomena may be beneficial in the control of rejection of transplanted organs.

Studies of effects of PGs upon immune mechanisms have shown conflicting results. Generally PGE_1 and PGE_2 seem to inhibit T cell and possibly B cell function, while at the same time acting as mediators of inflammation. Many experiments have used pharmacological doses of PGs rather than naturally occurring amounts,[26,31] and perhaps some of the inhibition has been due to nonspecific toxicity of the PGs acting upon lymphocytes. It is also possible that subtle balances between concentrations of antagonistic PGs control the overall outcome (in a similar way to the control of platelet activity by a balance between PGI_2 — prostacyclin — and TXA_2[32]), and that many of the in vitro experiments cannot be related to events occurring in vivo. Perhaps levels of PGs within cellular microcompartments are more important than overall tissue or culture-fluid levels, and perhaps short-lived PG endoperoxides or leukotrienes[33] are also important in the control of lymphocyte activity.

Moore and Jaffe[34] showed that at the time of rejection of heterotopic rat heart allografts, PGE levels in the grafts and in the host spleen and thymus were greatly increased. This suggested an involvement of PGE in the afferent and efferent arms of the immune response. Venous blood from the hearts also showed elevated PGE levels at the time of rejection.[35] Plasma PGE levels increased during rejection of human renal allografts and dog skin grafts.[36] It is possible that these increases in PGE production merely reflect concomitant inflammation during rejection; however, much effort has been spent in studying further effects of PGs upon immunocompetent cells, and some of the results will now be reviewed.

A. Evidence that Prostaglandins Inhibit Immune Functions

PG precursors such as polyunsaturated fatty acids have a specific inhibitory action on lymphocyte transformation induced by phytohemagglutinin (PHA) or purified protein derivative of tubercle (PPD),[37] and precursor supply is generally regarded as the rate-limiting step in PG production. Linoleic acid and arachidonic acid prolong skin allograft survival in mice.[38] PGs of the E series suppress human T cell mitogenesis,[39] and PGE_1 inhibits T cell proliferation and renal disease in MRL/1 mice.[40] PGE_2 inhibits E rosette formation by human T cells,[41] and PGE_1 and PGE_2 inhibit PHA stimulation of human lymphocytes, probably via an increase in intracellular cAMP.[42] PG inhibition of T cell proliferation appears to be mediated at two levels,[43] by inhibiting both lymphokine production[44] and action. PGE secreted by an adherent cell population appears to inhibit the production of human interleukin (IL) 2,[45] while PG synthetase inhibitors raised IL-2 production above normal levels. Macrophage migration inhibitory factor (MIF) is inhibited by PGE₁ and PGE₂,[46] and these PGs inhibit interferon-activated macrophages of mice.[47] Perhaps PGE₁ and PGE₂ act locally in negative feedback inhibition to limit macrophage activity.[47] Macrophages synthesize and release PGs in response to inflammatory stimuli.[48] In mixed lymphocyte culture, PGE₂ inhibited proliferation and generation of specific cytotoxicity.[49] PG synthesis inhibitors enhanced proliferation and cytotoxicity.

There is accumulating evidence that PGs stimulate suppressor cells. Goodwin, Bankhurst, and Messner[39] identified a population of glass adherent mononuclear cells that suppress T cell mitogenic activity through production of PGs of the E series. Webb and Nowowiejski[50] showed that glass-wool-adherent lymphocytes could be stimulated directly by the addition of PGE₂ to become suppressor cells and to release a soluble suppressor product. They also showed that macrophages can activate suppressor cells via PGs.[51] Fischer, Durandy, and Griscelli[52] showed that human monocytes can activate short-lived suppressor lymphocytes through secretion of PGE₂. Fulton and Levy[53] described the in vitro induction of suppressor cell activity by the exogenous addition of PGE₁ to normal mouse spleen cells. Gualde and Goodwin[54] showed that PGE₂ inhibits OKT4⁺ (helper/inducer) cells and stimulates OKT8⁺ (suppressor/cytotoxic) cells in their response to PHA. Rogers et al.[55] described the activity of a PG-induced T cell-derived suppressor (PITSβ) that has a protein or peptide component. This factor inhibited mixed-lymphocyte reactions and antibody responses to both T-dependent and -independent antigens.

Zurier and Quagliata[56] showed that when rats are treated with PGE₁, adjuvant arthritis is prevented and suppressed. Orally active PGs were also effective.[57] PGs have also been shown to inhibit cytolytic activity of mouse lymphocytes acting upon tumor cells,[58] and this was related to increased intracellular cAMP levels. Hemolytic plaque formation by splenic leukocytes from immunized mice was similarly inhibited.[59] PGE₁ inhibits antibody production to sheep red blood cells in rats,[56] but Braun and Ishizuka[60] showed that different doses of agents increasing cellular cAMP may enhance or reduce antibody formation.

Leung and Mihich[61] studied PG modulation of cell-mediated immunity in culture, using spleen cell response to allogeneic mastocytoma cells. PGE₁ and PGE₂ inhibited lymphocyte activity, while indomethacin augemented ³H-thymidine incorporation and lytic activity. PGI₂ inhibited the cytolytic activity of effector cells from immunized mice, while the PGI₂ synthetase inhibitor tranylcypromine augmented the development of cell-mediated immunity. It was suggested that PGI₂ may be an inhibitory regulator of development of cell-mediated immunity, while TXA₂ may be an augmentative regulator, and that the relative concentrations of PGI₂, TXA₂, and PGs may determine the magnitude of the immune response.

B. Evidence that Prostaglandins Stimulate Immune Functions

Mertin and Stackpoole[62] have produced good evidence that antibodies against PGE₁ can suppress cell-mediated immunity in vivo. Anti-PGE₁ antiserum raised in Lewis rats, and given subcutaneously to Lewis rats receiving guinea pig brain stem and spinal cord material emulsified in complete Freund's adjuvant, suppressed the development of experimental allergic encephalomyelitis in rats. The antiserum also suppressed both host-vs.-graft and graft-vs.-host reactions in mice. Inhibition was greatest when the antiserum was given early in the development of an immune response. This would suggest that PGE is required as an augmentative mediator substance during the induction phase of cell-mediated immunity. It was also suggested that the effect of PGE was governed by a bell-shaped, dose-response relationship. Although small amounts of PGE are necessary for the induction of an immune response, larger amounts of PGE could still act in an inhibitory capacity, perhaps limiting the extent of the response.

Zurier, Dore-Duffy, and Viola[63] showed enhancement by PGE_1 of adherence of human peripheral blood lymphocytes to measles-infected cells. PGE_1 given to Freund's complete adjuvant sensitized rats enhanced the delayed hypersensitivity response to PPD, measured following transfer of donor lymph node cells into syngeneic recipients,[64] while in mice passive transfer of delayed hypersensitivity to sheep red blood cells was reduced by PGE_1. Ceuppens and Goodwin[65] showed that in vitro endogenous PGE_2 enhances polyclonal immunoglobulin production by tonically inhibiting T suppressor cell activity. Low concentrations of PGE_2 were involved (3×10^{-9} to 3×10^{-8} *M*). It was postulated that suppressor cell function might be pharmacologically enhanced by blocking endogenous PGE_2 production. Favalli et al.[66] showed that 16,16-dimethyl-PGE_2-methyl ester was mildly immunosuppressive in normal mice, but when given to animals immunosuppressed by thymectomy plus antithymocyte serum the drug augmented the humoral and cellular responses to B-16 melanoma cells.

Glucocorticoids probably act at several points on the immune system to suppress it, and it is therefore impossible to imply that because they generally lead to a reduction in PG production, it is this reduced PG supply that leads to immunosuppression. However, the discovery that steroids stimulate the production of macrocortin[67] or lipomodulin,[68] a protein which inhibits phospholipase and leukotriene production, may lead to the discovery of further pathways of control of PG metabolism by steroids. It is also possible that leukotrienes are involved in the inflammatory component of graft rejection, and that some of the beneficial actions of steroids in transplantation are related to the production of macrocortin.

This conflicting evidence for inhibition and stimulation of immune mechanisms by PGs in different systems is probably related to the great differences between in vivo and in vitro conditions, and the effects of widely varying PG concentrations on different combinations of cell populations. There is, however, enough evidence for a role of endogenous PGs in the intercellular control of immune mechanisms for attempts to be made to study the effects of interference with PG metabolism upon the rejection of organ allografts.

Figure 1 shows some of the mechanisms by which PGs of the E group might be involved in the coordination of rejection of transplanted organs. This emphasizes the general inhibitory effects of PGE upon the immune mechanisms, but does not include the evidence of Mertin and Stackpoole[62] that small amounts of PGE are necessary for the induction of the immune response.

The exact role of inflammation during rejection has never been determined, and as PGs are powerful inflammatory mediators it is possible that attempts to reduce any inflammatory component by inhibiting PG production may be beneficial to graft survival. There are therefore cases to be made for studying both PG inhibition and stimulation in graft rejection, as well as the effects of PGs controlling platelet activity.

V. THERAPEUTIC USES OF PROSTAGLANDINS IN TRANSPLANTATION

Having discussed the reasons for studying the effects of drugs affecting PG metabolism in transplantation, this section details experiments relating to this field.

A. Organ Procurement

Mundy et al.[69] studied the role of PGI_2 in the harvesting of kidneys in experimental canine transplantation. Intra-aortic infusion of PGI_2, 0.25 μg/kg/min gave a 52.6% increase in renal blood flow prenephrectomy despite inducing a 23% drop in mean arterial pressure. The fall in renal vascular resistance was 50.2%. The flow of flushing solution through the kidney after nephrectomy and red blood cell washout was im-

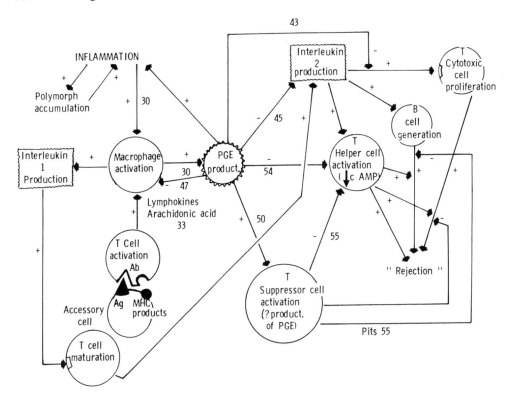

FIGURE 1.   Diagrammatic schedule for possible regulation of immune mechanisms by PGE. Numbers on pathway arrows indicate references to relevant data.

proved when heparin and PGI$_2$ were used together in pretreatment. When a warm ischemia time of 45 min was introduced, autotransplanted kidneys in dogs pretreated with PGI$_2$ (0.25 µg/kg/min, given intravenously for 15 min before clamping the renal artery) had normal renal function within 48 hr as judged by the serum creatinine, whereas untreated dogs had permanent impairment of function.

In similar experiments Bradley et al.[70] showed improved perfusion of pig kidneys when PGI$_2$ was infused during nephrectomy, and the peak serum creatinine after surgery was reduced by PGI$_2$ pretreatment of donors.

Casey et al.[71] studied alterations of postischemic renal pathology by PGE$_1$ and PGI$_2$ infusions. After 1 hr of warm ischemia to the kidneys, dogs were treated with PGE$_1$ 1.0 µg/kg/min or PGI$_2$ 0.3 µg/kg/min, or saline by intravenous infusion for 1 hr. Histology of the kidneys showed more extensive proximal tubular damage and eosinophilia in the saline-treated controls than in the treated groups. Although cellular protection seemed to have been provided by the PG infusion, serum creatinine levels did not demonstrate any improvement in the functional defect.

B. Organ Preservation

Monden and Fortner[72] preserved canine livers by simple hypothermic storage using modified Sack's solution, and then transplanted the livers orthotopically. When PGI$_2$ was added to the perfusion solution to a concentration of 100 µg/ℓ, 5 of 6 and 3 of 5 livers preserved for 24 and 48 hr, respectively, were able to sustain life for more than 5 days. Only 1 of 5 livers preserved for 24 hr without PGI$_2$ sustained life for over 5 days. There was less histological evidence of liver damage when PGI$_2$ was used in the preservation fluid.

We have performed similar experiments using rat hearts perfused and preserved at 4°C with Marchall's solution, followed by heterotopic transplantation into syngeneic rats. PGI_2 in concentrations up to 500 $\mu g/\ell$ did not improve heart preservation when compared with control solution lacking PGI_2. However, it is quite possible that a more alkaline hyperosmolar solution would give better results; this remains to be studied.

C. Hyperacute and Xenograft Rejection

Kakita et al.[73] studied hamster-to-rat cardiac xenografts. Untreated control grafts lost electrical activity after a median time of 73.5 hr. PGE_1 injections, 2 mg/kg daily, prolonged median time to loss of activity to 94 hr, and suppressed the hemagglutination titer to hamster red cells at the time of rejection.

Mundy et al.[74] investigated the effects of PGI_2 upon hyperacute renal allograft rejection in presensitized dogs. Control kidneys were all rejected by 4 hr, with blood flow ceasing at 70 to 220 min. When PGI_2 was infused into the aorta of recipient dogs at 0.25 $\mu g/kg/min$, graft failure had not occurred by 4 hr. PGI_2-treated kidneys had normal or above normal blood flow rates at 4 hr, were producing urine, and were similar histologically to 4-hr autografts. Control kidneys were shown to accumulate platelets from the perfusing blood until cessation of circulation. In the PGI_2 treated group there was no decrease in the venous platelet count compared to the arterial count throughout the perfusion time.

Mundy[75] also showed prolongation of cat to dog renal xenograft survival with PGI_2. Untreated dogs rejected cat kidneys, as determined by cessation of blood flow to the kidneys, within 25 min. This rejection was accompanied by platelet accumulation within the graft, and histological studies showed widespread glomerular and tubular damage with interstitial hemorrhage. When PGI_2 was infused into the aorta of recipient dogs at 1.0 $\mu g/kg/min$, blood flow to the kidneys was maintained within normal limits for at least 8 hr apart from a drop and slow return to normal at about 20 min, which corresponded to the time rejection occurred in untreated kidneys. Histology of the PGI_2-treated kidneys showed only mild patchy peritubular congestion and tubular dilation.

The author has transplanted guinea-pig hearts heterotopically to DA rats and studied the effect of PGI_2 infusions in this model. When the recipients were given infusions of glycine buffer (pH 10.5) 10 min before graft circulation commenced, cessation of graft beat occurred between 6 and 14 min after clamp removal. When PGI_2 was added to the glycine buffer and infused at doses up to 12 $\mu g/kg/min$, maximum duration of graft beat was prolonged to only 20 min. Prior to cessation of graft beat the hearts showed evidence of interstitial hemorrhage, and at the time of cessation of graft beat the coronary circulation persisted. It is likely that in this model the severe mismatch between graft and recipient enabled antibody-mediated vascular damage to lead to graft failure without the necessary involvement of platelet degranulation and activation of the clotting cascade within the vessels.

Other investigators have studied the effects of anticoagulants in hyperacute and xenograft rejection. Amery et al.[9] found that heparin infusion delayed but did not prevent hyperacute rejection in dog renal allografts. Thrombus formation was not seen in renal vessels in either the control or heparin-treated group, and it was suggested that thrombus formation is a secondary phenomenon occurring after the rejection phase. MacDonald et al.[76] studied the effects of Arvin in hyperacute canine renal allograft and sheep-to-dog xenograft rejection. Fibrin deposition was absent or diminished in Arvin-treated recipients, but the profound anticoagulation did not lead to a reduction in the severity of graft rejection.

D. Acute Rejection

1. Prostaglandin Administration

Pausescu et al.[77] studied effects of PGE_2 and $PGF_{2\alpha}$ upon antibody-mediated damage to rat hearts in vivo and in vitro. PGE_2 administered intraperitoneally at a dose of 100 $\mu g/kg$ or $PGF_{2\alpha}$ at 75 $\mu g/kg$ prevented myocardial lesions caused by intraperitoneal injection of anti-rat serum. Isolated perfused rat hearts were damaged by addition of anti-rat serum to the perfusate, but the damage was prevented by the addition of PGE_2 (3 $\mu g/\ell$) or $PGF_{2\alpha}$ (2.5 $\mu g/\ell$) to the perfusate.

Favalli et al.[66] showed that 16,16-dimethyl-PGE_2-methyl ester augmented the growth of transplanted B-16 melanoma in mice. Quagliata et al.[78] investigated PGE_1 in skin graft rejection in mice. When 200 μg were injected subcutaneously twice daily into recipient mice, there was no prolongation of allograft survival; however, when PGE_1 was added to procarbazine treatment, the PGE_1 led to longer graft survival than that obtained when procarbazine alone was used. One serious problem with the use of PGs of the E group is their short half-life in vivo. Strom et al.[79] synthesized PG derivatives with longer biological half-lives and tested the action of these in rat kidney allografts. L-619,375 (8-acetyl-12-hydroxyheptadecanoic acid) and L-630,523 (8-methylsulfonyl-12-hydroxyheptadecanoic acid) given by intraperitoneal injection greatly improved survival of bilaterally nephrectomized Lewis rats receiving Lewis × Brown Norway F_1 renal grafts and was associated with improvements in renal function 7 days after transplantation.

PGI_2 was tested in acute rejection of human kidney transplants by Sinzinger et al.[80] Early studies have shown reduced platelet deposition when PGI_2 was used and this may be associated with improvement in renal function.[81] Shaw[82] has investigated the effect of PGI_2 infusions in rat heart allograft rejection. PGI_2 was infused at 250 ng/kg/min into the inferior vena cava of PVG ($RT1^c$) rats that received hearts from DA ($RT1^a$) rats. When PGI_2 was infused from day 5 median, graft survival time was prolonged from a control of 7.8 days to 9.3 days ($p < 0.05$). When PGI_2 was infused from day 1, graft survival time was prolonged from a control of 7.4 days to 8.6 days ($p < 0.05$). Apart from the instability of PGI_2, another problem with the use of PGI_2 is the decreased sensitivity of tissues during long-term infusion.[83] If PGI_2 proved to be of use in clinical transplant rejection it would presumably have to be reserved for episodes of rejection rather than for prophylaxis of rejection.

2. Stimulation of Prostaglandin Production

Precursor availability seems to be one of the rate-limiting steps in PG production. PG production may be increased by providing extra precursors or by shifting precursor entry from another PG synthetic pathway into the pathway of interest (for example, TX synthetase inhibition may stimulate PGI_2 production). Studies of such mechanisms in graft rejection have so far been limited, but Santiago-Delpin and Szepsenwol[84] reported prolonged survival of skin and tumor allografts in mice fed on high-fat diets. McHugh et al.[85] undertook a double-blind controlled trial to assess the value of a preparation containing polyunsaturated fatty acids in human cadaveric renal transplantation. Graft survival during the first 4 months after transplantation was significantly better in the polyunsaturated fatty acid group than in controls, but by 6 months the difference between the groups was no longer significant. It is quite possible that some of the beneficial effects of drugs like salicylate are due to selective inhibition of parts of the PG synthetic pathways with precursor shift toward other pathways.

3. Inhibition of Prostaglandin Production

As already discussed, some of the beneficial effects of steroids in transplantation may be related to inhibition of leukotriene production via phospholipase inhibition.

Moore and Hoult[86] studied anti-inflammatory steroids in rats and showed that prednisolone produced a dose-related decrease in acitivity of microsomal PG synthetase and increased the activity of PG-metabolizing enzymes. Belldegrun et al.[87] studied effects of hydrocortisone and PG synthesis inhibitors upon survival of mouse skin allografts. Neither hydrocortisone nor indomethacin or flufenamate alone prolonged graft survival, but hydrocortisone in combination with indomethacin or flufenamate prolonged skin graft survival from 11.4 days to over 20 days. Jamieson et al.[88] showed that sodium salicylate and azathioprine together led to long-term survival of rat heart allografts. Shaw[89] showed that sodium salicylate in combination with very low doses of Cyclosporin A gave prolonged graft survival when DA (RT1^a) rat hearts were transplanted to PVG (RT1^c) rats. When sodium salicylate was compared with aspirin in this model, sodium salicylate alone given by subcutaneous injection at a dose of 200 mg/kg/day, gave a median graft survival of 10.5 days, with 1 out of 12 grafts beating for 63 days and another beating well at 6 months. Studies of aspirin and sodium salicylate effects on ADP-induced aggregation of platelets in these rats showed that salicylate was about 13 times weaker than aspirin in inhibiting platelet aggregation, and it cylate effects on ADP-induced aggregation of platelets in these rats showed that salicylate was about 13 times weaker than aspirin in inhibiting platelet aggregation, and it seems likely that the beneficial effect of salicylate in prolongation of graft survival is mediated by mechanisms other than by inhibition of platelet aggregation. Whether this involves changes in PG metabolism remains the subject of further investigation.

4. Prostaglandin Antagonism

Mertin and Stackpoole[62] raised anti-PGE$_1$ antibodies in Lewis rats by injection of a conjugate of PGE$_1$ and bovine serum albumin emulsified in complete Freund's adjuvant. When these antibodies were administered to mice by subcutaneous injection, host vs. graft reactions to infection of allogeneic cells as measured by a lymph node assay system were suppressed. It was suggested that small amounts of PGE$_1$ might be necessary for induction of an immune response.

We have used this rat anti-PGE$_1$ antiserum, kindly supplied by Mertin, in the DA to PVG rat heart allograft model. Initial experiments used 0.2 mℓ of antiserum injected intravenously into recipients 12 hr before transplantation, with 0.2 mℓ injected subcutaneously 30 min before transplantation, followed by daily subcutaneous injections of 0.2 mℓ antiserum. In this model the anti-PGE$_1$ antiserum led to earlier rejection of transplanted hearts. Anti-PGE$_1$ antiserum treated rats rejected hearts at a median time of 6.0 days, while controls rejected at 7.2 days (Wilcoxon $p<0.05$). This would support the idea discussed above that PGE might act as a physiological feedback mechanism to limit the severity of cell-mediated immune attack.

Studies are at present in progress to assess the effects of drugs inhibiting particular parts of the PG and leukotriene biosynthetic pathways in the rat heart allograft model. At present the results have been disappointing, with sodium salicylate remaining by far the most effective of drugs of this type. Figure 2 shows some of the points at which control of PG biosynthesis may be attempted.

5. Other Drugs Affecting Platelets and Anticoagulants

Shehadeh et al.[90] studied renal allograft rejection in rats. Aspirin and sodium salicylate were used to modify platelet behavior, and heparin and bishydroxycoumarin were used to inhibit fibrin deposition. Aspirin given orally, 100 mg/kg/day, led to a reduction in platelet aggregates in peritubular capillaries and fibrin deposition in glomerular capillaries. On day 7 effective renal plasma flow (ERPF) was 0.38 mℓ/min/100 g. When 50 mg/kg/day aspirin was used, ERPF was 0.11 mℓ/min/100 g. Both doses of aspirin led to slight reduction in cellular infiltrate on day 7. Sodium salicylate,

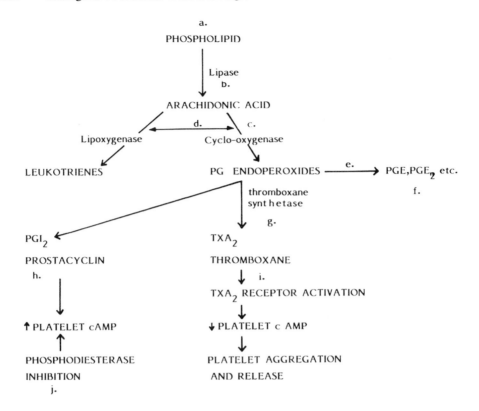

FIGURE 2.   Possible points for pharmacological manipulation of PG biosynthetic pathway and platelet behavior. (a) Control of precursor supply; (b) inhibited by steroids; (c) inhibited by aspirin; (d) inhibited by BW 755C (Wellcome); (e) inhibited by Surgam (Roussel); (f) inhibited by specific antibodies; (g) inhibited by UK-38485 (Pfizer); (h) addition of exogenous PGI₂ (Upjohn); (i) EIP (Upjohn) inhibition; and (j) phosphodiesterase inhibition by dipyridamole (Boehringer-Ingelheim).

100 mg/kg/day and 50 mg/kg/day, led to mean day 7 ERPF of 0.60 mℓ/min/100 g and 0.58 mℓ/min/100 g, respectively, and to less cellular infiltration than in the aspirin-treated group. Heparin, 400 units given subcutaneously every 12 hr, killed 10 out of 11 rats at days 4 to 6. The surviving rat on day 7 had ERPF of 1.0 mℓ/min/100 g, minimal cellular infiltrate, and no platelet or fibrin deposition. Bishydroxycoumarin, 10 mg/kg/day, had no beneficial effect.

George et al.[91] investigated aspirin, dypyridamole, and heparin in dog renal allografts. There was no improvement in platelet destruction or graft survival when compared with control animals, and there was a high incidence of hemorrhage after heparin treatment. Kauffman et al.[92] compared aspirin, 10 mg/day, with dipyridamole, 400 mg/day, in human kidney allografts. Dipyridamole produced a reduction in the incidence of postanastomotic transplant renal artery stenosis and aspirin caused a high incidence of GI bleeding, but neither drug led to improvements in graft survival or function at 6 months. Laden[93] showed that dipyridamole had no effect on rat cardiac allografts. Jamieson[94] found that promethazine, an antihistamine that reduces platelet aggregation, when given intraperitoneally prevented rejection of rat cardiac allografts. Cyproheptadine has been studied by Burrows et al.[95] in rat kidney allografts and in human renal transplant recipients. This treatment prolonged mean survival time of rat renal allografts from a control of 13.5 to 84 days. Initial studies in humans suggested that the use of this drug reduced the severity of rejection episodes, but Jessing et al.[96] in a larger study were unable to demonstrate any beneficial effect from the use of cyproheptadine in human kidney allografts. Kostakis et al.[97] showed prolongation of rat cardiac and renal allograft survival by the use of pentoxifylline, which decreases blood viscosity.

McMillan[98] found that heparin improved the function of human kidney allografts in a small series of cases; however, Griffin and Salaman[99] undertook a controlled trial of heparin in renal transplant rejection and showed no benefit from the use of this drug.

Kincaid-Smith[100,101] studied heparin and phenindione anticoagulation together with dipyridamole in human kidney transplant rejection. These drugs appeared to prevent thrombosis of vessels in acute rejection and also the progressive narrowing of vessels seen in chronic rejection. However, results of a prospective, controlled trial of anti-coagulation and dipyridamole,[102] despite confirming a beneficial effect on the histological appearance of glomeruli and blood vessels, showed no significant difference in graft function between treated and control groups. Barnes et al.[103] showed that warfarin anticoagulation did not improve the function of human renal allografts and was associated with a high incidence of complications. Soper et al.[104] showed that heparin may be useful in the treatment of acute rejection with mild vascular changes, but that anti-coagulation was associated with a high morbidity and did not prevent chronic rejection.

6. Diagnosis of Acute Rejection

Changes in PG metabolism at the time of acute rejection may be useful to differentiate acute rejection from other causes of graft failure. Foegh et al. showed that in rejection of kidneys[18] and hearts[19] urinary immunoreactive TXB_2 levels are elevated. This could be an important tool for differentiating between acute rejection of renal allografts and Cyclosporin A-induced nephrotoxicity.

E. Chronic Rejection

Lurie et al.[7] studied graft arteriosclerosis in rat heart allografts treated with Cyclosporin A. This condition was prevented by treatment with dipyridamole but not by sulfinpyrazone.

Leithner et al.[105] have used PGI_2 in chronic rejection of human renal allografts. Continuous infusion of PGI_2 at a dose of 5 ng/kg/min led to a decrease in platelet deposition and a prolongation of platelet survival, with reduction in serum creatinine.

VI. CONCLUSIONS

The study of protection of transplanted organs by the use of PG modulation is in its infancy, but evidence reviewed above would suggest a possible role for the PGs in the procurement and storage of organs for transplantation and perhaps in the suppression of acute and chronic rejection. Investigation into this field is complicated by several factors. First, there is a great difference in preservation characteristics between different organs, and a formula that proves satisfactory in preservation of a dog liver, for example, may not necessarily prove to be useful for storage of human liver or hearts. Second, the exact mechanism of rejection of transplanted organs is far from clear as is the role of endogenous PGs in this process. Results of studies of the control of rejection in rat heart or kidney allografts cannot necessarily be extrapolated to events occurring in rejection of organs in dogs and humans. Experiments in large numbers of dogs or primates are very expensive, but there must be good evidence from animal studies that a new protocol is beneficial before it is introduced into a clinical transplantation program.

The short biological half-life of many PGs makes their clinical use difficult, yet when an analogue with greater stability is developed, it is quite possible that other biological activities of the PG molecule will also differ from that of the parent compound. When drugs affecting the PG biosynthetic pathway are studied, the particular selectivities of action of the various drugs depend upon the dose range and the species under investigation. Tampering with one part of the pathway may lead to shift of precursors toward the synthesis of other PGs, perhaps antagonistic to those produced by the inhibited pathway.

A further problem results from changes in clinical immunosuppression. It is likely that rejection seen when Cyclosporin A is used differs in several ways from that seen with conventional immunosuppression. Therefore, many of the drugs used to suppress secondary phenomena occurring in graft microvasculature during rejection might be beneficial when used with Cyclosporin A, even if clinical trials have not shown them to be beneficial with conventional immunosuppression. Despite these difficulties, it is hoped that further investigation into the field of PGs in preservation and control of rejection of transplanted organs will prove to be helpful to the quality of life of organ recipients.

REFERENCES

1. Weil, R., Clarke, D. R., Iwaki, Y., Porter, K. A., Koep, L. J., Paton, B. C., Terasaki, P. I., and Starzl, T. E., Hyperacute rejection of a transplanted human heart, *Transplantation*, 32, 71, 1981.
2. White, D. J. G. and Calne, R. Y., The use of Cyclosporin A immunosuppression in organ grafting, *Immunol. Rev.*, 65, 115, 1982.
3. Calne, R. Y., Rolles, K., White, D. J. G., Thiru, S., Evans, D. B., McMaster, P., Dunn, D. C., Craddock, G. N., Henderson, R., G., Aziz, S., and Lewis, P., Cyclosporin A initially as the only immunosuppressant in 34 recipients of cadaveric organs: 32 kidneys, 2 pancreases, and 2 livers, *Lancet*, 2, 1033, 1979.
4. Starzl, T. E., Hakala, T. R., Rosenthal, J. T., Iwatsuki, S., and Shaw, B. W., Variable convalescence and therapy after cadaveric renal transplantation under Cyclosporin A and steroids, *Surg. Gynecol. Obstet.*, 154, 819, 1982.
5. Calne, R. Y., White, D. J. G., Thiru, S., Evans, D. B., McMaster, P., Dunn, D. C., Craddock, G. N., Pentlow, B. D., and Rolles, K., Cyclosporin A in patients receiving renal allografts from cadaver donors, *Lancet*, 2, 1323, 1978.
6. Klintmalm, G., Bergstrand, A., Ringden, O., Collste, H., Lundgren, G., Wilczek, H., and Groth, C. G., Graft biopsy for the differentiation between nephrotoxicity and rejection in Cyclosporin A treated renal transplant recipients, *Abstr. 9 Int. Congr. Transplant. Soc.*, 1982, p 12.3
7. Lurie, K. G., Billingham, M. E., Jamieson, S. W., Harrison, D. C., and Reitz, B. A., Pathogenesis and prevention of graft arteriosclerosis in an experimental heart transplant model, *Transplantation*, 31, 41, 1981.
8. Bergentz, S. E., Brunius, U., Gelin, L. E., and Lewis, D. H., Operative blood flow measurement in transplanted human kidneys and subsequent rejection, *Ann. Surg.*, 174, 44, 1971.
9. Amery, A. H., Pegrum, G. D., Risdon, R. A., and Williams, G., Nature of hyperacute (accelerated second set) rejection in dog renal allografts and effects of heparin on rejection process, *Br. Med. J.*, 1, 455, 1973.
10. Lowenhaupt, R. and Nathan, P., Platelet accumulation observed by electron microscopy in the early phase of renal allotransplant rejection, *Nature (London)*, 220, 822, 1968.
11. Forbes, R. D. C., Kuramochi, T., Guttmann, R. D., Klassen, J., and Knaack, J., A controlled sequential morphologic study of hyperacute cardiac allograft rejection in the rat, *Lab. Invest.*, 33, 280, 1975.
12. Rosenberg, J. C., Broersma, R. J., Bullemer, G., Mammen, E. F., Lenaghan, R., and Rosenberg, B. F., Relationship of platelets, blood coagulation, and fibrinolysis to hyperacute rejection of renal xenografts, *Transplantation*, 8, 152, 1969.
13. Mowbray, J. F., Methods of suppression of immune responses, *Excerpta Med. Int. Congr. Ser.*, 137, 106, 1966.
14. Porter, K. A., Rejection in treated renal allografts, *J. Clin. Pathol.*, 20 (Suppl), 518, 1967.
15. Porter, K. A., Dossetor, J. B., Marchioro, T. L., Peart, W. S., Rendall, J. M., Starzl, T. E., and Terasaki, P. I., Human renal transplants, *Lab. Invest.*, 16, 153, 1967.

16. Kincaid-Smith, P., The pathogenesis of the vascular and glomerular lesions of rejection in renal allografts and their modification by antithrombotic and anticoagulant drugs, *Aust. Ann. Med.,* 19, 201, 1970.

17. Smith, N., Chandler, S., Hawker, R. J., Hawker, L. M., and Barnes, A. D., Indium-labelled autologous platelets as diagnostic aid after renal transplantation, *Lancet,* 2, 1241, 1979.

18. Foegh, M. L., Winchester, J. F., Zmudka, M., Helfrich, G. B., Cooley, C., Ramwell, P. W., and Schreiner, G. E., Urine i-TXB$_2$ in renal allograft rejection, *Lancet,* 2, 431, 1981.

19. Foegh, M. L., Goldman, M. H., Barnhart, G. R., Lower, A. A., Szentpietery, S., and Ramwell, P. W., Urine immunoreactive thromboxane B$_2$ in human heart transplant rejection, *Abstr. 5th Int. Conf. Prostaglandins,* 1982, 634.

20. Capitanio, A., Ponticelli, C., D'Angelo, A., and Mannucci, P. M., Platelet abnormalities in renal transplantation, *Proc. EDTA,* 18, 375, 1981.

21. Nachman, R. L. and Weksler, B., The platelet as an inflammatory cell, *Ann. N. Y. Acad. Sci.,* 201, 131, 1972.

22. Batchelor, J. R., The riddle of kidney graft enhancement, *Transplantation,* 26, 139, 1978.

23. Hansson, L. O., The influence of thrombocyte aggregation on renal circulation. An experimental study in the cat, *Acta Chir. Scand. Suppl.* 345, 1965.

24. Leithner, C., Sinzinger, H., Angelberger, P., and Syre, G., Indium-111 labelled platelets in chronic kidney transplant rejection, *Lancet,* 2, 213, 1980.

25. Goodwin, J. S. and Webb, D. R., Regulation of the immune response by prostaglandins, *Clin. Immunol. Immunopathol.,* 15, 106, 1980.

26. Pelus, L. M. and Strausser, H. R., Prostaglandins and the immune response, *Life Sci.,* 20, 903, 1977.

27. Webb, D. R. and Osheroff, P. L., Antigen stimulation of prostaglandin synthesis and control of immune responses, *Proc. Natl. Acad. Sci. U.S.A.,* 73, 1300, 1976.

28. Stenson, W. F. and Parker, C. W., Prostaglandins, macrophages, and immunity, *J. Immunol.,* 125, 1, 1980.

29. Bourne, H. R., Lichtenstein, L. M., Melmon, K. L., Henney, C. S., Weinstein, Y., and Shearer, G. M., Modulation of inflammation and immunity by cyclic AMP, *Science,* 184, 19, 1974.

30. Humes, J. L., Bonney, R. J., Pelus, L., Dahlgren, M. E., Sadowski, S. J., Kuehl, F. A., and Davies, P., Macrophages synthesise and release prostaglandins in response to inflammatory stimuli, *Nature (London),* 269, 149, 1977.

31. Ceuppens, J. L. and Goodwin, J. S., Endogenous prostaglandin E$_2$ enhances polyclonal immunoglobulin production by tonically inhibiting T suppressor cell activity, *Cell. Immunol.,* 70, 41, 1982.

32. Moncada, S., Gryglewski, R., Bunting, S., and Vane, J. R., An enzyme isolated from arteries transforms prostaglandin endoperoxides to an unstable substance that inhibits platelet aggregation, *Nature (London),* 263, 663, 1976.

33. Hughes, R., Theis, G., and Wong, P. Y. K., Oxygenation of arachidonic acid ([^{14}C]-AA) by lipoxygenase in rat and mouse spleen lymphocytes, *Abstr. 5th Int. Conf. Prostaglandins,* 1982, 616.

34. Moore, T. C. and Jaffe, B. M., Prostaglandin E levels of heterotopic rat heart allografts and host lymphoid tissues at intervals post-grafting, *Transplantation,* 18, 383, 1974.

35. Jaffe, B. M. and Moore, T. C., Elevation in prostaglandin-E activity of rat heart allograft coronary sinus venous blood, *IRCS Med. Sci.,* 2, 1417, 1974.

36. Anderson, C. B., Newton, W. T., and Jaffe, B. M., Circulating prostaglandin E and allograft rejection, *Transplantation,* 19, 526, 1975.

37. Mertin, J. and Hughes, D., Specific inhibitory action of polyunsaturated fatty acids on lymphocyte transformation induced by PHA and PPD, *Int. Arch. Allergy Appl. Immunol.,* 48, 203, 1975.

38. Mertin, J. and Stackpoole, A., Prostaglandin precursors and the cell-mediated immune response, *Cell. Immunol.,* 62, 293, 1981.

39. Goodwin, J. S., Bankhurst, A. D., and Messner, R. P., Suppression of human T-cell mitogenesis by prostaglandin, *J. Exp. Med.,* 146, 1719, 1977.

40. Kelley, V. E., Winkelstein, A., Izui, S., and Dixon, F. J., Prostaglandin E$_1$ inhibits T-cell proliferation and renal disease in MRL/1 mice, *Clin. Immunol. Immunopathol.,* 21, 190, 1981.

41. Teti, D. V., Misefari, A., and Teti, G., Effect of cytochalasin A on E rosette formation and inhibition by prostaglandin E$_2$, *IRCS Med. Sci.,* 10, 517, 1982.

42. Smith, J. W., Steiner, A. L., and Parker, C. W., Human lymphocyte metabolism. Effects of cyclic and non-cyclic nucleotides on stimulation by phytohemagglutinin, *J. Clin. Invest.,* 50, 442, 1971.

43. Baker, P. E., Fahey, J. V., and Munck, A., Prostaglandin inhibition of T-cell proliferation is mediated at two levels, *Cell. Immunol.,* 61, 52, 1981.

44. Gordon, D., Bray, M. A., and Morely, J., Control of lymphokine secretion by prostaglandins, *Nature (London),* 262, 401, 1976.

45. Rappaport, R. S. and Dodge, G. R., Prostaglandin E inhibits the production of human interleukin 2, *J. Exp. Med.,* 155, 943, 1982.

46. Koopman, W. J., Gillis, M. H., and David, J. R., Prevention of MIF activity by agents known to increase cellular cyclic AMP, *J. Immunol.*, 110, 1609, 1973.

47. Schultz, R. M., Pavlidis, N. A., Stylos, W. A., and Chirigos, M. A., Regulation of macrophage tumoricidal function: a role for prostaglandins of the E series, *Science,* 202, 320, 1978.

48. Humes, J. L., Bonney, R. J., Pelus, L., Dahlgren, M. E., Sadowski, S. J., Kuehl, F. A., and Davies, P., Macrophages synthesise and release prostaglandins in response to inflammatory stimuli, *Nature (London)* 269, 149, 1977.

49. Darrow, T. L. and Tomar, R. H., Prostaglandin-mediated regulation of the mixed lymphocyte culture and generation of cytotoxic cells, *Cell. Immunol.,* 56, 172, 1980.

50. Webb, D. R. and Nowowiejski, I., Mitogen-induced changes in lymphocyte prostaglandin levels: a signal for the induction of suppressor cell activity, *Cell. Immunol.,* 41, 72, 1978.

51. Webb, D. R. and Nowowiejski, I., Control of suppressor cell activation via endogenous prostaglandin synthesis; the role of T cells and macrophages, *Cell. Immunol.,* 63, 321, 1981.

52. Fischer, A., Durandy, A., and Griscelli, C., Role of prostaglandin E_2 in the induction of non-specific T lymphocyte suppressor activity, *J. Immunol.,* 126, 1452, 1981.

53. Fulton, A. M. and Levy, J. G., The induction of non-specific T suppressor lymphocytes by prostaglandin E_1, *Cell. Immunol.,* 59, 54, 1981.

54. Gualde, N. and Goodwin, J. S., Effects of prostaglandin E_2 and preincubation on lectin-stimulated proliferation of human T cell subsets, *Cell. Immunol.,* 70, 373, 1982.

55. Rogers, T. J., Campbell, L., Calhoun, K., Nowowiejski, I., and Webb, D. R., Suppression of B-cell and T-cell responses by the prostaglandin-induced T-cell-derived suppressor (PITS), *Cell. Immunol.,* 66, 269, 1982.

56. Zurier, R. B. and Quagliata, F., Effect of prostaglandin E_1 on adjuvant arthritis, *Nature (London),* 234, 304, 1971.

57. Kunkel, S. L., Ogawa, H., Conran, P. B., Ward, P. A., and Zurier, R. B., Suppression of acute and chronic inflammation by orally administered prostaglandins, *Arthritis Rheum.,* 24, 1151, 1981.

58. Henney, C. S., Bourne, H. R., and Lichtenstein, L. M., The role of cyclic 3′, 5′ adenosine monophosphate in the specific cytolytic activity of lymphocytes, *J. Immunol.,* 108, 1526, 1972.

59. Melmon, K. L., Bourne, H. R., Weinstein, Y., Shearer, G. M., Kram, J., and Bauminger, S., Hemolytic plaque formation by leukocytes in vitro, *J. Clin. Invest.,* 53, 13, 1973.

60. Braun, W. and Ishizuka, M., Antibody formation: reduced responses after administration of excessive amounts of non-specific stimulation, *Proc. Natl. Acad. Sci. U.S.A.,* 68, 1114, 1971.

61. Leung, K. H. and Mihich, E., Prostaglandin modulation of development of cell-mediated immunity in culture, *Nature (London),* 288, 597, 1980.

62. Mertin, J. and Stackpoole, A., Anti-PGE antibodies inhibit *in vivo* development of cell-mediated immunity, *Nature (London),* 294, 456, 1981.

63. Zurier, R. B., Dore-Duffy, P., and Viola, M. V., Adherence of human peripheral blood lymphocytes to measles-infected cells, *N. Engl. J. Med.,* 296, 1443, 1977.

64. Parnham, M. J., Schoester, G. A P., and Van der Kwast, T. H., Enhancement by prostaglandin E_1 and essential fatty acid deficiency of the passive transfer of delayed hypersensitivity to PPD in rats, *Int. J. Immunopharmacol.,* 1, 119, 1979.

65. Ceuppens, J. L. and Goodwin, J. S., Endogenous prostaglandin E_2 enhances polyclonal immunoglobulin production by toxically inhibiting T suppressor cell activity, *Cell. Immunol.,* 70, 41, 1982.

66. Favalli, C., Mastino, A., Jezzi, T., Rinaldi, C., Garaci, E., and Jaffe, B. M., Influence of PGE on immune response in normal and immunosuppressed mice, *Abstr. 5th Int. Conf. Prostaglandins,* 1982, 638.

67. Blackwell, G. J., Carnuccio, R., Di Rosa, M., Flower, R. J., Parente, L., and Persico, P., Macrocortin: a polypeptide causing the anti-phospholipase effect of glucocorticoids, *Nature (London),* 287, 147, 1980.

68. Hirata, F., Schiffmann, E., Venkatasubramanian, K., Salomon, D., and Axelrod, J., A phospholipase A_2 inhibitory protein in rabbit neutrophils induced by glucocorticoids, *Proc. Natl. Acad. Sci. U.S.A.,* 77, 2533, 1980.

69. Mundy, A. R., Bewick, M., Moncada, S., and Vane, J. R., Experimental assessment of prostacyclin in the harvesting of kidneys for transplantation, *Transplantation,* 30, 251, 1980.

70. Bradley, J. W., Cho, S. I., Murray, J. C., Baker, K., Bush, H. L. and Nabseth, D. C., The use of prostacyclin for pretreatment of kidney donors, *Abstr. 9th Int. Congr. Transplant. Soc.,* 1982, F17.6.

71. Casey, K. F., Machiedo, G. W., Lyons, M. J., Slotman, G. J., and Novak, R. T., Alteration of postischemic renal pathology by prostaglandin infusion, *J. Surg. Res.,* 29, 1 1980.

72. Monden, M. and Fortner, J. G., Twenty-four and 48-hour canine liver preservation by simple hypothermia with prostacyclin, *Ann. Surg.,* 196, 38, 1982.

73. Kakita, A., Blanchard, J., and Fortner, J. G., Effectiveness of prostaglandin E_1 and procarbazine hydrochloride in prolonging the survival of vascularized cardiac hamster-to-rat xenograft, *Transplantation,* 20, 439, 1975.

74. Mundy, A. R., Bewick, M., Moncada, S., and Vane, J. R., Short term suppression of hyperacute renal allograft rejection in presensitized dogs with prostacyclin, *Prostaglandins,* 19, 595, 1980.

75. Mundy, A. R., Prolongation of cat to dog renal xenograft survival with prostacyclin, *Transplantation,* 30, 226, 1980.

76. MacDonald, A. S., Bell, W. R., Busch, G. J., Ghose, T., Chan, C. C., Falvey, C. F., and Merrill, J. P., A comparison of hyperacute canine renal allograft and sheep-to-dog xenograft rejection, *Transplantation,* 13, 146, 1972.

77. Pausescu, E., Laky, D., and Popescu, M. V., In vivo and in vitro morphological studies on the myocardial protection induced by PGE_2 and PGF_2 against the immune aggression, *Eur. Surg. Res.,* 13, 1 1981.

78. Quagliata, F., Lawrence, V. J. W., and Phillips-Quagliata, J. M., Prostaglandin E_1 as a regulator of lymphocyte function, *Cell. Immunol.,* 6, 457, 1973.

79. Strom, T. B., Carpenter, C. B., Cragoe, E. J., Norris, S., Devlin, R., and Perper, R. J., Suppression of in vivo and in vitro alloimmunity by prostaglandins, *Transplant. Proc.,* 9, 1075, 1977.

80. Sinzinger, H., Leithner, C., and Schwarz, M., Monitoring of human kidney transplants using quantification of autologous 111 Indium-oxine platelet label deposition-beneficial effect of PGI_2 treatment in acute and chronic rejection, *Thromb. Haemost.,* 46, 263, 1981.

81. Leithner, C., Sinzinger, H., Pohanka, E., and Schwarz, M., Treatment of acute and chronic kidney transplant rejection with prostacyclin, *Abstr. 5th Int. Conf. Prostaglandins,* 1982, 636.

82. Shaw, J. F. L., Prolongation of rat cardiac allograft survival by treatment with prostacyclin or aspirin during acute rejection, *Transplantation,* in press.

83. Sinzinger, H., Silberbauer, K., Horsch, A. K., and Gall, A., Decreased sensitivity of human platelets to PGI_2 during long-term intraarterial prostacyclin infusion in patients with peripheral vascular disease, *Prostaglandins,* 21, 49, 1981.

84. Santiago-Delpin, E. A. and Szepsenwol, J., Prolonged survival of skin and tumor allografts in mice on high-fat diets, *J. Natl. Cancer Inst.,* 59, 459, 1977.

85. McHugh, M. I., Wilkinson, R., Elliott, R. W., Field, E. J., Dewar, P., Hall, R. R., Taylor, R. M. R., and Uldall, P. R., Immunosuppression with polyunsaturated fatty acids in renal transplantation, *Transplantation,* 24, 263, 1977.

86. Moore, P. K. and Hoult, J. R. S., Anti-inflammatory steroids reduce tissue PG synthetase activity and enhance PG breakdown, *Nature (London),* 288, 269, 1980.

87. Belldegrun, A., Cohen, I. R., Frenkel, A., Serviado, C., and Zor, U., Hydrocortisone and inhibitors of prostaglandin synthesis, *Transplantation,* 31, 407, 1981.

88. Jamieson, S. W., Burton, N. A., Reitz, B. A., and Stinson, E. B., Survival of heart allografts in rats treated with azathioprine and sodium salicylate, *Lancet,* 1, 130, 1979.

89. Shaw, J. F. L., Combined effects of Cyclosporin A and sodium salicylate upon survival of rat heart allografts, *IRCS Med. Sci.,* 10, 827, 1982.

90. Shehadeh, I. H., Guttmann, R. D., Lindquist, R. R., and Rodriguez-Erdmann, F., Renal transplantation in the inbred rat, *Transplantation,* 10, 75, 1970.

91. George, C. R. P., Slichter, S. J., Quadracci, L. J., Kenny, G. M., Dennis, M. B., Striker, G. E., and Harker, L. A., The treatment of rejection, *Transplantation,* 20, 237, 1975.

92. Kauffman, H. M., Adams, M. B., Hebert, L. A., and Walczak, P. M., Platelet inhibitors in human renal homotransplantation: randomized comparison of aspirin versus dipyridamole, *Transplant. Proc.,* 12, 311, 1980.

93. Laden, A. M. K., The effects of treatment on the arterial lesions of rat and rabbit cardiac allografts, *Transplantation,* 13, 281, 1972.

94. Jamieson, S. W., Premethazine-HCL (Phenergan) in the treatment of rat cardiac allografts, *Transplantation,* 21, 69, 1976.

95. Burrows, L., Haimov, M., Aledort, L., Leiter, E., Nirmul, G., Shanzer, H., Taut, R., and Glabman, S., The platelet in the obliterative vascular rejection phenomenon, *Transplant. Proc.,* 5, 157, 1973.

96. Jessing, P., Agger, B., and Pedersen, F. B., Periactin (cyproheptadine hydrochloride) as a supplement to the immunosuppressive treatment in human cadaver kidney transplantation, *Scand. J. Urol. Nephrol.,* 10, 147, 1976.

97. Kostakis, A. J., Karayannacos, P. E., Pattakos, S., Nakopoulou, L., Karatzas, G., and Kouletianos, E., Prolongation of cardiac and renal allograft survival by pentoxifylline in rats, *IRCS Med. Sci.,* 10, 77, 1982.

98. McMillan, R., Heparin in delayed transplant function, *Lancet,* 1, 1178, 1968.

99. Griffin, P. J. A. and Salaman, J. R., A controlled trial of heparin in renal transplant rejection, *Transplantation,* 32, 306, 1981.

100. Kincaid-Smith, P., Modification of the vascular lesions of rejection in cadaveric renal allografts by dipyridamole and anticoagulants, *Lancet,* 2, 920, 1969.

101. Kincaid-Smith, P., The pathogenesis of the vascular and glomerular lesions of rejection in renal allografts and their modification by antithrombotic and anticoagulant drugs, *Aust. Ann. Med.,* 19, 201, 1970.
102. Mathew, T. H., Kincaid-Smith, P., Clyne, D. H., Saker, B. M., Nanra, R. S., Morris, P. J., and Marshall, V. C., A controlled trial of oral anticoagulants and dipyridamole in cadaveric renal allografts, *Lancet,* 2, 1307, 1974.
103. Barnes, A. D., Coles, G. A., and White, H. J. O., A controlled tiral of anticoagulants in cadaveric renal transplantation, *Transplantation,* 17, 491, 1974.
104. Soper, W. D., Pollak, R., Manaligod, J. R., Hau, T., Mozes, M. F., and Jonasson, O., Use of anticoagulation in cadaver renal transplants, *J. Surg. Res.,* 32, 370, 1982.
105. Leithner, C., Sinzinger, H., and Schwarz, M., Treatment of chronic kidney transplant rejection with prostacyclin, *Prostaglandins,* 22, 783, 1981.

Hemostasis and Thrombosis and Other Sites of Action

Chapter 11

PLASMA LIPOPROTEINS AND PROSTAGLANDIN BIOSYNTHESIS

Lloyd N. Fleisher, Alan R. Tall, Larry D. Witte, and Paul J. Cannon

TABLE OF CONTENTS

I. INTRODUCTION

Until quite recently there was little that could be said about interrelationships between plasma lipoproteins and prostaglandin (PG) biosynthesis. Today, a convincing body of evidence exists indicating that PG production is influenced by plasma lipoproteins (i.e., low density lipoproteins or LDL and high density lipoproteins or HDL). Furthermore, interactions between plasma lipoproteins and PGs may have important implications for our concepts of hemostasis and the atherosclerotic process. Particular interest has centered upon the effect of LDL and HDL on the synthesis of prostacyclin (PGI$_2$) by the vascular endothelium. PGI$_2$ is the predominant PG synthesized by the vascular endothelium[1-4] and produces vasodilation and especially potent inhibition of platelet aggregation.[1,5] In contrast thromboxane A$_2$ (TXA$_2$), which is synthesized by platelets, exhibits actions opposite to PGI$_2$, producing vasoconstriction and increased platelet aggregation.[1,2] The opposing actions of these two prostanoids has led to the proposal by Moncada and Vane[1,2] that a proper balance between PGI$_2$ and TXA$_2$ production is important for the maintenance of vascular integrity.

PGs are not stored in cells, but are found in precursor forms as polyunsaturated fatty acids esterified to membrane phospholipids. These fatty acids include dihomo-γ-linolenic acid (C20:3ω6), arachidonic acid (C20:4ω6), and eicosapentaenoic acid (C20:5ω3), the precursors of the 1, 2, and 3 series of PGs, respectively.[1,5-7] In response to a variety of mechanical and hormonal stimuli arachidonic acid can be hydrolyzed off the phospholipids, enter the "arachidonic acid cascade", and give rise to PGs of the 2 series. In most cells (including endothelial cells) phospholipase A$_2$ is thought to initiate the cascade by catalyzing the hydrolysis of arachidonic acid from the 2 position of phosphatidylcholine.[8-11] In platelets, arachidonic acid arises by a different mechanism. Through the sequential actions of phospholipase C, a diglyceride lipase and a monoglyceride lipase, arachidonic acid is released from the second glyceryl carbon of phosphatidylinositol.[12-15] Regardless of the tissue of origin, arachidonic acid is rapidly converted to the PG endoperoxide, PGG$_2$, by the enzyme cyclooxygenase.[16] PGG$_2$ is converted to PGH$_2$ which isomerizes enzymatically or nonenzymatically to PGE$_2$, PGD$_2$, and PGF$_{2\alpha}$, and also to PGI$_2$ and TXA$_2$ through the actions of PGI$_2$ synthetase and TX synthetase, respectively (Figure 1). Both PGI$_2$ and TXA$_2$ are highly unstable at physiologic pH and rapidly convert to 6-keto-PGF$_{1\alpha}$ and TXB$_2$. Arachidonic acid can also be peroxidized by various lipoxygenases to unstable hydroperoxides. The hydroperoxides rapidly break down into hydroxy acids and can be further metabolized to the leukotrienes.[5,17] The leukotrienes are important chemotactic agents and mediators of inflammation.

Arachidonic acid can be obtained in the diet or can be synthesized from the essential fatty acid, linoleic acid (C18:2ω6). The biosynthesis involves desaturation to γ-linolenic acid, chain elongation to dihomo-γ-linolenic acid and another desaturation to arachidonic acid (Figure 2). The levels of free arachidonic acid circulating in the plasma are very low; most of the plasma arachidonic acid is found in the lipoproteins as esters of phospholipids, cholesterol, and triglycerides. Thus, vascular endothelium is exposed to a milieu low in free arachidonic acid but rich in arachidonate esters. This situation is especially interesting in light of the observation by Spector et al.[18] that human umbilical vein endothelial cells grown in tissue culture were unable to convert linoleic acid to arachidonic acid. This was due to a deficiency of Δ^6-desaturase, the enzyme that catalyzes the first step in the 3-step process from linoleic to arachidonic acid. This raises the possibility that endothelial cells may require an exogenous source of arachidonic acid in order to maintain adequate intracellular stores of this compound. In the following sections evidence will be presented from our laboratory and others supporting the hypothesis that HDL may provide a source of extracellular ar-

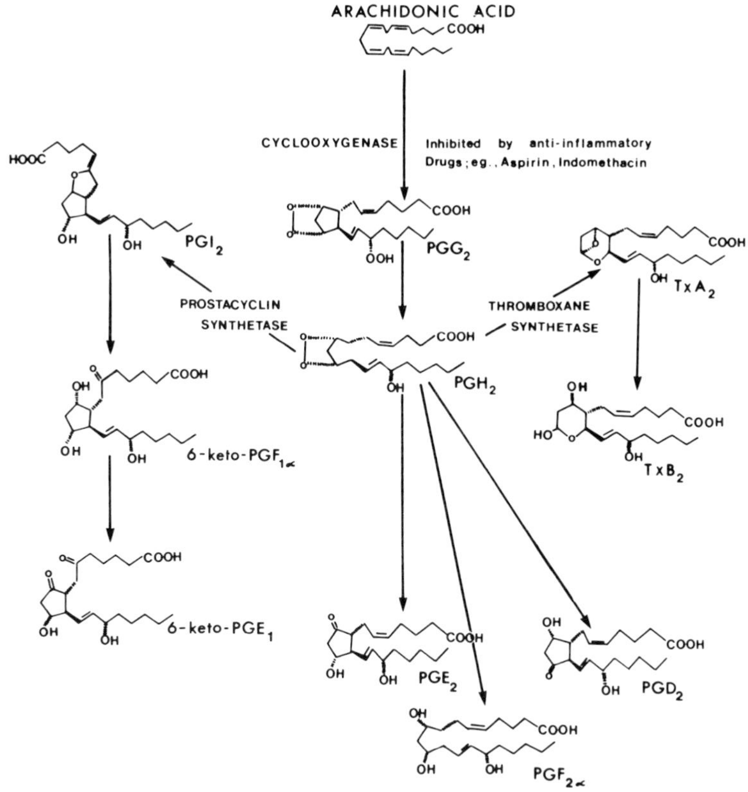

ARACHIDONIC ACID

CYCLOOXYGENASE | Inhibited by anti-inflammatory Drugs;eg., Aspirin, Indomethacin

HOOC

PGI$_2$

PROSTACYCLIN SYNTHETASE

PGG$_2$

THROMBOXANE SYNTHETASE

TxA$_2$

6-keto-PGF$_{1\alpha}$

PGH$_2$

TxB$_2$

6-keto-PGE$_1$

PGE$_2$

PGD$_2$

PGF$_{2\alpha}$

FIGURE 1.   Biosynthesis of PGs and TXs.

achidonic acid for endothelial cells and increase the utilization of intracellular stores. Before doing this a discussion of the properties of the plasma lipoproteins is in order.

II. STRUCTURE AND PROPERTIES OF PLASMA LIPOPROTEINS

The plasma lipoproteins represent nature's solution to the problem of the immiscibility of oil and water. By encapsulating an apolar core of cholesteryl esters and triglycerides within a stabilizing monolayer of hydrophilic apoproteins and polar lipids (phospholipids and unesterified cholesterol),[19-21] the highly water-insoluble cholesteryl esters and triglycerides can be transported through the aqueous environment of the plasma, hydrolyzed to free cholesterol and fatty acids, and utilized by cells for a variety of functions. Normal human plasma contains five general types of lipoproteins: the chylomicrons, very low density lipoprotein, intermediate density lipoprotein, low density lipoprotein, and high density lipoprotein, which can be differentiated on the basis of particle size, composition, and density (Table 1). The largest and least dense are the chylomicrons (d. <0.95), which are formed in the intestinal wall following the ingestion of dietary lipids and enter the circulation via the thoracic duct. Chylomicrons are rich in triglycerides, the fatty acids of which are delivered to tissues that either store or oxidatively metabolize fatty acids, such as adipose tissue and muscle. This is accomplished by the action of lipoprotein lipase, an enzyme bound to the luminal surface of endothelial cells in the capillaries of these tissues. The resulting triglyceride-depleted chylomicrons (chylomicron remnants) are then rapidly removed from the circulation by the liver.[22-26] The very low density lipoproteins (VLDL; d. 0.95 to 1.006) are another group of triglyceride-rich particles. They are synthesized primarily in the liver and

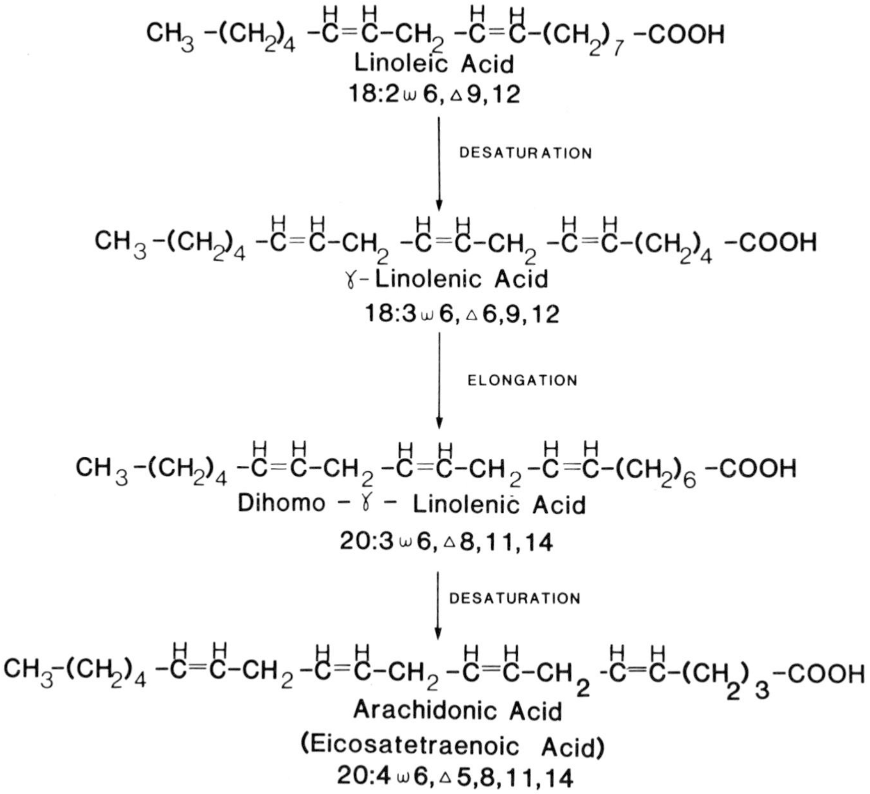

$$CH_3-(CH_2)_4-\overset{H}{C}=\overset{H}{C}-CH_2-\overset{H}{C}=\overset{H}{C}-(CH_2)_7-COOH$$

Linoleic Acid

18:2 ω6, Δ9,12

↓ DESATURATION

$$CH_3-(CH_2)_4-\overset{H}{C}=\overset{H}{C}-CH_2-\overset{H}{C}=\overset{H}{C}-CH_2-\overset{H}{C}=\overset{H}{C}-(CH_2)_4-COOH$$

γ-Linolenic Acid

18:3 ω6, Δ6,9,12

↓ ELONGATION

$$CH_3-(CH_2)_4-\overset{H}{C}=\overset{H}{C}-CH_2-\overset{H}{C}=\overset{H}{C}-CH_2-\overset{H}{C}=\overset{H}{C}-(CH_2)_6-COOH$$

Dihomo – γ – Linolenic Acid

20:3 ω6, Δ8,11,14

↓ DESATURATION

$$CH_3-(CH_2)_4-\overset{H}{C}=\overset{H}{C}-CH_2-\overset{H}{C}=\overset{H}{C}-CH_2-\overset{H}{C}=\overset{H}{C}-CH_2-\overset{H}{C}=\overset{H}{C}-(CH_2)_3-COOH$$

Arachidonic Acid

(Eicosatetraenoic Acid)

20:4 ω6, Δ5,8,11,14

FIGURE 2.   Biosynthesis of arachidonic acid from linoleic acid.

transport cholesterol and fatty acids to extrahepatic tissues. The triglycerides are handled similarly to those in the chylomicrons through the action of lipoprotein lipase. As a result of the attrition of the triglyceride core the density increases and VLDL is gradually transformed first into intermediate density lipoprotein (IDL; d. 1.006 to 1.019) and then into LDL (d. 1.019 to 1.063). In addition to the hydrolysis of the triglyceride core the cholesteryl ester content also increases, presumably through the action of the plasma enzyme lecithin, cholesterol acyltransferase (LCAT), which esterifies cholesterol by transferring a fatty acid from the 2-position of lecithin (phosphatidylcholine) to cholesterol.[27] It is LDL that actually delivers cholesterol to extrahepatic tissues through a receptor-mediated endocytosis of the LDL particle.[19-28] The LDL is incorporated into lysosomes where the protein and cholesteryl esters are hydrolyzed, thus making free cholesterol available to the cell. The cholesterol released from the lysosomes regulates the number of LDL receptors and the activity of 3-hydroxy-3-methylglutaryl CoA reductase, a key enzyme in the *de novo* synthesis of cholesterol. The free cholesterol either is utilized by the cell, leaves the cell, or is esterified by cytoplasmic acyl CoA, cholesterol acyltransferase.

The HDL are a heterogeneous group of lipoprotein particles (d. 1.063 to 1.21) in terms of composition, synthesis, and disposition. They occupy a pivotal role in the regulation of apoprotein metabolism, triglyceride catabolism, and cholesteryl ester synthesis. Although there is not complete agreement on exactly how HDL are formed, one widely accepted scheme describes a maturation process whereby disc-shaped particles consisting of phospholipid, some free cholesterol, and apoprotein (nascent HDL) are secreted by the liver[29,30] and intestine[31] and gradually tansformed into less dense HDL₃ and HDL₂. Discoidal HDL may be converted into the mature spherical form of the lipoprotein as a result of the LCAT reaction.[32] It appears that free cholesterol, phospholipids, and apoproteins are transferred from triglyceride-rich lipoproteins to HDL during lipoprotein lipase-catalyzed lipolysis.[32-34] The enrichment of the HDL core with cholesteryl esters is a consequence of LCAT-catalyzed transfer of an unsaturated fatty acid from the 2-position of lecithin to cholesterol located on the surface of the HDL particle.[27] The hydrophobic cholesteryl ester is subsequently internalized in the lipoidal core allowing for the insertion of another free cholesterol molecule on the HDL surface. The free cholesterol is probably dervied from other lipoproteins and from cellular membranes.[35-38] Recent evidence suggests that HDL cholesteryl esters are not simply delivered to the liver, but undergo bidirectional transfer with other lipoproteins, such as VLDL and LDL.[39] This process, mediated by cholesteryl ester transfer protein,[40,41] provides a mechanism whereby cholesteryl esters can be equilibrated among HDL, LDL, and VLDL.

The ability of HDL to accept free cholesterol from cells is of particular interest since it may be related to the protective role played by HDL in coronary heart disease.[42] The inverse relationship between HDL-cholesterol concentration and the incidence of coronary heart disease has been amply demonstrated in a number of studies.[43-47] Since extrahepatic tissues (with the exceptions of the adrenal and the gonads) are unable to catabolize cholesterol, the assumption has been that by facilitating the exit of cholesterol from these tissues HDL tends to reduce cholesteryl ester accumulation, and in consequence the atherosclerotic process. Indeed, HDL has been shown to facilitate the removal of cholesterol from cultured fibroblasts and vascular smooth muscle cells,[36,48] and from atherosclerotic tissue in vitro.[49] The mechanism by which HDL accomplishes cellular cholesterol efflux is poorly understood although it is thought to involve the LCAT reaction. HDL can also combine with cholesterol resulting in the formation of soluble macromolecular complexes called liposomes. These liposomes could play a role in vivo in the removal of cholesterol deposits.[50,51] In the remaining portion of this chapter evidence will be presented supporting the hypothesis that HDL and LDL alter the synthesis of PGI_2 and that the effects of this alteration on platelet function and vascular dynamics may have important consequences upon the atherosclerotic process.

III. LDL, HDL, AND THE VASCULAR ENDOTHELIUM

In many regards, LDL and HDL exert opposing actions. Elevated plasma HDL-cholesterol is associated with decreased coronary risk; however, elevated plasma LDL-cholesterol is associated with increased risk of atherosclerosis and ischemic heart disease.[44-47,52,53] Perhaps the most striking demonstration of this is seen in patients with familial hypercholesterolemia. Homozygous individuals exhibit LDL-cholesterol levels 4 to 6 times above normal and severe heart disease is common before the age of 20. Heterozygotes are less severely affected; LDL-cholesterol is elevated 2- to 3-fold above normal and severe heart disease is usually delayed until 40 or 50 years of age.[19] Furthermore, in terms of cholesterol utilization by extrahepatic tissues, LDL supplies cholesterol whereas HDL is thought to facilitate its removal. Similar types of relationships are seen between lipoproteins, vascular endothelium, and platelets. Lipid peroxides have been shown to inhibit G-PGI_2 synthetase,[54-56] block the anti-aggregatory activity of the vascular endothelium,[57] and accumulate in atherosclerotic lesions[58] and in the LDL (but not the HDL) of hypercholesterolemic patients.[59,60] This accumulation of lipid peroxides may explain why PGI_2 synthesis is reduced in atherosclerotic blood vessels from humans and experimental animals[61-64] and in cultured smooth muscle cells from hypercholesterolemic animals with early atherosclerotic lesions.[65] Lipid peroxide accumulation may also be related to age-related decreases in PGI_2 synthesis observed in porcine arteries[66] and in cultured smooth muscle cells from aortae of old rats.[67]

Table 1

HUMAN PLASMA LIPOPROTEINS

Property	Chylomicrons	Very low density	Intermediate density	Low density	High density
Density (g/mℓ)	<0.95	0.95—1.006	1.006—1.019	1.019—1.063	1.063—1.210
Flotation range (Sf)	>400	60—400	12—60	0—12	
Diameter (nm)	100—500	30—100	25—30	20—25	10—15
Origin	Intestine	Liver	VLDL catabolism	IDL catabolism	Liver, intestine
Lipid composition	Mainly triglyceride	Triglyceride, some phospholipid, cholesterol	Triglyceride, cholesterol, some phospholipid	Mainly cholesterol, some phospholipid	Phospholipid, cholesterol
Apoproteins	A, B, C	B, C, E	B, C, E	B	A, C, E
					Small amounts of D, F

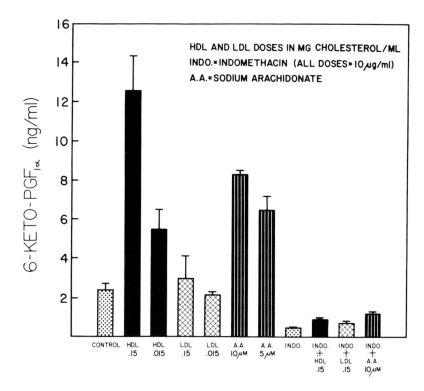

FIGURE 3.   Effect of HDL, LDL, and sodium arachidonate on PGI_2 biosynthesis by subconfluent porcine aortic endothelial cells.

Similarly, decreases in PGI_2 synthesis (and increases in PGE_2 synthesis) reported for repeatedly subcultured bovine smooth muscle and endothelial cells,[68] may be secondary to extensive lipid peroxidation. The ability of HDL to prevent some of these deleterious actions of LDL has been demonstrated in a number of studies. Henriksen et al.[69] have shown that LDL damaged human endothelial cells grown in culture and this process could be retarded by HDL. Tauber et al.[70] found LDL to be cytotoxic, but HDL to be mitogenic for low density vascular endothelial cell cultures. Nordoy et al.[71] demonstrated that the ability of human endothelial cell monolayers, grown in culture, to inhibit ADP- or collagen-induced platelet aggregation was inhibited by LDL. HDL had no such effect and offered some protection from the LDL effect. Whole plasma had a similar protective effect. Beitz and Forster[72] found that the capacity to convert PGH_2 to PGI_2 by porcine microsomes was negatively correlated with LDL-cholesterol, but positively correlated with HDL-cholesterol in the incubation medium. Szczeklik et al.[73] showed that LDL inhibited PGI_2 synthesis by rat aortic slices and ascribed this to the accumulation of lipid peroxides occurring during fractionation and dialysis of the lipoproteins. However, LDL obtained from 25% of their patients was relatively peroxide-free, yet still inhibited PGI_2 synthesis by more than 50%. Fleisher et al.[74,75] have studied the effects of LDL, HDL, and delipidated HDL on the synthesis of PGI_2 by porcine aortic endothelium grown in tissue culture. Human HDL produced a dose-dependent increase in PGI_2 synthesis (as measured by radioimmunoassay of the stable metabolite, 6-keto-PGF_{1a}), which was continuous over a 24 hr period of incubation and could be blocked by indomethacin. In contrast, human LDL had no significant effect on PGI_2 synthesis (Figure 3). The stimulation of PGI_2 synthesis by HDL did not appear to involve interaction with the specific LDL receptor-mediated uptake system (for which an apo-E-rich subspecies of HDL has very high affinity[76,77]), since co-incubation of the cells with HDL and varying concentrations of LDL did not alter the degree of HDL-induced stimulation. The mechanism by which HDL stimulates endothelial cell PGI_2 synthesis remains to be elucidated, but two additional observations may supply significant clues. HDL that had been delipidated by ethanol/ether extraction still retained some capacity to stimulate endothelial cell PGI_2 synthesis, and intact rat HDL produced four times more stimulation of PGI_2 synthesis than intact human HDL at equal protein concentrations. Rat HDL is known to contain a higher content of arachidonic acid in its cholesteryl esters than human HDL,[29] thus raising the possibility that HDL may supply endothelial cells with substrate for PGI_2 synthesis. This is a tempting speculation in light of the deficient capacity of endothelial cells to convert linoleic acid to arachidonic acid.[18] Rat HDL also differs from human HDL in its apoprotein composition with more apo-E and apo-A-IV, but less apo-A-II.[78] When rat HDL was depleted of its apo-E fraction by heparin-Sepharose® chromatography,[79] no change was observed in its capacity to stimulate endothelial cell PGI_2 synthesis.[80] Furthermore, when rat apo-HDL was compared to human apo-HDL at equal protein concentrations, the capacity of each to stimulate endothelial cell PGI_2 synthesis was essentially equal.[75] These results suggest that the greater stimulation produced by rat HDL is not due to differences in apoprotein composition, but is a consequence of the higher content of arachidonic acid in its cholesteryl esters. The precise mechanism may be complex, involving both the apoprotein and lipid moieties. The fact that HDL, but not LDL, stimulated PGI_2 synthesis suggests that the specificity resides in the apoprotein moeity since these lipoproteins do not differ greatly in fatty acid composition. One possiblity is that HDL could interact with the cell through apo-A-I-specific binding sites (apo-A-I is present in rat and human HDL, but absent in LDL) with eventual transfer of HDL lipids to the cell.

IV. HDL RECEPTORS

A variety of HDL receptors, separate from the LDL receptor, have been described and could provide a mechanism by which HDL lipid becomes accessible to the cell. In the rat, HDL receptors are found in the adrenal, testes, and ovary and appear to be part of a system by which HDL cholesterol can be used for the synthesis of steroid hormones.[81-84] The receptors on rat adrenal cells are specific, saturable, and ACTH-dependent. Furthermore, the utilization of the HDL cholesterol did not appear to require endocytosis and lysosomal degradation of the entire HDL particle.[81] In contrast to LDL receptor binding, the HDL binding was resistant to proteolytic digestion and glycosaminoglycans displacement.[82] Tauber et al.[85] have described HDL binding sites on endothelial cells distinct from the LDL receptor and not dependent on apo-E. These receptors were not down-regulated in the presence of excess LDL, yet LDL was as effective as HDL in competing for the binding sites. Cellular uptake of ^{125}I-LDL was rapid, chloroquine-sensitive, and relatively resistant to inhibition by excess cold HDL. In contrast, HDL uptake and degradation was only 5 to 10% of that seen for LDL, resistant to chloroquine, and could be accounted for by fluid pinocytosis and associated nonspecific adsorptive endocytosis. Thus, there appear to be binding sites on endothelial cells with which HDL can interact. Perhaps occupancy of these sites is coupled to transfer of HDL lipids into the cell without internalization of the particle, or if internalization does occur then subsequent nonlysosomal degradation of the HDL particle.

The entry of HDL lipids into cells need not be limited to receptor-mediated processes; nonreceptor mediated mechanisms for lipoproteins have also been described. In two studies[86,87] endothelial cells have been shown to remove cholesteryl esters from chylomicron remnants via an uptake system independent of receptor-mediated endocytosis. Ritter and Scanu[88] found that leukocytes could modify HDL_3 without any requirement for lipoprotein uptake. In this study there was specific degradation of apo-A-II (but not apo-A-I) and the formation of lysophosphatidylcholine, suggesting the existence of cell surface phospholipases and specific proteinases.

It is apparent from these studies that a variety of mechanisms exist by which endothelial cells can interact with HDL and utilize HDL lipids. In order to determine just how HDL lipids are actually involved in the stimulation of endothelial cell PGI_2 synthesis, it will be necessary to label the arachidonate in the cholesteryl esters and phospholipids of HDL and monitor its incorporation in the cellular lipid pool and its eventual appearance as arachidonic acid metabolites. Investigations are currently being carried out to address these issues.

V. HDL AND PROTECTION FROM ATHEROGENESIS

Elevated plasma HDL levels are associated with reduced risk of cardiovascular disease and it has been proposed that this is due, at least in part, to increased synthesis and release of PGI_2. Does this mean that in the presence of high levels of HDL the vascular endothelium exhibits a continuous elevated release of PGI_2, or do HDL-induced increases in PGI_2 synthesis occur only at crucial periods, for example, during injury to the endothelial lining? Although this question cannot be answered definitively, there is some evidence suggesting that the latter alternative is more probable. The HDL-induced stimulation of PGI_2 synthesis demonstrated with cultured aortic endothelial cells was only observed when subconfluent cell populations were used.[74,75] When cultures reached confluence PGI_2 synthesis in the presence of HDL was virtually indistinguishable from control values. Tauber et al.[70] reported that HDL had a mitogenic effect on low-density vascular endothelial cell cultures over a 2- to 5-day period in serum-free media. The effect of LDL was biphasic, being weakly mitogenic at low concentration, but cytotoxic at physiological concentrations. Although it is tempting to speculate that PGI_2 played some role in HDL-induced endothelial cell mitogenicity, there is no direct data to support this suggestion. However, these results do suggest that HDL stimulates PGI_2 production and endothelial cell growth only before a continuous monolayer of cells has formed. If the damaged vascular endothelium is analogous to the subconfluent culture, then the influence of HDL on PGI_2 production and endothelial cell growth in vivo would be most pronounced during damage to the endothelial lining.

The synthesis of PGI_2 is greatest at the intimal surface of a blood vessel and decreases toward the adventitia.[89] Consequently, de-endothelialization of rabbit aorta with a balloon catheter virtually abolished PGI_2 production. The recovery of PGI_2 production was slow, occurring over a 70-day period and was due predominantly to the elaboration of increasing quantities of PGI_2 by proliferating smooth muscle cells of the neointima. The development of the muscular neointima and the recovery of PGI_2 production preceded the regrowth of vascular endothelium and were probably responsible for the recovery of thromboresistance by the de-endothelialized aortic wall.[90] Diet-induced hypercholesterolemia inhibited the recovery of PGI_2 production in de-endothelialized and re-endothelialized aorta.[91] Cholesteryl esters increased in injured aortae and preferentially accumulated in re-endothelialized areas.[92] The accumulation of cholesteryl esters was inversely correlated with the activity of acid cholesteryl ester hydrolase, a lysosomal enzyme responsible for cholesteryl ester hydrolytic activity. A decrease in hydrolase activity was also observed in de-endothelialized aortae of hypercholesterolemic rabbits.[93] Hajjar et al.[94] found that PGI_2 and two of its metabolites, 6-keto-$PGF_{1\alpha}$ and 6-keto-PGE_1, stimulated the activity of acid cholesteryl ester hydrolase in cultures of rabbit smooth muscle cells. This effect was apparently mediated by cyclic AMP (cAMP) and was not seen with PGE_1 or PGE_2. Furthermore, PGI_2 and its two metabolites appeared to enhance the efflux of cholesterol from these cells over a period of 14 days.

Based upon these studies it is consistent to speculate that HDL may afford anti-atherogenesis in two rather novel ways. First, by enhancing the rate of proliferation of endothelial cells in damaged areas it would hasten the re-endothelialization of injured vascular areas. This may or may not be PGI_2-dependent; the hypothesis remains to be tested. Second, through the stimulation of PGI_2 synthesis by neointimal smooth muscle cells, acid cholesteryl ester hydrolase activity would increase and cholesteryl ester accumulation would be reduced. The HDL-dependent increase in PGI_2 production would also decrease platelet aggregation and provide vasodilation, both effects favoring increased vascular thromboresistance. It remains to be demonstrated which of these in vitro actions of HDL actually occur in vivo. The chain of events by which elevated plasma HDL levels decrease the atheroslcerotic process is still largely speculative. It is quite possible that there is no causal relationship between these two phenomena; however, if PGI_2 should prove to be a chemical trigger by which HDL exerts a palliative influence on the atherosclerotic process, then it would be reasonable to consider the therapeutic potential of increasing plasma HDL levels by dietary and pharmacological means.

REFERENCES

1. Moncada, S. and Vane, J. R., Pharmacology and endogenous roles of prostaglandin endoperoxides, thromboxane A_2 and prostacyclin, *Pharmacol. Rev.*, 30, 293, 1979.
2. Moncada, S. and Vane, J. R., Arachidonic acid metabolites and the interactions between platelets and blood vessel walls, *N. Engl. J. Med.*, 300, 1142, 1979.
3. Weksler, B. B., Marcus, A. J., and Jaffe, E. A., Synthesis of prostaglandin I_2 (prostacyclin) by cultured human and bovine endothelial cells, *Proc. Natl. Acad. Sci. U.S.A.*, 74, 3922, 1977.
4. MacIntyre, D. E., Pearson, J. D., and Gordon, J. L., Localization and stimulation of prostacyclin production in vascular cells, *Nature (London)*, 271, 549, 1978.
5. Vane, J. R., Bunting, S., and Moncada, S., Prostacyclin physiology and pathophysiology, in *International Review of Experimental Pathology*, Vol. 23, Richter, G. W. and Epstein, M. A., Eds., Academic Press, New York, 1982, 293.
6. Smith J. B., The prostanoids in hemostasis and thrombosis, *Am. J. Pathol.*, 99, 743, 1980.
7. Ramwell, P. W., Leovey, E. M. K., and Sinetetos, A. L., Regulation of arachidonate cascade, *Biol. Reprod.*, 16, 70, 1977.
8. Lands, W. E. M. and Samuelsson, B., Phospholipid precursors of prostaglandins, *Biochim. Biophys. Acta*, 164, 426, 1968.
9. Kunze, J. and Vogt, W., Significance of phospholipase A for prostaglandin formation, *Ann. N.Y. Acad. Sci.*, 180, 123, 1971.
10. Vonkeman, H. and Van Dorp, D. A., The action of prostaglandin synthetase on 2-arachidonyl lecithin, *Biochim. Biophys. Acta*, 164, 430, 1968.
11. Bills, T. K., Smith, J. B., and Silver, M. J., Selective release of arachidonic acid from the phospholipids of human platelets in response to thrombin, *J. Clin. Invest.*, 60, 1, 1977.
12. Rittenhouse-Simmons, S., Production of diglyceride from phosphatidylinositol in activated human platelets, *J. Clin. Invest.*, 63, 580, 1979.
13. Bell, R. L., Kennerly, D. A., Stanford, N., and Majerus, P. W., Diglyceride lipase: a pathway for arachidonate release from human platelets, *Proc. Natl. Acad. Sci. U.S.A.*, 76, 3238, 1979.
14. Bell, R. L. and Majerus, P. W., Thrombin-induced hydrolysis of phosphatidylinositol in human platelets, *J. Biol. Chem.*, 255, 1790, 1980.
15. Manco, G., Chap, H., and Douste-Blazy, L., Characterization and properties of a phosphatidylinositol phosphodiesterase (phospholipase C) from platelet cytosol, *FEBS Lett.*, 100, 367, 1979.
16. Hamberg, M., Svensson, J., and Samuelsson, B., Prostaglandin endoperoxides: a new concept concerning the mode of action and release of prostaglandins, *Proc. Natl. Acad. Sci. U.S.A.*, 71, 3824, 1974.

17. Samuelsson, B., The leukotrienes: an introduction, in *Advances in Prostaglandin, Thromboxane, and Leukotriene Research,* Vol. 9, Samuelsson, B. and Paoletti, R., Eds., Raven Press, New York, 1982, 1.

18. Spector, A. A., Kaduce, T. L., Hoak, J. C., and Fry, G. L., Utilization of arachidonic and linoleic acids by cultured human endothelial cells, *J. Clin. Ivest.,* 68, 1003, 1981.

19. Goldstein, J. L. and Brown, M. S., The low density lipoprotein pathway and its relation to atherosclerosis, *Ann. Rev. Biochem.,* 46, 897, 1977.

20. Tall, A. R. and Small, D. M., Body cholesterol removal: role of plasma high density lipoproteins, *Adv. Lipid Res.,* 17, 1, 1980.

21. Bradley, W. A. and Gotto, A. M., Jr., Structure of intact human plasma lipoproteins, in *Disturbances in Lipid and Lipoprotein Metabolism,* Dietschy, J. M., Gotto, A. M., Jr., and Ontko, J. A., Eds., American Physiological Society, Bethesda, Md., 1978, 111.

22. Bergman, E. N., Havel, R. J., Wolfe, B. M., and Bohmer, T., Quantitative studies of the metabolism of chylomicron triglycerides and cholesterol by liver and extrahepatic tissues of sheep and dogs, *J. Clin. Invest.,* 50, 1831, 1971.

23. Felts, J. M., Itakura, H., and Crane, R. T., The mechanism of assimilation of constituents of chylomicrons, very low density lipoproteins and remnants - a new theory, *Biochem. Biophys. Res. Commun.,* 66, 1467, 1975.

24. Noel, S., Dolphin, P. J., and Rubinstein, D., An in vitro model for the catabolism of rat chylomicrons, *Biochem. Biophys. Res. Commun.,* 63, 764, 1975.

25. Quarfordt, S. H. and Goodman, D. S., Metabolism of doubly-labeled chylomicron cholesteryl esters in the rat, *J. Lipid Res.,* 8, 264, 1967.

26. Redgrave, T. G., Formation of cholesteryl ester-rich particulate lipid during metabolism of chylomicrons, *J. Clin. Invest.,* 49, 465, 1970.

27. Glomset, J. A., The plasma lecithin: cholesterol acyltransferase reaction, *J. Lipid Res.,* 9, 155, 1968.

28. Goldstein, J. L., Anderson, R. G. W., and Brown, M. S., Coated pits, coated vesicles and receptor mediated endocytosis, *Nature (London),* 279, 679, 1979.

29. Hamilton, R. L., Williams, M. C., Fielding, C. J., and Havel, R. J., Discoidal bilayer structure of nascent high density lipoproteins from perfused rat liver, *J. Clin. Invest.,* 58, 667, 1976.

30. Felker, T. E., Fainaru, M., Hamilton, R. L., and Havel, R. J., Secretion of the arginine rich and A-1 apolipoproteins by the isolated perfused rat liver, *J. Lipid Res.,* 18, 465, 1977.

31. Green, P. H. R., Tall, A. R., and Glickman, R. M., Rat intestine secretes discoid high density lipoprotein, *J. Clin. Invest.,* 61, 528, 1978.

32. Tall, A. R. and Small, D. M., Plasma high density lipoproteins, *N. Engl. J. Med.,* 299, 1232, 1978.

33. Patsch, J. R., Gotto, A. M., Jr., Olivecrona, T., and Eisenberg, S., Formation of high density lipoprotein-like particles during lipolysis of very low density lipoproteins in vitro, *Proc. Natl. Acad. Sci. U.S.A.,* 75, 4519, 1978.

34. Redgrave, T. G. and Small, D. M., Quantitation of the transfer of surface phospholipid of chylomicrons to the high density lipoprotein fraction during the catabolism of the chylomicrons, *J. Clin. Invest.,* 63, 162, 1979.

35. Bondjers, G., Gustafson, A., Kral, J., Schersten, T., and Sjostrom, L., Cholesterol content in arterial tissue in relation to serum liopoproteins in man, *Artery,* 2, 200, 1976.

36. Stein, O., Vanderhock, J., and Stein, Y., Cholesterol content and sterol synthesis in human skin fibroblasts and rat aortic smooth muscle cells exposed to lipoprotein-depleted serum and high density lipoprotein phospholipid mixtures, *Biochim. Biophys. Acta,* 431, 347, 1976.

37. Miller, N. E., Nestel, P. J., and Clifton-Bligh, P., Relationships between plasma lipoprotein cholesterol concentrations and the pool size and metabolism of cholesterol in man, *Atherosclerosis,* 23, 535, 1976.

38. Miller, N. E., Weinstein, D. B., and Steinberg, D., Uptake and degradation of high density lipoprotein: comparison of fibroblasts from normal subjects and from homozygous familial hypercholesterolemic subjects, *J. Lipid Res.,* 19, 644, 1978.

39. Lally, J. I. and Barter, P. J., The in vivo metabolism of esterified cholesterol in the plasma high-density lipoproteins of rabbits, *J. Lab. Clin. Med.,* 93, 570, 1979.

40. Pattnaik, N. M., Montes, A., Highes, L. B., and Zilversmit, D. B., Cholesteryl ester exchange protein in human plasma. Isolation and characterization, *Biochim. Biophys. Acta,* 530, 428, 1978.

41. Pattnaik, N. M. and Zilversmit, D. B., Interaction of cholesteryl ester exchange protein with human plasma proteins and phospholipid vesicles, *J. Biol. Chem.,* 254, 2782, 1979.

42. Miller, G. J. and Miller, N. E., Plasma-high-density lipoprotein concentration and development of ischaemic heart disease, *Lancet,* 1, 16, 1975.

43. Castelli, W. P., Doyle, J. T., Gordon, T., Hames, C. G., Hjortland, M. C., Hulley, S. B., Kogan, A., and Zukel, W. J., HDL cholesterol and other lipids in coronary heart disease - the Cooperative Lipoprotein Phenotyping Study, *Circulation,* 55, 767, 1977.

44. Gordon, T., Castelli, W. P., Hjortland, M. C., Kannel, W. B., and Dawber, T. R., High density lipoprotein as a protective factor against coronary heart disease — the Framingham Study, *Am. J. Med.*, 62, 707, 1977.

45. Miller, N. E., Forde, O. H., Thelle, D. S., and Mjos, O. D., The Tromso Heart Study — High density lipoprotein and coronary heart disease: a prospective case-control study, *Lancet*, 1, 965, 1977.

46. Enger, S. C., Hjermann, I., Foss, O. P., Helgeland, A., Holme, I., Loren, P., and Norum, K. R., High density lipoprotein cholesterol and myocaradial infarction or sudden coronary death. A prospective case-control study in middle-aged men of the Oslo Study, *Artery*, 5, 170, 1979.

47. Goldbourt, V. and Medalie, J. H., High density lipoprotein cholesterol and incidence of coronary heart disease. The Israeli Ischemic Heart Disease Study, *Am. J. Epidemiol.*, 109, 296, 1979.

48. Stein, Y., Glangeaud, M. C., Fainaru, M., and Stein, O., The removal of cholesterol ester from aortic smooth muscle cells in culture and Landschutz ascites cells by fractions of high density lipoprotein, *Biochim. Biophys. Acta*, 380, 106, 1975.

49. Bondjers, G., and Bjorkerud, S., Cholesterol transfer between arterial smooth muscle tissue and serum lipoproteins in vitro, *Artery*, 1, 3, 1974.

50. Adams, C. W. M. and Abdulla, Y. H., The action of human high density lipoprotein on cholesterol crystals. I. Light-microscopic observations, *Atherosclerosis*, 31, 465, 1978.

51. Abdulla, Y. H. and Adams, C. W. M., The action of human high density lipoprotein on cholesterol crystals. II. Biochemical observations, *Atherosclerosis*, 31, 474, 1978.

52. Medalie, J. H., Kahn, H. A., Neufeld, H. N., Riss, E., and Goldbourt, V., Myocardial infarction over a two-year period. I. Prevalence, incidence and mortality experience, *J. Chronic Dis.*, 26, 63, 1973.

53. Kannel, W. B., Castelli, W. P., and Gordon, T., Cholesterol in the prediction of atherosclerotic disease, *Ann. Intern. Med.*, 90, 85, 1979.

54. Bunting, S., Gryglewski, R., Moncada, S., and Vane, J. R., Arterial walls generate from prostaglandin endoperoxides a substance (prostaglandin X) which relaxes strips of mesenteric and coeliac arteries and inhibits platelet aggregation, *Prostaglandins*, 12, 897, 1976.

55. Gryglewski, R. J., Bunting, S., Moncada, S., Flower, R. J., and Vane, J. R., Arterial walls are protected against deposition of platelet thrombi by a substance (prostaglandin X) which they make from prostaglandin endoperoxides, *Prostaglandins*, 12, 685, 1976.

56. Moncada, S., Gryglewski, R. J., Bunting, S., and Vane, J. R., A lipid peroxide inhibits the enzyme in blood vessel microsomes that generates from prostaglandin endoperoxides the substance (prostaglandin X) which prevents platelet aggregation, *Prostaglandins*, 12, 715, 1976.

57. Bunting, S., Moncada, S., and Vane, J. R., Antithrombotic properties of vascular endothelium, *Lancet*, 2, 1075, 1977.

58. Glavind, J., Hartmann, S., Clemmesen, J., Jessen, K. E., and Dam, H., Studies on the role of lipoperoxides in human pathology. II. The presence of peroxidized lipids in the atherosclerotic aorta, *Acta Pathol. Microbiol. Scand.*, 30, 1, 1952.

59. Szczeklik, A. and Gryglewski, R. J., Low density lipoproteins (LDL) are carriers for lipid peroxides and inhibit prostacyclin (PGI$_2$) biosynthesis in arteries, *Artery*, 7, 488, 1980.

60. Gryglewski, R. J. and Szczeklik, A., Prostacyclin and atherosclerosis, in *Clinical Pharmacology of Prostacyclin*, Lewis, P. J. and O'Grady, J., Eds., Raven Press, New York, 1981, 89.

61. Dimbinska-Kiec, A., Gryglewska, T., Zmuda, A., and Gryglewski, R. J., The generation of prostacyclin by arteries and by the coronary vascular bed is reduced in experimental atherosclerosis in rabbits, *Prostaglandins*, 14, 1025, 1977.

62. D'Angelo, V. D., Villa, S., Mysliwiec, M., Donati, M. B., and De Gaetano, G., Defective fibrinolytic and prostacyclin-like activity in human atheromatous plaques, *Thromb. Diath. Haemorrh.*, 39, 535, 1978.

63. Sinzinger, H., Silberbauer, K., Feigl, W., Wagner, O., Winter, M., and Auerswald, W., Prostacyclin activity is diminished in different types of morphologically controlled human atherosclerotic lesions, *Thromb. Haemostas. (Stuttgart)*, 42, 803, 1979.

64. Sinzinger, H., Feigl, W., and Silberbauer, K., Prostacyclin generation in atherosclerotic arteries, *Lancet*, 2, 469, 1979.

65. Larrue, J., Rigaud, M., Daret, D., Demond, J., Durrand, J., and Bricaud, H., Prostacyclin productions by cultured smooth muscle cells from atherosclerotic rabbit aorta, *Nature (London)*, 285, 480, 1980.

66. Kent, R. S., Kitchell, B. B., Shand, D. G., and Whorton, A. R., The ability of vascular tissue to produce prostacyclin decreases with age, *Prostaglandins*, 21, 483, 1981.

67. Chang, W. C., Murota, S. I., Nakao, J., and Orimo, H., Age-related decrease in prostacyclin biosynthetic activity in rat aortic smooth muscle cells, *Biochim. Biophys. Acta*, 620, 159, 1980.

68. Ager, A., Gordon, J. L., Moncada, S., Pearson, J. D., Salmon, J. A., and Trevethick, M. A., Effects of isolation and culture on prostaglandin synthesis by porcine aortic endothelial and smooth muscle cells, *J. Cell. Physiol.*, 110, 9, 1982.

69. Henriksen, T., Evensen, S. A., and Carlander, B., Injury to human endothelial cells in culture induced by low density lipoproteins, *Scand. J. Clin. Lab. Invest.,* 39, 361, 1979.

70. Tauber, J. P., Cheng, J., and Gospodarowicz, D., Effect of high and low density lipoproteins on proliferation of cultured bovine vascular endothelial cells, *J. Clin. Invest.,* 66, 696, 1980.

71. Nordoy, A., Svensson, B., Wiebe, D., and Hoak, J. C., Lipoproteins and the inhibitory effect of human endothelial cells on platelet function, *Circ. Res.,* 43, 527, 1978.

72. Beitz, J. and Forster, W., Influence of human low density and high density lipoprotein-cholesterol on the in vitro prostaglandin I$_2$ synthetase activity, *Biochim. Biophys. Acta,* 620, 352, 1980.

73. Szczeklik, A., Gryglewski, R. J., Domegala, B., Zmuda, A., Hartwich, J., Wozny, E., Grzzwacz, M., Madej, J., and Gryglewska, T., Serum lipoproteins, lipid peroxides and prostacyclin biosynthesis in patients with coronary heart disease, *Prostaglandins,* 22, 795, 1981.

74. Fleisher, L. N., Tall, A. R., Witte, L. D., Miller, R. W., and Cannon, P. J., Stimulation of arterial endothelial cell prostacyclin synthesis by high density lipoproteins, *J. Biol. Chem.,* 257, 6653, 1982.

75. Fleisher, L. N., Tall, A. R., Witte, L. D., and Cannon, P. J., Effects of high-density lipoprotein and the apoprotein of high-density lipoprotein on prostacyclin synthesis by endothelial cells, in *Advances in Prostaglandin, Thromboxane, and Leukotriene Research,* Samuelsson, B., Paoleti, R., and Ramwell, P. W., Eds., Raven Press, New York, 1983, 475.

76. Mahley, R. W. and Innerarity, T. L., Interaction of canine and swine lipoproteins with the low density lipoprotein receptor of fibroblasts correlated with heparin manganese precipitability, *J. Biol. Chem.,* 252, 3980, 1977.

77. Innerarity, T. L., Mahley, R. W., Weisgraber, K. H., and Bersot, T. P., Apoprotein (E-A-11) complex of human plasma lipoproteins. II. Receptor binding activity of a high density lipoprotein subfraction modulated by the apo (E-A-11) complex, *J. Biol. Chem.,* 253, 6289, 1978.

78. Swaney, J. B., Braithwaite, F., and Elder, H. A., Characterization of the apolipoproteins of rat plasma lipoproteins, *Biochemistry,* 16, 271, 1977.

79. Weisgraber, K. H. and Mahley, R. W., Subfractionation of human high density lipoproteins by heparin-sepharose affinity chromatography, *J. Lipid Res.,* 21, 316, 1980.

80. Fleisher, L. N., Tall, A. R., Witte, L. D., and Cannon, P. J., Mechanisms of stimulation of arterial endothelial cell prostacyclin synthesis by high density lipoproteins, *Circulation,* 66(2), 39, 1982.

81. Gwynne, J. T. and Hess, B., The role of high density lipoproteins in rat adrenal cholesterol metabolism and steroidogenesis, *J. Biol. Chem.,* 255, 10875, 1980.

82. Ohashi, M., Carr, B. C., and Simpson, E. R., Binding of high density lipoproteins to human fetal adrenal membrane fractions, *Endocrinology,* 109, 783, 1981.

83. Chen, Y. D., Kraemer, F. B., and Reaven, G. M., Identification of specific high density lipoprotein-binding sites in rat testis and regulation of binding by human chorionic gonadotropin, *J. Biol. Chem.,* 255, 9162, 1980.

84. Shemesh, M., Bensdoun, A., and Hansel, W., Lipoprotein lipase activity in the bovine corpus luteum during the estrous cycle and early pregnancy, *Proc. Soc. Biol. Med.,* 151, 667, 1976.

85. Tauber, J. P., Goldminz, D., Vlodavsky, I., and Gospodarowicz, D., The interaction of the high-density lipoprotein with cultured cells of bovine vascular endothelium, *Eur. J. Biochem.,* 119, 317, 1981.

86. Fielding, C. J., Vlodavsky, I., Fielding, P. E., and Gospodarowicz, D., Characteristics of chylomicron binding and lipid uptake by endothelial cells in culture, *J. Biol. Chem.,* 254, 8861, 1979.

87. Chajek-Shaul, T., Friedman, G., Halperin, G., Stein, O., and Stein, Y., Uptake of chylomicron ^{3}H-3-cholesteryl linoleyl ether by mesenchymal rat heart cell cultures, *Biochim. Biophys. Acta,* 666, 147, 1981.

88. Ritter, M. C. and Scanu, A. M., Structural changes in human serum high-density lipoprotein -3 attending incubations with blood leukocytes, *J. Biol. Chem.,* 255, 3763, 1980.

89. Moncada, S., Herman, A. G., Higgs, E. A., and Vane, J. R., Differential formation of prostacyclin (PGX or PGI$_2$) by layers of the arterial wall. An explanation for the anti-thrombotic properties of the vascular endothelium, *Thromb. Res.,* 11, 323, 1977.

90. Eldor, A., Falcone, D. J., Hajjar, D. P., Minick, C. R., and Weksler, B. B., Recovery of prostacyclin production by deendothelialized rabbit aorta. Critical role of neointimal smooth muscle cells, *J. Clin. Invest.,* 67, 735, 1981.

91. Eldor, A., Falcone, D. J., Hajjar, D. P., Minick, C. R., and Weksler, B. B., Diet-induced hypercholesterolemia inhibits the recovery of prostacyclin production by injured rabbit aorta, *Am. J. Pathol.,* 107, 186, 1982.

92. Falcone, D. J., Hajjar, D. P., and Minick, C. R., Enhancement of cholesterol and cholesteryl ester accumulation in re-endothelialized aorta, *Am. J. Pathol.,* 99, 81, 1980.

93. Hajjar, D. P., Falcone, D. J., Fowler, S., and Minick, C. R., Endothelium modifies the altered metabolism of the injured aortic wall, *Am. J. Pathol.,* 102, 28, 1980.

94. Hajjar, D. P., Weksler, B. B., Falcone, D. J., Hefton, J. M., Tack-Goldman, K., and Minick, C. R., Prostacyclin modulates cholesteryl ester hydrolytic activity by its effect on cyclic adenosine monophosphate in rabbit aortic smooth muscle cells, *J. Clin. Invest.*, 70, 479, 1982.

Chapter 12

PROSTACYCLIN IN VASCULAR DISEASES

Ryszard J. Gryglewski

TABLE OF CONTENTS

I. INTRODUCTION

Prostacyclin (PGI$_2$) was discovered in 1976[1-4] and its first administration into healthy human volunteers took place in 1978.[5,6] Among pharmacological properties of PGI$_2$ which might be useful in the treatment of vascular disease, the best known are its effects on blood vessels and on blood platelets.

II. CARDIOVASCULAR ACTION OF PROSTACYCLIN

In vitro PGI$_2$ relaxes most vascular strips, e.g., bovine coronary artery,[7] rabbit mesenteric artery,[1] human and baboon cerebral arteries,[8] lamb ductus arteriosus,[9] and canine renal artery.[10] Human and rat venous strips are not relaxed by PGI$_2$.[11]

In dogs single bolus i.v. injection of PGI$_2$ (1 to 3 μg/kg) or i.v. infusion (0.02 to 1.0 μg/kg/min) causes a drop in systemic and pulmonary blood pressure as well as a decrease in peripheral resistance.[12,13] Renal and cerebral vascular beds are particularly sensitive to this action of PGI$_2$.[12] In the feline and canine pulmonary circulation PGI$_2$ produces a vasodilatory response.[14,15] PGI$_2$ also lowers pulmonary vascular resistance in patients with primary and secondary hypertension.[16] During i.v. infusion of PGI$_2$ in humans,[5,6,17] monkeys,[18] and cats,[19] a modest increase in heart rate is a typical response to be expected. Bradycardia may occur in anesthetized dogs[20,21] and in humans when high doses of PGI$_2$ (>20 ng/kg/min i.v.) are used.[5,6] In humans an increase in heart rate is reflected by an increase in cardiac output; however, stroke volume is not changed and thus it may be concluded that in humans PGI$_2$ does not affect cardiac contractility.[5,6] Intracoronary injection (30 to 500 ng) or topical application of PGI$_2$ (20 to 100 μg) onto canine epicardium results in coronary vasodilation;[21-23] however, administered systemically to dogs PGI$_2$ hardly increases coronary blood flow,[23,24] although several authors do not agree with this statement.[25,26] Therefore, the protective action of PGI$_2$ on myocardial ischemia both in laboratory animals[27] and in humans[28] must seek another explanation.

Apart from antiplatelet, fibrinolytic,[29] cytoprotective,[27,30] and oxygen-sparing[31] actions of PGI$_2$ that may contribute to its beneficial effects in myocardial ischemia[27,28] as well as in ischemia associated with arteriosclerosis obliterans,[32,33] Raynaud's syndrome,[34] retinal vein occlusion,[35] ischemic stroke,[36] and endotoxic[37,38] and traumatic[39,40] shocks, one has to take into account the effect of PGI$_2$ on microcirculation, local redistribution of blood, and on arterial anastomoses. PGI$_2$ reduces peripheral resistance in humans[5] and in animals.[22] It causes a dose-dependent dilation of arterioles whereas the postcapillary venules remain insensitive to PGI$_2$.[41,42] Hallenbeck and Furlow[43] have shown that PGI$_2$ (30 to 180 μg/kg/min i.v.) increases nutrient perfusion in cortex and white matter of dog brain in the postischemic period. These experimental data fit very well with the proposed effects of PGI$_2$ on microcirculation in humans.[5,44] In humans, vessels of head, neck, and palms are highly susceptible to the dilatory action of PGI$_2$. Erythema and feeling of warmth in these regions consistently occur in patients to whom PGI$_2$ is administered intravenously.

III. EFFECTS OF PROSTACYCLIN ON PLATELET FUNCTION

PGI$_2$ at concentrations of 2 to 20 nM inhibits platelet aggregation in platelet-rich plasma of humans, dogs, cats, rats, guinea pigs, rabbits, sheep, and horses,[45] and it is effective against aggregation induced by ADP, collagen, thrombin, arachidonic acid, TXA$_2$, and platelet-activating factor (PAF).[46] Like PGD$_2$ and PGE$_1$, which also inhibit platelet aggregation, PGI$_2$ elevates intraplatelet cyclic AMP (cAMP) levels.[47,48] In human platelet rich plasma the anti-aggregatory effect of PGI$_2$ is 20 and 40 times more potent than those of PGD$_2$ and PGE$_1$, respectively.[45]

PGI$_2$ seems to act on the same platelet receptor site as PGE$_1$ but on a different receptor site than that for PGD$_2$.[45,49-51] Phosphodiesterase inhibitors potentiate, and dibutyryl-cAMP mimics[52] the effects of PGI$_2$ on platelets. The experiments in vitro have shown that PGI$_2$ is able to suppress all forms of platelet activation such as spreading,[53] shape change,[54,55] adhesion,[56,57] aggregation,[2] mobilization of platelet membrane binding sites for fibrinogen,[58] the release reaction from dense bodies and α-granules,[52] as well as the release of procoagulant factors.[54,55] Most likely all these activities of PGI$_2$ are mediated by cAMP. It is no wonder that PGI$_2$ affects platelet function in vivo. When infused intravenously into humans,[5,6,17,59] PGI$_2$ reduces platelet aggregability, dissipates circulating platelet aggregates, and prolongs template bleeding time. In animals PGI$_2$ prevents white thrombi formation in small[60] and large[61] arteries as well as in pulmonary[62,63] and in coronary arteries.[64,65] PGI$_2$ disaggregates white thrombi in an extracorporeal system where blood of animals[66] or humans[67,68] is being superfused over collagen strips.

This property of PGI$_2$ enabled us to demonstrate that angiotensin II,[69,70] chemoreceptor stimulants,[71] nicotinic acid derivatives,[72] choline esters,[67] and thromboxane (TX) synthetase inhibitors[72] release PGI$_2$ into the circulation. The release of PGI$_2$ into the circulation in humans was confirmed using physicochemical methods.[73,74] American[64,65,75,76] and Japanese[77,78] authors reported that intravenous infusions of PGI$_2$ or of its stable analogues[76] effectively interrupted cyclic declines in myocardial blood flow or cerebral blood flow after partial occlusion of coronary or carotid arteries in anesthetized dogs. The first group of investigators pointed to the anti-aggregatory action of PGI$_2$ while the second group believes that its vasodilatory properties are responsible for its beneficial action. TX synthetase inhibitors release endogenous PGI$_2$.[72] Therefore, these drugs protect myocardial and cerebral blood flow against disturbances caused by partial occlusion of the blood-supplying arteries.[75,78]

IV. CLINICAL TRIALS

So far most clinical trials with PGI$_2$ have been open clinical trials. The first open clinical trial with PGI$_2$ was successfully completed in patients with peripheral vascular disease[32] and confirmed in a double-blind study.[79] Open clinical trials are necessary to formulate the claims for therapeutical effectiveness of PGI$_2$ whereas controlled clinical trials confirm or reject these claims.

Although PGI$_2$ is a powerful pharmacological agent by itself (see above), I presume that the rationale for its clinical use is to be searched for in pathophysiological situations when PGI$_2$ deficiency is suspected. Our hypothesis is that atherosclerosis is this kind of disease.[80-82] Indeed, a diminished generation of PGI$_2$ has been observed not only in arteries of animals with experimental atherosclerosis,[80-83] but also in human atherosclerotic arteries;[84] treatment with PGI$_2$ was claimed to prevent the development of experimental atherosclerosis.[85] Thus, we assume that the clinical use of PGI$_2$ in atherosclerosis is a substitutional therapy of this disease. Consequently, we have introduced PGI$_2$ rather than PGE$_1$ for the treatment of peripheral vascular disease. A number of pharmacological similarities exist between PGI$_2$ and PGE$_1$,[44] and there is a distinct possibility of biotransformation of PGI$_2$ to 6-keto-PGE$_1$.[86-88] No wonder then that PGE$_1$ was also successfully used in the treatment of peripheral vascular disease,[89-92] and in Raynaud's syndrome,[93] ischemic heart failure,[94] and unstable angina pectoris.[95]

So far over 300 patients have been treated with PGI$_2$ in the clinics of Copernicus Academy of Medicine in Cracow. This experience tells us that we cannot share the view that "the frequency and severity of side effects of PGI$_2$ have diverted attention to PGE$_1$."[93] Side effects that may occur during i.v. infusion of PGI$_2$ are mild and easy to avoid by adjusting the dose of the drug.[44,96,97] The choice between PGI_2 and PGE_1 must not be motivated by differences in their side effects or in their chemical stability since neither pose a serious clinical problem. In contrast to PGE_1, PGI_2 is a physiological product of vascular endothelium that is not removed from the circulation when passing through the lungs.[98] This may be the decisive argument for those who use PGI_2 in clinical trials.

We have looked for possible therapeutic actions of PGI_2 in patients with various types of illness that are associated with atherosclerosis.

A. Peripheral Vascular Disease

We started to use PGI_2 in the treatment of peripheral vascular disease of the lower extremities as early as 1979,[32] and reports on an increasing number of treated patients were published.[44,97,99] Presently, we have on record 218 patients with diagnosed arteriosclerosis obliterans (177 patients) and thrombangiitis obliterans (41 patients). One hundred twenty-nine (129) patients showed ischemic symptoms at rest, i. e., rest pain, ulcers, or necrosis and 89 patients suffered from intermittent claudication.

Epoprostenol (sodium salt of PGI_2, Wellcome Research Laboratores, Beckenham, U.K., and The Upjohn Company, Kalamazoo, Mich.) was infused i.v. at an average dose of 7 ng/kg/min (2 to 10 ng/kg/min) for 72 to 84 hr. If any side effects occurred (headache, hypotension), the dose was lowered to a level that was tolerated by the patient and the period of infusion prolonged. The observation period following the therapy was from 3 months to 3 years.

Relief of rest pain was the most consistent effect of the therapy. It appeared at the end of the PGI_2 infusion or 1 to 2 days later and it could last either for the whole observation period or for several weeks only. Of 73 patients with ischemic ulcers (at least of 3 months duration) 20 patients did not respond to the PGI_2 therapy and underwent amputation; in another 22 patients a short-term improvement could not be sustained, even though they received repeated courses of the PGI_2 treatment with a periodicity of 1 to 12 weeks. In the remaining 31 patients ulcers either healed completely or decreased markedly in size. In 19 of those patients the observation period has been longer than 1 year. Twenty-two (22) patients with dry black gangrene of the great toe or of other parts of the foot showed no response to the therapy and soon underwent amputation. Of 34 patients who suffered from rest pain without ulcerations, in 22 patients the alleviation of pain was sustained longer than 3 months after therapy with PGI_2. Walking distance improved in 59 of 89 patients with intermittent claudication. We found that the better responders to PGI_2 therapy were the patients with distal rather than proximal localization of atherosclerotic occlusion. For example, Larische's syndrome hardly improved after the infusion of PGI_2. Prentice's group has recently shown that in the PGI_2-treated group of patients with severe arterial disease vs. the placebo group of patients there was a significant improvement as measured by severity of rest pain and frequency of operative intervention.[79] Apart from this double-blind trial there are other uncontrolled studies[93,100-102] which confirm our original observation of beneficial effects of PGI_2 in the treatment of peripheral vascular disease. There are also studies that do not support our finding.[103] Controlled clinical trials are essential since the efficacy of therapy with PGI_2 in uncontrolled trials depends critically on the selection of patients.[44] Patients with spontaneous platelet aggregation[104] or with the occlusion of proximal axial limb artery,[101,104] as well as patients with gangrene[44] will not respond to treatment with PGI_2; those patients should be excluded from a controlled trial. Duration of the PGI_2 infusion may be of importance. Initial suppression of platelet aggregation[44,105] is followed by a paradoxical enhancement of platelet activity that appears toward the end of a prolonged infusion of PGI_2 into patients with peripheral vascular disease.[106-108] The initial activation by PGI_2 of the fibrinolytic system also tends to disappear.[29] Paradoxical behavior of platelets is probably caused by desensitization of platelet adenylate cyclase subsequent to its protracted exposure to PGI_2 at pharmacological concentrations.[108,109] Because of these findings we have recently decided to administer PGI_2 in 5- to 6-hr courses separated by 6- to 18-hr breaks. It seems that this regime of PGI_2 therapy avoids the "rebound phenomenon" of a 72-hr infusion.

B. Raynaud's Syndrome

There are few reports on the beneficial effect of PGI_2 in the treatment of patients with Raynaud's syndrome.[93,110-112] The most recent is a double-blind study[113] in which patients received PGI_2 at a dose of 7.5 ng/kg/min in 5-hr courses given weekly for 3 weeks. In patients treated with PGI_2 a marked clinical improvement compared to the control group was observed. Frequency and duration of attacks of vasospasm decreased and ischemic skin lesions healed for up to 6 weeks after the last infusion of PGI_2.

As in the case of the long-term beneficial effects of PGI_2 in arteriosclerosis of the lower extremities,[44,97,99] the long-term clinical improvement in patients with Raynaud's syndrome is hard to explain by known pharmacological actions of PGI_2 — a compound that will not survive in the circulation several minutes after its infusion is completed.

C. Pulmonary Hypertension

In patients with secondary pulmonary hypertension, PGI_2 at doses of 2.5 to 10.0 ng/kg/min i.v. for 30 min was found to significantly reduce pulmonary wedge resistance and total pulmonary resistance. The duration of this effect was limited to the period of infusion.[16,44] A similar pharmacological effect in patients with secondary pulmonary hypertension was reported for PGE_1.[114] Infusions of PGI_2 in patients with mitral stenosis undergoing cardiac surgery might be expected to lower the raised pulmonary pressure and, in consequence, reduce the risk of operation. PGI_2 or PGE_1 were also successfully used in children with idiopathic pulmonary artery stenosis or vasoconstriction.[115,116] Pharmacological manipulations of neonatal circulation with PGI_2, PGE_1, and PGE_2 as well as with cyclooxygenase inhibitors have been reviewed.[117,118]

D. Extracorporeal Circulation

In a series of clinical trials with PGI_2 in cardiopulmonary bypass in man[119-124] it has been shown that PGI_2 does significantly preserve platelet count and function as well as potentiate the anticoagulant action of heparin when extracorporeal circulation is being maintained. These two effects of PGI_2 may well lead to reduction of postoperative blood loss and to the prevention of formation of microemboli. The cardiovascular effects of PGI_2 are easily managed during surgery and the hypotensive properties of PGI_2 may be useful in controlling intrabypass hypertension.[125] The heparin-sparing effect of PGI_2 led to the idea of using PGI_2 alone during hemodialysis in dogs.[126-127] PGI_2 prevented platelet loss and coagulation. No heparin was needed. This amazing effect was confirmed in 15 patients[128,129] in whom PGI_2 was infused intravenously for 10 min before dialysis and into the arterial line during dialysis.

E. Kidney Transplants

Leithner et al.[130] have recently treated 8 patients with chronic kidney transplant rejection with PGI_2 (5 ng/kg/min, i.v. for 5 days). In the majority of cases this treatment improved the function of the transplant. In presensitized dogs PGI_2 suppressed the hyperacute allograft rejection[131] and in rats PGI_2 had a definite beneficial effect in prolonging the survival of the cardiac allografts.[132] The mechanism of this action is not clear, but inhibition of the platelet release reaction and suppression of platelet clumping in microcirculation of grafts might be of importance.

F. Central Retinal Vein Occlusion

Central retinal vein occlusion (CRVO) shows up as hemorrhage or ischemic unilateral retinopathy that causes loss of vision in half the affected patients. Late complications of CRVO include secondary glaucoma, maculopathy, proliferation of new blood vessels, and atrophy of the optic nerve disc. Frequency of the disease is estimated at 50/10,000 population. PGI_2 (2.5 to 5.0 ng/kg/min) was infused intravenously for 72 to 120 hr in 3 patients[35] and then in 17 patients with CRVO (Table 1). The effectiveness of this therapy was compared with the routine treatment of CRVO (i.e., heparin, ascorbic acid, hydergine, anti-inflammatory drugs) in an age-matched group of 10 other patients. PGI_2, when administered within the first 5 days after occlusion of the retinal blood vessel, was the most effective. A fast and long-lasting improvement (regression of edema, hemorrhages, tortuosity of retinal blood vessels, and other signs of damage of eye fundus (see Table 1) was observed in 70 and 50% of PGI_2-treated patients, respectively, whereas the conventional treatment produced improvement in 20% of patients (Table 1). The observation period in both groups of patients is 6 to 30 months. So far the percentage of late complications of CRVO is lower in the PGI_2-treated patients (23%) as compared to the conventional treatment (40%). We consider PGI_2 as the drug of choice for the treatment of the acute phase of CRVO.

G. Sudden Deafness of Unknown Origin

This disease consists of a severe sensorineuronal hearing loss that usually occurs only in one ear with a frequency of 2:10,000 persons. The sudden onset suggests thrombovascular etiology, although viral etiology seems more likely in children and young adults. Seventeen (17) patients aged 12 to 55 years were treated with PGI_2 at a dose of 5 ng/kg/min i.v. in 5-hr courses over 6 consecutive days.[133] The therapy began 2 to 20 days after hearing loss had been reported by patients. In 7 patients complete recovery occured within 2 weeks. In 8 patients only partial improvement was found during tone and speech audiometric examination within 6 weeks. In one patient no improvement was recorded. All of the treated patients reported a subjective relief resulting from disappearance of buzzing in the ear. A double-blind study is required.

H. Angina Pectoris

The therapeutic significance of PGI_2 in ischemic heart disease has not yet been assessed adequately. At the early stage of development of experimental atherosclerosis in rabbits the generation of PGI_2 by their coronary arteries is heavily suppressed.[81] In dogs PGI_2 protects against myocardial ischemia.[27] It also protects against the cyclic reductions of coronary blood flow following partial occlusion of the circumflex artery. This action of PGI_2 may be ascribed to its antagonism with TXA_2 at the level of platelets[75,76] or at the vascular level.[134] Transcardiac TXB_2 concentration is increased in patients with unstable angina who experience chest pain within 24 hr of study, whereas it is not elevated in patients with atherosclerotic coronary artery disease without pain for 96 hr.[135] This finding of Hirsch et al.[135] is of great interest when compared with the therapeutic reports of Szczeklik et al.[28,44,97] on the effectiveness of PGI_2 in unstable angina and its lack of effect in the treatment of exercise angina.

In the first group of 7 patients with effort angina and coronary atherosclerosis (as evidenced by coronary angiography) cardiac ischemia was precipitated by atrial pacing (100 to 170 beats per minute). The occurrence of chest pain, ischemic changes in ECG, pulmonary pressure indexes, and cardiac output were also recorded.

PGI_2 (5 to 10 ng/kg/min, i.v.) infused for various periods of time had no protective

Table 1

COMPARISON OF EFFICACY OF PGI$_2$ THERAPY WITH
CONVENTIONAL TREATMENT OF CRVO ASSESSED AT 3RD
MONTH AFTER COMPLETION OF THERAPY[a]

		Effect of pharmacological treatment						
		Eye fundus[b]				Visual acuity[b]		
Type of pharmacological treatment	Total no. of patients	++	+	∅	−	+	∅	−
PGI$_2$	17	6	6	5	0	9	5	3
Conventional	10	0	2	5	3	2	3	5

[a] See text.
[b] ++: Improvement, +: modest improvement, ∅: no change, and −: worsening.

effect against pain and cardiac ischemia which were induced by atrial pacing, although PGI$_2$ increased the ratio of cardiac index to pulmonary artery end-diastolic pressure. Bergman et al.[136] observed prolongation of atrial pacing time during infusion of PGI$_2$ in patients with angina.

The second group consisted of 11 patients with unstable angina that had begun 5 days to 3 months before admission. After 5 days of observation, during which nitroglycerine intake varied from 1 to 7 tablets daily, PGI$_2$ (5 ng/kg/min) was infused intravenously for 24 to 72 hr. Six of 11 patients remained free of angina for the subsequent 12-week period. In the remaining 5 patients nitroglycerine intake was only insignificantly reduced for various periods of time. PGE$_1$ (10 to 20 ng/kg/min, i.v.) was also effective in patients with unstable angina, even those who had been resistant to maximal doses of beta-adrenolytic agents and nitroglycerine.[95]

In conclusion PGI$_2$, while ineffective in effort angina, is effective in some patients with unstable angina in whose coronary bed an overproduction of TXA$_2$ by platelets may correctly be suspected.[135] The group of patients with "unstable angina" is still heterogenous and the response to PGI$_2$ may help in understanding the etiopathological background of this disease. The safety of intravenous[28,136] and intracoronary infusions of PGI$_2$ in patients with coronary artery disease has been established.

I. Thrombotic Microangiopathy

PGI$_2$ deficiency has been reported not only in atherosclerosis,[81] but also in thrombotic thrombocytopenic purpura (TTP),[138] hemolytic uremic syndrome (HUS),[139] preeclampsia,[140-142] and systemic lupus erythematosus (SLE).[143] The term "thrombotic microangiopathy" has been used to describe TTP and HUS as well as the complications of preeclampsia and SLE.[135] Remuzzi and Perico[142] proposed that an imbalance between PGI$_2$ and TXA$_2$ in thrombotic microangiopathy could result from the presence of inhibitory plasma factors or the absence of stimulatory plasma factors for the generation of PGI$_2$. Intravenous infusions of PGI$_2$ in HUS[144] and in preeclampsia[145-147] produced beneficial effects in patients. The reports on the response of patients with TTP to therapy with PGI$_2$ are conflicting. PGI$_2$ infusion into two patients with TTP did not correct their platelet count;[138,148] however, when PGI$_2$ was infused during 18 days in another patient with TTP an increase in platelet count and an improvement in the neurological status of the patient was observed.[149] Reports on these few patients suggest that controlled clinical trials with PGI$_2$ in thrombotic microangiopathy are required.

J. Ischemic Stroke

We have recently published a paper[36] on administration of PGI$_2$ to 10 patients with ischemic stroke. Patients were relatively young (53 ± 6 years old, 7 men and 3 women) with no previous history of transient ischemic attacks (TIA), although two of them suffered from effort angina pectoris in the past.

PGI_2 (2.5 to 5 ng/kg/min in 6-hr courses separated by 6-hr breaks) was administered not earlier than 1 day and not later than 5 days after ischemic stroke was completed. In all but two patients carotid angiography showed total or partial occlusion of one or more cranial or extracranial arteries. In the remaining 2 patients a generalized atherosclerosis of cerebral arteries was seen. As early as during the first few hours of the PGI_2 infusion the first signs of regression of hemiplegia in affected extremities, clearing of consciousness, and subsidence of the electroencephalographic changes typical of brain edema were observed. In the course of the next 4 to 8 weeks 6 patients were released from the hospital with a trace of asymmetry in reflexes and no sign of the aphasia that had been present in 3 of them on admission. Three patients still suffered from a rudimentary paresis in the upper limbs. One patient died 2 weeks after the termination of the therapy with PGI_2 because of a sudden occlusion of the contralateral carotid artery. Seven months later none of the remaining 9 patients suffered a second stroke or even TIA. All of them felt efficient physically and mentally, although two of them were treated pharmacologically for arterial hypertension and one for angina pectoris.

A comparison of control and post-treatment angiography in two patients of the first group was against our working hypothesis that PGI_2, because of its disaggregatory[66] or fibrinolytic[29] actions, had disintegrated thrombus in carotid or cerebral arteries and let blood into the ischemic area. PGI_2 is supposed to be a dilator of cerebral blood vessels.[8,150,152] Cerebral ischemia is associated with a release of vasoconstrictor prostanoids in the ischemic regions,[153,155] which may be responsible for postischemic hypoperfusion,[43,156] recurring decline in cerebral blood flow (CBF),[78,157] and neuronal hypermetabolism.[158] Cyclooxygenase inhibitors,[43,78,159] TXA_2 synthetase inhibitors,[78] and PGI_2[43,78,160] protect against experimental postischemic brain damage.

Perhaps in the patients studied PGI_2 increased cerebral blood flow through ischemic regions selectively, since PGI_2 would selectively lower tone in those cerebral arteries contracted by $PGF_{2\alpha}$ or 5-HT.[150,151] Selective vasodilatation by PGI_2 in a damaged hemisphere might be reinforced by inhibition of the release of TXA_2 and 5-HT from platelets[52] which are activated at the site of arterial stenosis. Finally, administration of PGI_2 is consistently associated with facial flush, headache, restlessness, fidgeting, lightheadedness, drowsiness,[32,44,59,96] extrapyramidal involuntary movements, paresthesia, melalgia, and suppression of epileptic episodes (unpublished data). This suggests that PGI_2 not only increases blood perfusion through facial skin capillaries, but may also have a similar action on intracranial blood vessels.

Our clinical observations strongly support the experimentally deduced concept of Hallenbeck, Furlow, and others[43,156,161,162] that the combination of PGI_2 and a cyclooxygenase inhibitor may protect against postischemic cerebral hypoperfusion and promote postischemic neuronal recovery. Because of our clinical experience we are not convinced about the importance of the third partner, heparin.[162] A combination of TXA_2 synthetase inhibitor[78] and PGI_2 might be an alternative to a PGI_2-indomethacin combination in the next series of clinical trials (see also Chapter 15).

In controlled clinical trials Fields et al.[163,164] and the Canadian Cooperative Study Group[165] have shown that aspirin at a high dose of 1.3 g daily reduces the risk of stroke and stroke-related mortality in patients with TIA. In these studies attention was focused on the anti-aggregatory action of aspirin.[163,166] It might well be that aspirin at the doses that were used eliminated not only TXA_2 from platelets, but also vasoconstrictor PGs[151,167-170] from ischemic cerebral areas, thereby protecting patients with TIA against threatening stroke.

Too often an acute stroke is regarded as an end stage illness without any chance for pharmacological treatment. Indeed, the clinical literature does not allow us to be overly enthusiastic about the pharmacotherapy of stroke.[171-176] We believe that our data on PGI$_2$ in ischemic stroke certainly encourage further controlled studies.

V. SIDE EFFECTS OF PGI$_2$ THERAPY

Of the side effects which may occur during intravenous infusion of PGI$_2$, headache is one of the most common. It usually appears at doses higher than 5 ng/kg/min. If the infusion rate is reduced, headache disappears. Some patients can tolerate PGI$_2$ at a dose of 10 ng/kg/min without headache. The most consistent but less annoying effect is facial flush, which occurs in practically all patients treated with PGI$_2$ given by intravenous, intra-arterial, or by inhalatory routes. Flushing of palms and a feeling of warmth are also quite common. Restlessness, uneasiness, and drowsiness are experienced by some patients. Typical cardiovascular effects of PGI$_2$ consist of a modest hypotension and blunted tachycardia. Overdosage of PGI$_2$ (50 ng/kg/min) may result in a sudden drop of arterial blood pressure associated with bradycardia and fainting, which actually occurred when the author infused PGI$_2$ for the first time into healthy volunteers. We have never seen this side effect in patients who were treated for various reasons with PGI$_2$ in doses of 2 to 10 ng/kg/min intravenously. A paradoxical rise in arterial blood pressure was observed in 6 out of 167 patients receiving PGI$_2$. Three of these subjects had a history of untreated severe arterial hypertension. In patients with a history of myocardial ischemic disease infusions of PGI$_2$ may cause chest pain and ectopic beats may appear in their ECG. Cardiac side effects of PGI$_2$ were relatively rare and appeared in 9 of our patients. In patients with ischemic ulceration pain may occur during the period of infusion of PGI$_2$, although ultimately PGI$_2$ will relieve patients of rest pain.

Another local pain which is quite frequently evoked by PGI$_2$ is the jaw articular pain that is aggravated by chewing. The hyperglycemic effect of PGI$_2$ on carbohydrate metabolism is readily reversible after termination of the infusion of PGI$_2$. We hardly observed in our patients any GI disturbances during intravenous infusions of PGI$_2$ apart from the rare occurrence of nausea.

The highest rate of intravenous infusion of PGI$_2$ that is presently being used in our studies is 7.5 ng/kg/min, although most frequently doses of 2.5 to 5.0 ng/kg/min are sufficient to obtain a therapeutic effect. In the vast majority of patients the above side effects of PGI$_2$, if they appear, are readily tempered by adjustment of the rate of the drug infusion.

The above side effects which may occur in the course of administration of PGI$_2$ to man are listed on the basis of our published[5,7,44,59,61,97,177] and unpublished clinical observations, as well as those of the Wellcome group.[178]

Side effects of therapy with PGI$_2$ do not constitute serious clinical problems, although an experienced and highly qualified staff is no doubt required for the running of these clinical trials.

VI. CONCLUSIONS

PGI$_2$ prevents blood platelets from adhesion and aggregation. The release of TXA$_2$, 5-HT, ADP, β-thromboglobulin, coagulation factors, and destructive enzymes from platelets is also reduced by PGI$_2$. Thus, PGI$_2$ has not only antiaggregatory, but also anticoagulant properties. PGI$_2$ dissipates the preformed platelet thrombi and disintegrates circulating platelet aggregates. PGI$_2$ stimulates the plasma fibrinolytic system by converting plasminogen proactivator to the activator. Apart from the above thrombolytic properties, PGI_2 is one of the most potent vasodilators in renal, cerebral, pulmonary, and coronary vascular beds. PGI_2 releases renin from the kidney. On the other hand angiotensin II releases PGI_2 from the lungs. This positive feedback loop is controlled by additional mechanisms that affect the release of PGI_2 through stimulation of endothelial cholinergic receptors, renal beta-adrenergic receptors, and aortic chemoreceptors. Pharmacological interference with these mechanisms may lead to a substantial rise in blood levels of circulating PGI_2.

Clinical usefulness of PGI_2 is based mainly on an assumption that atherosclerosis is a disease of PGI_2 deficiency as is thrombotic microangiopathy. Therefore, PGI_2 was used as the substitution therapy in peripheral vascular disease (e.g., arteriosclerosis obliterans), angina pectoris, central retinal vein occlusion, sudden deafness, ischemic stroke, thrombotic thrombocytopenic purpura, hemolytic uremic syndrome, and preeclampsia. Other indications for PGI_2 in clinical trials included diseases in which overproduction of a vasoconstrictor TXA_2 could be suspected, e.g., in Raynaud's syndrome, primary pulmonary hypertension, coronary bypass, kidney transplants, and unstable angina. In all these instances PGI_2 was administered as a therapeutic agent. Peripheral vascular disease, Raynaud's syndrome, and extracorporeal circulation during heart surgery benefit from therapy with PGI_2, as has been demonstrated in both uncontrolled and controlled clinical trials. Other indications for therapy with PGI_2 must await double-blind studies.

Looking to the future one may say that the pioneer clinical trials with PGI_2 have opened the clinic door to stable analogues of PGI_2, to releasers of endogenous PGI_2, and to TX synthetase inhibitors.

REFERENCES

1. Bunting, S., Gryglewski, R., Moncada, S., and Vane, J. R., Arterial walls generate from prostaglandin endoperoxides a substance (Prostaglandin X) which relaxes strips of mesenteric and coeliac arteries and inhibits platelet aggregation, *Prostaglandins*, 12, 897, 1976.
2. Gryglewski, R. J., Bunting, S., Moncada, S., Flower, R. J., and Vane, J. R., Arterial walls are protected against deposition of platelet thrombi by a substance (Prostaglandin X) which they make from prostaglandin endoperoxides, *Prostaglandins*, 12, 685, 1976.
3. Moncada, S., Gryglewski, R. J., Bunting, S., and Vane, J. R., A lipid peroxide inhibits the enzyme in blood vessel microsomes that generates from prostaglandin endoperoxides the substance (Prostaglandin X) which prevents platelet aggregation, *Prostaglandins*, 12, 715, 1976.
4. Moncada, S., Gryglewski, R. J., Bunting, S., and Vane, J. R., An enzyme isolated from arteries transforms prostaglandin endoperoxides to an unstable substance that inhibits platelet aggregation, *Nature (London)*, 263, 663, 1976.
5. Szczeklik, A. and Gryglewski, R. J., Actions of prostacyclin in man, in *Prostacyclin*, Vane, J. R. and Bergstrom, S., Eds., Raven Press, New York, 1979, 393.
6. Szczeklik, A., Gryglewski, R. J., Niżankowski, R., Musial, J., Pietoń, R., and Mruk, J., Circulatory and antiplatelet effects of intravenous prostacyclin in healthy men, *Pharmacol. Res. Commun.*, 10, 545, 1978.
7. Dusting, G. J., Moncada, S., and Vane, J. R., Prostacyclin (PGX) is the endogenous metabolite responsible for relaxation of coronary arteries induced by arachidonic acid, *Prostaglandins*, 13, 3, 1977.
8. Boullin, D. J., Bunting, S., Blaso, W. P., Hunt, T. M., and Moncada, S., Response of human and baboon arteries to prostaglandin endoperoxide and biologically generated and synthetic prostacyclin: their relevance to arterial cerebral spasm in man, *Br. J. Clin. Pharmacol.*, 7, 139, 1979.
9. Coceani, F., Bishai, J., White, E., Badach, E., and Olley, P. M., Action of prostaglandin endoperoxides and thromboxanes on the lamb ductus arteriosus, *Am. J. Physiol.*, 234, 1117, 1978.

10. Sintetos, A. L., Bogler, P. M., and Ramwell, P. W., Effects of prostacyclin on isolated canine renal artery and vein, in *Prostacyclin*, Vane, J. R. and Bergstrom, S., Eds., Raven Press, New York, 1979, 269.
11. Levy, S. V., Contractile responses to prostacyclin (PGI$_2$) of isolated human saphenous and rat venous tissue, *Prostaglandins*, 16, 93, 1978.
12. Weeks, J. R. and DuCharme, S., The cardiovascular pharmacology of prostacyclin (PGI$_2$) in the dog and rat, in *Abstr. 1st Sov. Union Conf. Prostaglandins Exp. Clin. Med.*, Moscow, 1978, 76.
13. Armstrong, J. M., Chapple, D. J., Dusting, G. J., Hughes, R., Moncada, S., and Vane, J. R., Cardiovascular actions of prostacyclin in chloralose anaesthetized dogs, *Br. J. Pharmacol.*, 62, 125, 1978.
14. Kadovitz, P. J., Chapnick, B. M., Feigen, L. P., Hyman, A. L., Nelson, P. K., and Spannhake, E. W., Pulmonary and systemic vasodilatory effects of the newly discovered prostaglandin PGI$_2$, *J. Appl. Physiol.*, 45, 408, 1978.
15. Kadovitz, P. J., She, S. S., McNamara, D. B., Spannhake, E. W., and Hyman, A. L., Arachidonic acid transformation in the lung, in *Cardiovascular Pharmacology in Prostaglandins*, Herman, A. G., Vanhoutte, P. M., Denolin, S., and Goossens, A., Eds., Raven Press, New York, 1982, 287.
16. Szczeklik, J., Szczeklik, A., and Nizankowski, R., Prostacyclin for pulmonary hypertension, *Lancet*, 2, 1076, 1980.
17. O'Grady, J., Warrington, S., Moti, J., Bunting, S., Flower, R. J., Fowle, A. S. E., Higgs, E. A., and Moncada, S., Effect of intravenous infusion of prostacyclin in man, *Prostaglandins*, 19, 319, 1980.
18. Fletcher, J. R. and Ramwell, P. W., Comparison of the cardiovascular effects of prostacyclin with those of prostaglandins E$_2$ in the Rhesus monkey, in *Prostacyclin*, Vane, J. R. and Bergstrom, S., Eds., Raven Press, New York, 1979, 259.
19. Lefer, A. M., Ogletree, M. L., Smith, J. B., Silver, M. J., Nicolau, K. C., Barnette, W. E., and Gasic, G. P., Prostacyclin: a potentially valuable agent for preserving myocardial tissue in acute myocardial ischaemia, *Science*, 200, 52, 1978.
20. Hintze, T. H., Kaley, G., Martin, E. H., and Messiha, E. J., PGI$_2$ induces bradycardia in the dog, *Prostaglandins*, 15, 712, 1978.
21. Dusting, G. J., Chapple, D. J., Hughes, R., Moncada, S., and Vane, J. R., Prostacyclin induces coronary vasodilation in anaesthetized dogs, *Cardiovasc. Res.*, 12, 720, 1978.
22. Armstrong, J. M., Chapple, D. J., Dusting, G. J., Hughes, R., Moncada, S., and Vane, J. R., Cardiovascular actions of prostacyclin in chloralose anesthetized dogs, *Br. J. Pharmacol.*, 61, 136P, 1977.
23. Fiedler, V. R., Effects of prostacyclin on the coronary circulation in conscious dogs, in *Proc. 5th Int. Conf. Prostaglandins*, Fondazione Giovanni Lorenzini, Milan, 1982, 273.
24. Jentzer, J. H., Snnenblick, E. H., and Kirk, E. S., Coronary and systemic vasomotor effects of prostacyclin: implication for ischemic myocardium, in *Prostacyclin*, Vane, J. R. and Bergstrom, S., Eds., Raven Press, New York, 1979, 323.
25. Smirnov, J. E., Mentz, P. R., and Markov, C. M., Effect of prostacyclin on coronary blood flow and cardiac activity in normotensive and spontaneously hypertensive rats, in *Advances in Prostaglandin Thrombosis Research*, Vol. 7, Samuelsson, B., Ramwell, P. W., and Paoletti, R., Eds., Raven Press, New York, 1980, 631.
26. Ito, T., Ogawa, K., Enomoto, J., Hasimoto, H., Kai, J., and Satake, T., Comparison of the effects of PGI$_2$ and PGE$_1$ on coronary and systemic hemodynamics and coronary arterial cyclic nucleotide levels in dogs, in *Advances in Prostaglandin Thrombosis Research*, Vol. 7, Samuelsson, B., Ramwell, P. W., and Paoletti, R., Eds., Raven Press, New York, 1980, 641.
27. Lefer, A. M. and Smith, E. F., III, Protective action of prostacyclin in myocardial ischemia and trauma, in *Prostacyclin*, Vane, J. R. and Bergstrom, S., Eds., Raven Press, New York, 1979, 339.
28. Szczeklik, A., Szczeklik, J., Niżankowski, R., and Głuszko, P., Prostacyclin for unstable angina, *N. Engl. J. Med.*, 303, 881, 1980.
29. Dembińska-Kieć, A., Kostka-Trąbka, E., and Gryglewski, R. J., Effects of prostacyclin on fibrinolytic activity in patients with arteriosclerosis obliterans, *Thromb. Haemostas.*, 47, 190, 1982.
30. Araki, H. and Lefer, A. M., Cytoprotective actions of prostacyclin during hypoxia in the isolated perfused cat liver, *Am. J. Physiol.*, 238, H176, 1980.
31. Glessen, W. J. and Verdouw, P. D., Oxygen-sparing effect of prostacyclin is a possible mechanism for myocardial salvage, in *Proc. 5th Int. Conf. Prostaglandins*, Fondazione Giovanni Lorenzini, Milan, 1982, 274.
32. Szczeklik, A., Niżankowski, R., Skawiński, S., Głuszko, P., and Gryglewski, R. J., Successful therapy of advanced arteriosclerosis obliterans with prostacyclin, *Lancet*, 1, 1111, 1979.

33. Belch, J. J. F., McKay, A. J., Lowe, C. D. O., McLaren, M., Leiberman, G. P., Pollock, J. G., Forbes, C. D., and Prentice, C. R. M., A controlled trial of intravenous prostacyclin in the management of severe peripheral arterial disease, in *Proc. 5th Int. Conf. Prostaglandins,* Fondazione Giovanni Lorenzini, Milan, 1982, 292.

34. Belch, J. J. F., Newman, P., Drury, J. K., Capell, H., Leiberman, P., Forbes, C. D., and Prentice, C. R. M., A double-blind controlled clinical trial of prostacyclin in the treatment of Raynaud's syndrome, in *Proc. 5th Int. Conf. Prostaglandins,* Fondazione Giovanni Lorenzini, Milan, 1982, 291.

35. Żygulska-Mach, H., Kostka-Trąbka, E., Nitoń, A., and Gryglewski, R. J., Prostacyclin in central retinal vein occlusion, *Lancet,* 2, 1075, 1980.

36. Nowak, S., Kostka-Trąbka, E., and Gryglewski, R. J., Clinical use of prostacyclin (PGI$_2$) in ischaemic stroke, *Pharmacol. Res. Commun.,* 14, 879, 1982.

37. Lefer, A. M., Tabas, J., and Smith, E. F., Salutary effects of prostacyclin in endotoxic shock, *Pharmacology,* 21, 206, 1980.

38. Krausz, M. M., Utsunomiya, T., Feuerstein, G., Shepro, D., and Hechtman, H. B., Reversal of lethal endotoxemia with prostacyclin, *Surg. Forum,* 31, 37, 1980.

39. Lefer, A. M., Sollott, S. L., and Galvin, M. J., Beneficial actions of prostacyclin in traumatic shock, *Prostaglandins,* 17, 761, 1979.

40. Bult, H. and Herman, A. G., Prostaglandins and circulatory shock, in *Cardiovascular Pharmacology in Prostaglandins,* Herman, A. G., Vanhoutte, P. W., Denolin, G., and Goossens, A., Eds., Raven Press, New York, 1982, 327.

41. Messina, E. J. and Kaley, G., Microcirculatory responses to prostacyclin and PGE$_2$ in rat cremaster muscle, in *Advances in Prostaglandin Thrombosis Research,* Vol. 7, Samuelsson, B., Ramwell, P. W., and Paoletti, R., Eds., Raven Press, New York, 1980, 719.

42. Higgs, G. A., Prostaglandins and the microcirculation, in *Cardiovascular Pharmacology in Prostaglandins,* Herman, A. G., Vanhoutte, P. W., Denilin, G., and Goossens, A., Eds., Raven Press, New York, 1982, 315.

43. Hallenbeck, J. M. and Furlow, T. W., Jr., Prostaglandins influence nutrient perfusion in brain during the postischemic period, in *Prostacyclin,* Vane, J. R. and Bergstrom, S., Eds., Raven Press, New York, 1979, 299.

44. Szczeklik, A. and Gryglewski, R. J., Prostaglandins as therapeutic agents in cardiovascular disease, in *Cardiovascular Pharmacology in Prostaglandins,* Herman, A. G., Vanhoutte, P. W., Denolin, G., and Goossens, A., Eds., Raven Press, New York, 1982, 347.

45. Whittle, B. J. R., Moncada, S., and Vane, J. R., Comparison of the effects of prostacyclin, prostaglandin E$_1$ and D$_2$ on platelet aggregation of different species, *Prostaglandins,* 16, 373, 1978.

46. Bussolino, F. and Camussi, G., Effect of prostacyclin on platelet activating factor induced platelet aggregation, *Prostaglandins,* 20, 781, 1980.

47. Tateson, J. E., Moncada, S., and Vane, J. R., Effects of prostacyclin (PGX) on cyclic AMP concentrations in human platelets, *Prostaglandins,* 13, 389, 1977.

48. Gorman, R. R., Bunting, S., and Miller, O. V., Modulation of human platelet adenylate cyclase by prostacyclin (PGX), *Prostaglandins,* 13, 377, 1977.

49. MacIntyre, D. E. and Gordoy, J. L., Discrimination between platelet prostaglandin receptors with a specific antagonist of biosenoic prostaglandins, *Thromb. Res.,* 11, 705, 1977.

50. Miller, O. V. and Gorman, R. R., Evidence for distinct prostacyclin I$_2$ and D$_2$ receptors in human platelets, *J. Pharmacol. Exp. Ther.,* 210, 134, 1979.

51. Siegl, A. M., Smith, J. B., and Silver, M. J., Selective binding site for (^{3}H) prostacyclin in platelets, *J. Clin. Invest.,* 63, 215, 1979.

52. Karniguaian, A., Legrand, Y. J., and Caen, J. P., Prostaglandins: specific inhibition of platelet adhesion to collagen and relationship with cAMP level, *Prostaglandins,* 23, 437, 1982.

53. Repin, A., in *Abstr. 9th Int. Congr. Cardiol.,* Moscow, 1982.

54. Harsfalvi, J., Muszbek, L., Stadler, J., and Fesüs, L., Inhibition of platelet factor 3 availability by prostacyclin, *Prostaglandins,* 20, 935, 1980.

55. Ehrmann, H.L. and Jaffe, E.A., Prostacyclin (PGI$_2$) inhibits the development in human platelets of ADP and arachidonic acid-induced shape change and procoagulant activity, *Prostaglandins,* 20, 1103, 1980.

56. Fry, G. L., Czervionke, R. L., Hoak, J. C., Smith, J. B., and Haycraft, P. L., Platelet adherence to cultured vascular cells: influence of prostacyclin (PGI$_2$), *Blood,* 55, 271, 1980.

57. Higgs, E. A., Moncada, S., and Vane, J. R., Effect of prostacyclin (PGI$_2$) on platelet adhesion to rabbit arterial subendothelium, *Prostaglandins,* 16, 17, 1977.

58. Hawiger, J., Parkinson, S., and Timmons, S., Prostacyclin inhibits mobilization of fibrinogen-binding sites on human ADP and thrombin-treated platelets, *Nature (London),* 283, 195, 1980.

59. Gryglewski, R. J., Szczeklik, A., and Niżankowski, R., Antiplatelet action of intravenous infusion of prostacyclin in man, *Thromb. Res.,* 13, 153, 1978.

60. Higgs, E. A., Higgs, G. A., Moncada, S., and Vane, J. R., Prostacyclin (PGI$_2$) inhibits the formation of platelet thrombi in arterioles and venules of the hamster cheek pouch, *Br. J. Pharmacol.*, 63, 535, 1978.

61. Ubatuba, F. B., Moncada, S., and Vane, J. R., The effect of prostacyclin (PGI$_2$) on platelet behaviour, thrombus formation in vivo and bleeding time, *Thromb. Haemost.*, 41, 425, 1979.

62. Bayer, B. L., Blass, K. E., and Förster, W., Antiaggregatory effect of prostacyclin (PGI$_2$) in vivo, *Br. J. Pharmacol.*, 66, 10, 1979.

63. Utsunomiya, T., Krausz, M. M., Valeri, G. R., Shepro, D., and Hechtman, H. B., Treatment of pulmonary embolism with prostacyclin, *Surgery*, 88, 25, 1980.

64. Aiken, J. W., Gorman, R. R., and Shebuski, R. J., Prevention of blockage of partially obstructed coronary arteries with prostacyclin correlates with inhibition of platelet aggregation, *Prostaglandins*, 17, 483, 1979.

65. Aiken, J. W., Shebuski, R. J., and Gorman, R. R., Blockade of partially obstructed coronary arteries with platelet thrombi: comparison between its prevention with cyclooxygenase inhibitors versus prostacyclin, in *Advances in Prostaglandin Thrombosis Research*, Vol. 7, Samuelsson, B., Ramwell, P. W., and Paoletti, R., Eds., Raven Press, New York, 1980, 635.

66. Gryglewski, R. J., Korbut, R., and Ocetkiewicz, A., Generation of prostacyclin by lungs in vivo and its release into the arterial circulation, *Nature (London)*, 273, 765, 1978.

67. Brandt, R., Dembińska-Kieć, A., Korbut, R., Gryglewski, R. J., and Nowak, J., Release of prostacyclin from the human pulmonary vascular bed in response to cholinergic stimulation, *Acta Physiol. Scand.*, in press.

68. Nowak, J., Radomski, M., Kaijser, L., and Gryglewski, R. J., Conversion of exogenous arachidonic acid to prostaglandins in the pulmonary circulation in vivo, *Acta Physiol. Scand.*, 112, 405, 1981.

69. Gryglewski, R. J., Spławiński, J., and Korbut, R., Endogenous mechanisms that regulate prostacyclin release, in *Advances in Prostaglandin Thrombosis Research*, Vol. 7, Samuelsson, B., Ramwell, P. W., and Paoletti, R., Eds., Raven Press, New York, 1980, 777.

70. Dusting, G. J., Mullins, E. M., and Doyle, A. E., Angiotensin-induced prostacyclin release may contribute to the hypotensive action of converting enzyme inhibitors, in *Advances in Prostaglandin Thrombosis Research*, Vol. 7, Samuelsson, B., Ramwell, P. W., and Paoletti, R., Eds., Raven Press, New York, 1980, 815.

71. Gryglewski, R. J., Le poumon producteur de prostacycline, *Ann. Anesthesiol. Fr.*, 6, 613, 1980.

72. Gryglewski, R. J., Szczeklik, A., Kostka-Trąbka, E., and Żygulska-Mach, H., Prostacyclin-experimental and clinical approach, in *Proc. 5th Int. Conf. Prostaglandins*, Fondazione Giovanni Lorenzini, Milan, 1982, 595.

73. Ritter, J. M., Barrow, S. E., Blair, J. A., and Dollery, C. T., Release of prostacyclin in vivo and its role in man, *Lancet*, 1, 317, 1983.

74. Nowak, J., Brandt, R., Dembińska-Kieć, A., Gryglewski, R. J., and Korbut, R., A cholinergic agonist carbaminoylcholine stimulates the release of prostacyclin from the human pulmonary circulation in *Proc. 5th Int. Conf. Prostaglandins*, Fondazione Giovanni Lorenzini, Milan, 1982, 570.

75. Aiken, J. W., Shebuski, R. J., Miller, O. V., and Gorman, R., Endogenous prostacyclin contributes to the efficacy of a thromboxane synthetase inhibitor for preventing coronary artery thrombosis, *J. Pharmacol. Exp. Ther.*, 219, 299, 1981.

76. Aiken, J. W. and Shebuski, R. J., Comparison in anesthetized dogs of the antiaggregatory and hemodynamic effects of prostacyclin and a chemically stable prostacyclin analog 6 a-carba-PGI$_2$ (carbacyclin), *Prostaglandins*, 19, 629, 1980.

77. Uchida, Y. and Murao, S., Effect of prostaglandin I$_2$ on cyclical reductions of coronary blood flow, *Jpn. Circ. J.*, 43, 645, 1979.

78. Uchida, S. and Murao, S., Role of prostaglandin I$_2$ and thromboxane A$_2$ in recurring reduction of carotid and cerebral flow in dogs, *Stroke*, 12, 786, 1981.

79. Belch, J., McKay, A., McArdle, B., Leiberman, P., Pollock, Y. G., Lowe, G. O. O., Forbes, C. D., and Prentice, C. R. M., Epoprostenol (prostacyclin) and severe arterial disease, *Lancet*, 1, 315, 1983.

80. Dembińska-Kieć, A., Gryglewska, T., Żmuda, A., and Gryglewski, R. J., The generation of prostacyclin by arteries and by the coronary vascular bed is reduced in experimental atherosclerosis in rabbits, *Prostaglandins*, 14, 1025, 1977.

81. Gryglewski, R. J., Dembińska-Kieć, A., Żmuda, A., Chytkowski, A., and Gryglewska, T., Prostacyclin and thromboxane A$_2$ biosynthesis capacities of heart, arteries and platelets at various stages of experimental atherosclerosis in rabbits, *Atherosclerosis*, 31, 385, 1978.

82. Gryglewski, R. J., Prostaglandins, platelets and atherosclerosis, *CRC Rev. Biochem.*, 7, 291, 1980.

83. Gryglewski, R. J. and Szczeklik, A., Atherosclerosis and prostacyclin in *Cardiovascular Pharmacology in Prostaglandins*, Herman, A. G., Vanhoutte, P. W., Denolin, G., and Goossens, A., Eds., Raven Press, New York, 1982, 215.

84. Sinzinger, H., Silberbauer, K., and Feigl, W., Prostacyclin generation in atherosclerotic arteries, *Lancet*, 1, 469, 1979.

85. Makary, A., Pataki, M., Lusztig, G., Stadler, J., and Virag, S., Effect of prostacyclin (PGI₂) in experimental atherosclerosis in rabbits, in *Proc. 5th Int. Conf. Prostaglandins,* Fondazione Giovanni Lorenzini, Milan, 1982, 224.

86. McGiff, J. C., Spokas, E. G., and Wong, P. Y.-K., Stimulation of renin release by 6-oxo-prostaglandin E₁ and prostacyclin, *Br. J. Pharmacol.,* 75, 137, 1982.

87. Quilley, C. P., McGiff, J. C., Lee, W. H., Sun, F. F., and Wong, P. Y.-K., 6-Keto-PGE₁: a possible metabolite of prostacyclin having platelet antiaggregatory effects, *Hypertension,* 2, 524, 1980.

88. Wong, P. Y.-K., Lee, W. H., Chao, P. H. W., Reiss, R. F., and McGiff, J. C., Metabolism of prostacyclin by 9-hydroxy-prostaglandin dehydrogenase in human platelets, *J. Biol. Chem.,* 255, 9021, 1980.

89. Carlson, L. A., Prostaglandins: effect on the cardiovascular system in normal man and their use in peripheral vascular disease, in *Proc. 5th Int. Conf. Prostaglandins,* Fondazione Giovanni Lorenzini, Milan, 1982, 592.

90. Data, J. L., Intravenous prostaglandin E₁ (PGE₁): its use in peripheral vascular disease complications, in *Prostaglandins in Clinical Medicine,* Wu, K. K. and Rosse, E. C., Eds., Year Book Medical Publishing, Chicago, 1982, 205.

91. Olsson, A. G., Eriksson, G., and Eklund, A. E., Double-blind controlled study of the effect of prostaglandin E₁ on healing of ischemic ulcers of the lower limb, in *Prostaglandins in Clinical Medicine,* Wu, K. K. and Rossi, E. C., Eds., Year Book Medical Publishing Chicago, 1982, 225.

92. Olsson, A. G. and Carlson, L. A., Clinical, hemodynamic and metabolic effects of intraarterial infusion of prostaglandin E₁ in patients with peripheral vascular disease, in *Advances in Prostaglandin Thrombosis Research,* Vol. 1, Samuelsson, B. and Paoletti, R., Eds., Raven Press, New York, 1976, 429.

93. Pardy, B. J. and Eastcott, H. H. G., Prostaglandins and vasospasm, in *Prostaglandins in Clinical Medicine,* Wu, K. K. and Rossi, E. C., Eds., Year Book Medical Publishing, Chicago, 1982, 191.

94. Needham, K. E., Evenson, M. K., and Mason, D. T., Prostaglandin E₁ in ischaemic heart failure: demonstration of salutary actions on myocardial energetics and ventricular pump performance, in *Prostaglandins in Clinical Medicine,* Wu, K. K. and Rossi, E. C., Eds., Year Book Medical Publishing, Chicago, 1982, 289.

95. Nemerowski, M. and Shell, W., Prostaglandin E₁ therapy in unstable angina, in *Prostaglandins in Clinical Medicine,* Wu, K. K. and Rossi, E. C., Eds., Year Book Medical Publishing Chicago, 1982, 292.

96. Pickles, H. and O'Grady, J., Side effects occurring during administration of epoprostenol (prostacyclin PGI₂) in man, *Br. J. Pharmacol.,* 14, 177, 1982.

97. Szczeklik, A. and Gryglewski, R. J., Treatment of vascular disease with prostacyclin, in *Clinical Pharmacology of Prostacyclin,* Lewis, P. J. and O'Grady, J., Eds., Raven Press, New York, 1981, 159.

98. Dusting, G. J., Moncada, S., and Vane, J. R., Prostacyclin: its biosynthesis actions and clinical potential, in *Prostaglandins and the Cardiovascular System,* Oates, J. A., Ed., Raven Press, New York, 1982, 59.

99. Szczeklik, A., Gryglewski, R. J., Niżankowski, R., Skawiński, S., and Głuszko, P., Prostacyclin therapy of peripheral vascular disease, *Thromb. Res.,* 19, 191, 1980.

100. Hossman, V., Heinen, A., Anel, H., and Fitzgerald, G. A., A randomized placebo controlled trial of prostacyclin (PGI₂) in peripheral arterial disease, *Thromb. Res.,* 13, 153, 1981.

101. Pardy, B. J., Lewis, J. D., and Eastcott, H. H. G., Preliminary experience with prostaglandins E₁ and I₂ in peripheral vascular disease, *Surgery,* 88, 826, 1980.

102. Olsson, A. G., Intravenous prostacyclin for ischaemic ulcers in peripheral artery disease, *Lancet,* 2, 1076, 1980.

103. Vermylen, J., Chamone, D. A. F., Machin, S. Y., Defreyn, C. R., and Verstraete, M., Prostacyclin in inoperable ischemic rest pain, *Acta Ther.,* 6, 33, 1980.

104. Machin, S. J., Defreyn, G., Chamone, D. A. F., and Vermylen, J., Clinical infusions of prostacyclin in advanced arterial disease, in *Clinical Pharmacology of Prostacyclin,* Lewis, P. J. and O'Grady, J., Eds., Raven Press, New York, 1981, 173.

105. Fitzgerald, G. A., Hawiger, J., Oates, J. A., and Roberts, L. J., In vivo antiplatelet effect during low dose prostacyclin (PGI₂) in obstructive arterial disease, in *Proc. 5th Int. Conf. Prostaglandins,* Fondazione Giovanni Lorenzini, Milan, 1982, 308.

106. Sinzinger, H., Silberbauer, K., Horsch, A. K., and Gall, A., Decreased sensitivity of human platelets to PGI₂ during long-term intraarterial prostacyclin infusion in patients with peripheral vascular disease — a rebound phenomenon, *Prostaglandins,* 21, 49, 1981.

107. Dembińska-Kieć, A., Żmuda, A., Grodzińska, L., Bieroń, K., Basista, M., Kedzior, A., Kostka-Trąbka, E., Telesz, E., Żelazny, T., Increased platelet activity after treatment of prostacyclin infusion into man, *Prostaglandins,* 21, 827, 1981.

108. Silberbauer, K., Sinzinger, H., and Punzengruber, C., Long-term prostacyclin (PGI₂) therapy in peripheral vascular disease. Influence on some vascular and platelet regulation mechanisms, in *Prostaglandins in Clinical Medicine*, Wu, K. K. and Rossi, E. C., Eds., Year Book Medical Publishing, Chicago, 1982, 233.

109. Miller, O. V., Brown, W. P., Lund, J. E., and Gorman, R. R., Continuous infusion of prostacyclin in beagle dogs: desensitization of platelet adenylate cyclase and thrombocytopenia, in *Proc. 5th Int. Conf. Prostaglandins*, Fondazione Giovanni Lorenzini, Milan, 1982, 307.

110. Dieppe, P. A., Cliford, P. C., Martin, M. R. F., Whicker, J. T., and Baird, R. N., Intravenous infusions of prostaglandin E₁ and I₂ for the treatment of small artery ischemia and peripheral vasospasm, in *Prostaglandins in Clinical Medicine*, Wu, K. K. and Rossi, E. C., Eds., Year Book Medical Publishing, Chicago, 1982, 215.

111. Dowd, P. M., Martin, M. F. R., Cooke, E. D., Bowcock, S. A., Jones, R., Dieppe, P. A., and Kirby, J. D. T., Therapy of Raynaud's phenomenon by intravenous infusion of prostacyclin (PGI₂), *Br. J. Dermatol.*, 106, 81, 1982.

112. Belch, J. J. F., Newman, P., Drury, J. K., and Prentice, C. R. M., Successful treatment of Raynaud's syndrome with prostacyclin, *Thromb. Haemostas.*, 45, 255, 1981.

113. Belch, J. J. F., Drury, J. K., Capell, H., Forbes, C. D., Newman, P., McKenzie, F., Leiberman, P., and Prentice, C. R. M., Intermittent epoprostenol (prostacyclin infusion) in patients with Raynaud's syndrome. A double-blind trial, *Lancet*, 1, 313, 1983.

114. Szczeklik, J., Dubier, J. S., Mysik, M., Król, R., and Horzela, T., Effects of prostaglandin E₁ on pulmonary circulation in patients with pulmonary hypertension, *Br. Heart J.*, 40, 1397, 1978.

115. Lock, J. E., Olley, P. M., Coceani, F., Swyer, P. R., and Rowe, R. D., Use of prostacyclin in persistent foetal circulation, *Lancet*, 1, 1343, 1979.

116. Natkins, W. D., Peterson, M. P., Brone, R. K., Shannon, D. C., and Levine, L., Prostacyclin and prostaglandin E₁ for severe pulmonary artery hypertension, *Lancet*, 1, 1083, 1980.

117. Coceani, F. and Olley, P. M., Prostaglandins and the circulation at birth, in *Cardiovascular Pharmacology in Prostaglandins*, Herman, A. G., Vanhoutte, P. W., Denolin, G., and Goossens, A., Eds., Raven Press, New York, 1982, 303.

118. Friedman, W. F., Printz, M. P., Skidgel, R. A., Benson, L. N., and Zadnikova, M., Prostaglandins and the ductus arteriosus, in *Prostaglandins and the Cardiovascular System*, Oates, J. A., Ed., Raven Press, New York, 1982, 277.

119. Bunting, S., O'Grady, J., Fabiani, J. N., Terrier, E., Moncada, S., Vane, J. R., and Dubost, Ch., Cardiopulmonary bypass in man: effects of prostacyclin, in *Clinical Pharmacology of Prostacyclin*, Lewis, P. J. and O'Grady, J., Eds., Raven Press, New York, 1981, 181.

120. Walker, J. D., Davidson, J. F., Faichney, A., Wheatley, D., and Davidson, K., Prostacyclin in cardiopulmonary bypass surgery, in *Clinical Pharmacology of Prostacyclin*, Lewis, P. J. and O'Grady, J., Eds., Raven Press, New York, 1981, 195.

121. Bennett, J. G., Longmore, D. B., and O'Grady, J., Use of prostacyclin in cardiopulmonary bypass in man, in *Clinical Pharmacology of Prostacyclin*, Lewis, P. J. and O'Grady, J., Eds., Raven Press, New York, 1981, 201.

122. Chelly, J., Tricot, C., Garcia, A., Boucherie, J. C., Fabiani, J. N., Passalecq, J., and Dubost, C., Haemodynamic effects of prostacyclin infusion after coronary bypass surgery, in *Clinical Pharmacology of Prostacyclin*, Lewis, P. J. and O'Grady, J., Eds., Raven Press, New York, 1981, 209.

123. Longmore, D. B., Bennett, J. G., Hayle, P. M., Smith, M. A., Gregory, A., Osivand, T., and Jones, W. A., Prostacyclin administered during cardiopulmonary bypass in man, *Lancet*, 1, 800, 1981.

124. Radegran, K., Aren, C., Egberg, N., Papaconstatinou, C., and Teger-Nilsson, A. C., Experiences with use of prostacyclin in open heart surgery, in *Prostaglandins in Clinical Medicine*, Wu, K. K. and Rossi, C. E., Eds., Year Book Medical Publishing, Chicago, 1982, 379.

125. Kaye, M. P., Peterson, K. A., Noback, C. R., and Dewanjee, M. K., Hemodynamic and platelet-preserving effects of prostacyclin during cardiopulmonary bypass, in *Prostaglandins in Clinical Medicine*, Wu, K. K. and Rossi, E. C., Eds., Year Book Medical Publishing, Chicago, 1982, 371.

126. Woods, H. F., Ash, G., Weston, M. J., Bunting, S., Moncada, S., and Vane, J. R., Prostacyclin can replace heparin in hemodialysis in dogs, *Lancet*, 2, 1075A, 1980.

127. Longmore, D. B., Benett, G., Gueirrara, D., Smith, M., Bunting, S., Reed, P., Moncada, S., Read, N. G., and Vane, J. R., Prostacyclin: a solution to some problems of extracorporeal circulation, *Lancet*, 1, 1002, 1979.

128. Turney, J. H., Dodd, N. J., and Weston, M. J., Prostacyclin in extracorporeal circulation, *Lancet*, 1, 1101, 1981.

129. Zusman, R. M., Rubin, R. H., Cato, A. E., Cocchetto, D. M., Crow, J. W., and Tolkoff-Rubin, N., Hemodialysis using prostacyclin instead of heparin as the sole antithrombotic agent, *N. Engl. J. Med.*, 304, 934, 1981.

130. Leithner, C., Sinzinger, H., and Schwartz, M., Treatment of chronic kidney transplant rejection with prostacyclin: reduction of platelet deposition in the transplant, prolongation of platelet survival and improvement of transplant function, *Prostaglandins*, 22, 783, 1981.

131. Mundy, A. R., Bewick, M., Moncada, S., and Vane, J. R., Short-term suppression of hyperacute renal allograft rejection in presensitized dogs with prostacyclin, *Prostaglandins*, 19, 595, 1980.

132. Shaw, J. R. L., Influence of prostacyclin (PGI₂) infusion upon rejection of cardiac allografts in rats, in *Proc. 5th Conf. Prostaglandins*, Fondazione Giovanni Lorenzini, Milan, 1982, 637.

133. Sekuła, J., Olszewski, G., Kostka-Trąbka, E., and Gryglewski, R. J., Prostacyclin in sudden deafness of unknown origin, manuscript in preparation.

134. Uchida, Y., Yoshimoto, N., and Murao, S., Angiographic changes in the coronary artery associated with cyclical reductions of coronary blood pressure, *Jpn. Circ. J.*, 44, 163, 1980.

135. Hirsh, P. D., Hills, L. D., Campbell, W. B., Firth, B. G., and Willerson, J. T., Coronary prostacyclin and thromboxane levels in patients with coronary artery disease, in *Prostaglandins in Clinical Medicine*, Wu, K. K. and Rossi, E. C., Eds., Year Book Medical Publishing, Chicago, 1982, 273.

136. Bergman, G., Daly, R., Atkinson, L., Rothman, M., Richardson, J. P., Jackson, G., and Jawitt, D. E., Prostacyclin haemodynamic and metabolic effects in patients with coronary disease, *Lancet*, 1, 569, 1981.

137. Hall, R. J. C. and Dewar, H. A., Safety of coronary arterial prostacyclin infusion, *Lancet*, 1, 949, 1981.

138. Hensby, C. N., Lewis, P. J., Hilgard, P., Mufti, G. J., Hows, J., and Webster, J., Prostacyclin deficiency in thrombotic thrombocytopenic purpura, *Lancet*, 2, 748, 1979.

139. Webster, J., Rees, A. J., Lewis, P. J., and Hensby, C. N., Prostacyclin deficiency in haemolytic uraemic syndrome, *Br. Med. J.*, 281, 1980.

140. Bodzenta, A., Thomson, J. M., and Poller, L., Prostacyclin activity in amniotic fluid in pre-eclampsia, *Lancet*, 2, 650, 1980.

141. Downing, J., Shepherd, G. L., and Lewis, J. P., Reduced prostacyclin production in pre-eclampsia, *Lancet*, 2, 1374, 1980.

142. Remuzzi, G. and Perico, N., Prostacyclin in thrombotic thrombocytopenic purpura and hemolytic uremic syndrome, in *Prostaglandins in Clinical Medicine*, Wu, K.K. and Rossi, E.C., Eds., Year Book Medical Publishing, Chicago, 1982, 319.

143. Carreras, L. O., Defreyn, G., Machin, S. J., Vermylen, J., Deman, R., Spitz, B., and VanAsche A., Arterial thrombosis, intrauterine death and "lupus" anticoagulant detection of immunoglobulin interfering with prostacyclin formation, *Lancet*, 1, 244, 1981.

144. Webster, J., Borysiewicz, L. K., Rees, A. J., and Lewis, P. J., Prostacyclin therapy for haemolytic uraemic syndrome, in *Clinical Pharmacology of Prostacyclin*, Lewis, P. J. and O'Grady, J., Eds., Raven Press, New York, 1981, 77.

145. Fidler, J., Ellis, C., Bennett, M. J., deSwiet, M., and Lewis, P. J., Prostacyclin and preeclamptic toxaemia, in *Clinical Pharmacology of Prostacyclin*, Lewis, P. J. and O'Grady, J., Eds., Raven Press, New York, 1981, 141.

146. Fidler, J., Bermett, M. J., deSwiet, M., Ellis, C., and Lewis, P. J., Treatment of pregnancy hypertension with prostacyclin, *Lancet*, 2, 31, 1980.

147. Remuzzi, G., Marches, D., Mecca, G., Misiani, R., Rossi, E., Donati, M. B., and deGaetano, G., Reduction of fetal vascular prostacyclin activity in pre-eclampsia, *Lancet*, 2, 310, 1980.

148. Budd, G. T., Bukowski, R. M., Lucas, F. V., Cato, A. E., and Cocchetto, D. M., Prostacyclin therapy of thrombotic thrombocytopenic purpura, *Lancet*, 2, 915, 1980.

149. Fitzgerald, G. A., Roberts, L. J., Maas, D., Brash, A. R., and Oates, J. A., Intravenous prostacyclin in thrombotic thrombocytopenic purpura, in *Clinical Pharmacology of Prostacyclin*, Lewis, P. J. and O'Grady, J., Raven Press, New York, 1981, 81.

150. Chapleau, D. E. and White, R. P., Effects of prostacyclin on the canine isolated basilar artery, *Prostaglandins*, 17, 573, 1979.

151. Paul, K. S., Whalley, E. T., Forster, C., and Lye, R., Relaxant and contractile effects of prostanoids on human basilar artery in vitro, in *Proc. 5th Int. Conf. Prostaglandins*, Fondazione Giovanni Lorenzini, Milan, 1982, 787.

152. Pickard, J. D., Tamura, A., McGeorge, A., and Fitch, W., Prostacyclin reverses the effect of indomethacin on the cerebral circulation, in *Pathophysiological Pharmacotherapy for Cerebrovascular Disorders*, Betz, E., Ed., Gerhard Witzstrock, Baden-Baden, 1980, 56.

153. Abdel-Halim, M. S., Lunden, J., Cseh, G., and Anggard, E., Prostaglandin profiles in venous tissue and blood vessels of the brain of various animals, *Prostaglandins*, 19, 249, 1980.

154. Abdel-Halim, M. S., vonHolts, H., Meyerson, B., Sachs, C., and Anggard, E., Prostaglandin profiles in tissues and blood vessels from human brain, *J. Neurochem.*, 34, 1331, 1980.

155. Gaudet, R. J. and Levine, L., Transient cerebral ischaemia and brain prostaglandins, *Biochem. Biophys. Res. Commun.*, 86, 893, 1979.

156. Furlow, T. W., Jr. and Hallenbeck, J. M., Indomethacin prevents impaired perfusion of the dog's brain after global ischaemia, *Stroke*, 9, 591, 1978.

157. Uchida, Y. and Murao, S., Angiographic changes associated with recurrent reduction of carotid and cerebral blood flow with special reference to transient focal cerebral ischemic attacks, *Jpn. Circ. J.*, 45, 427, 1981.

158. Vincent, J. E., Zijlstra, F. J., and Dzdjie, M. R., Formation of prostaglandins in rat brain, lack of effect of enkephalin, in *Advances in Prostaglandin Thrombosis Research*, Vol. 8, Samuelsson, B., Ramwell, P. W., and Paoletti, R., Raven Press, New York, 1980, 12A.

159. Bhakoo, K. K., Lascelles, P. T., Crockard, H. A., and Avery, S. F., Brain prostaglandins and cerebral oedema following temporary vascular occlusion in gerbils, in *Proc. 5th Int. Conf. Prostaglandins*, Fondazione Giovanni Lorenzini, Milan, 1982, 796.

160. Borzeix, M. G. and Cahn, J., Effect of ZK 36 374 (PGI$_2$) on Na arachidonate induced cerebral infarct in hypertensive rats, in *Proc. 5 Int. Conf. Prostaglandins*, Fondazione Giovanni Lorenzini, Milan, 1982, 800.

161. Hallenbeck, J. M. and Furlow, T. W., Jr., Prostaglandin I$_2$ and indomethacin prevent impairment of postischemic brain reperfusion in the dog, *Stroke*, 10, 629, 1979.

162. Hallenbeck, J. M., Leitgh, D. R., Dutka, A. J., and Greenbaum, L. J., Jr., PGI$_2$ indomethacin and heparin promote postischemic neoronal recovery in dogs when administered therapeutically, in *Prostaglandins in Clinical Medicine*, Wu, K. K. and Rossi, E. C., Eds., Year Book Medical Publishing, Chicago, 1982, 335.

163. Fields, W. S., Present status of platelet-modulating therapy in cerebrovascular disease, in *Cardiovascular Pharmacology in Prostaglandins*, Herman, A. G., Vanhoutte, P. W., Denolin, G., and Goossens, A., Eds., Raven Press, New York, 1982, 391.

164. Fields, W. S., Lemak, N. A., Frankowski, R. F., and Hady, R. J., Controlled trail of aspirin in cerebral ischaemia, *Stroke*, 8, 301, 1977.

165. Barnett, H. J. M., A randomized trial of aspirin and sulfinpyrazone in threatened stroke, *N. Engl. J. Med.*, 299, 53, 1978.

166. Mustard, J. F. and Packam, M. A., Role of platelets in stroke and transient ischaemic attacks, in *Prostaglandins, Platelets, Lipids: New Developments in Atherosclerosis*, Conn, H. L., Ed., Elsevier-North Holland, New York, 1981, 95.

167. Allen, G. S., Gross, C. J., French, W. A., and Chou, S. N., Cerebral arterial spasm. V. In vitro contractile activity of vasoactive agents including human CCF on human basilar and anterior cerebral arteries, *J. Neurosurg.*, 44, 594, 1976.

168. Pennink, M., White, R. P., Crockarell, J. R., and Robertson, J. T., Role of prostaglandin F$_2$ in the genesis of experimental cerebral vasospasm, *J. Neurosurg.*, 37, 398, 1972.

169. Toda, N., Different resposiveness of a variety of isolated dog arteries to prostaglandin D$_2$, *Prostaglandins*, 23, 99, 1982.

170. White, R. P., Hagen, A. A., Morgan, H., Dawson, N. N., and Robertson, J. T., Experimental study on the genesis of cerebral vasospasm, *Stroke*, 6, 52, 1975.

171. Britton, M., DeFaire, V., Helmers, C., Miah, K., and Rane, A., A double-blind evaluation of theophylline infusion in acute cerebral infarction, in *Cerebral Vascular Disease*, Vol. 6, Meyer, J. S., Ed., Excerpta Medica, Amsterdam, 1981, 31.

172. Heiss, W. D., Effect of drugs on cerebral blood flow in man, in *Advances in Neurology*, Vol. 25, Goldstein, M. et al., Eds., Raven Press, New York, 1979, 95.

173. Hossmann, K. A., Experimental basis for the treatment of cerebral ischemia, in *Advances in Neurology*, Vol. 25, Goldstein, M. et al., Eds., Raven Press, New York, 1979, 253.

174. Mulley, G., Wilcox, R. G., and Mitchell, Y. R. A., Dexamethasone in acute stroke, *Br. Med. J.*, 2, 994, 1978.

175. Norris, J. W., Steriod therapy in acute cerebral infarction, *Arch. Neurol.*, 33, 69, 1976.

176. Scheinberg, P., Management of acute ischaemic stroke, *Advances in Neurology*, Vol. 25, Goldstein, M., Ed., Raven Press, New York, 1979, 263.

177. Szczeklik, A., Gryglewski, R. J., Niżankowska, E., Niżankowski, R., and Musiał, J., Pulmonary and anti-platelet effects of intravenous and inhaled prostacyclin in man, *Prostaglandins*, 16, 651, 1978.

178. O'Grady, J., Warrington, J., Moti, M. J., Bunting, S., Flower, R. J., Fowle, A. S. E., Wiggs, E. A., and Moncada, S., Effects of intravenous prostacyclin infusions in healthy volunteers — some preliminary observations, in *Prostacyclin*, Vane, J. R. and Bergstrom, S., Eds., Raven Press, New York, 1979, 409.

Chapter 13

PROSTAGLANDINS AND THE TREATMENT OF SEVERE ISCHEMIC PERIPHERAL VASCULAR DISEASE

Anders G. Olsson and Lars A. Carlson

TABLE OF CONTENTS

I. INTRODUCTION

The end stage of atherosclerotic peripheral artery disease (PAD) is a condition causing great trouble to the patient due to rest pain and ulceration. Also it is one of the most common causes of disability in the middle aged and elderly.[1] The development of these symptoms in an ischemic limb indicates a serious threat to the limb and urgent treatment is needed if amputation is to be avoided. Many patients are not suitable for reconstructive vascular surgery due to extensive arterial disease. Therefore, there is a great need for medical treatment which could relieve these severe symptoms.

II. PROSTAGLANDINS

In this situation two prostaglandins (PGs) are of particular interest:PGE_1 and PGI_2 (prostacyclin).

A. PGE_1

The interest was originally focused on PGE_1 because of its vasodilatory potency.[2] On a weight basis it is one of the most powerful vasodilatory substances known. It also has other properties which might be of value in the treatment of PAD, e.g., platelet aggregation inhibition.[3]

B. PGI_2

PGI_2 is an extremely potent anti-aggregatory substance[4] and has the unique capability of dissolving existing platelet aggregates. According to a hypothesis proposed by Moncada et al.,[4] PGI_2 is responsible for keeping the endothelium free from platelet aggregation. Its potential role as a therapeutic agent in a number of diseases involving thrombotic complications, including atherosclerosis, is evident.

III. PROSTAGLANDINS IN PERIPHERAL VASCULAR DISEASE

The use of PGs for the treatment of the end stage of PAD was introduced by Carlson and Eriksson in 1973. In a number of studies during the last 10 years, PGE_1 and later PGI_2 have been investigated with regard to their capacity for diminishing end stage symptoms and lesions of PAD. We will review the literature on what has been done to date in this context with the two PGs and conclude by summarizing what remains to be done with them.

A. PGE_1
1. Uncontrolled Observations
Ten years ago we reported on the first four cases of advanced end stage peripheral artery disease successfully treated with PGE_1 intraarterially.[5] In these cases there was no additional conservative or reconstructive treatment that could be offered to the patients. PGE_1 was infused into a catheter placed in the femoral artery in a dose of 1 ng/kg/min for 10 min every hour for 24 to 72 hr. In three patients the rest pain in the legs completely disappeared in response to the infusion. No definite effect was reported by the fourth patient. In all cases there was a considerable improvement in rest pain. The gangrene in two cases healed. The vasodilatory action of PGE_1 as well as its effects on metabolism and platelet aggregation were mentioned as possible causes of the remarkably beneficial action of PGE_1 in these four patients. During our subsequent work with PGE_1 we have reported striking effects with intravenous administration.[6,7] Following our original observations good experience with PGE_1 treatment in atherosclerotic PAD has been reported in open studies in a number of investigations.[8-12]

2. Controlled Studies

Both ischemic pain and ulcers due to atherosclerotic PAD are subject to a great "spontaneous" variability during the course of the disease. In addition, considerable placebo effect occurs in studies of this kind, which has been documented for ischemic pain by Lowe et al.[13] and for ulcer healing by the authors.[14] Therefore, controlled studies are necessary to correctly assess the beneficial effects of PGs in PAD.

For PGE_1 the most convincing study is that performed by Sakaguchi et al.[15] (double-blind). Patients with intractable ischemic ulcers were randomly treated with PGE_1 intraarterially at either a high or a low dose or by inositol nicotinate. The high dose was 0.15 ng/kg/min close to the original mean dose used by the authors[5] of 0.17 ng/kg/min. All together 65 patients were treated and the results blindly evaluated by an elected Evaluation Committee. In the three groups, high and low PGE_1 and niacinate, 68, 44, and 39%, respectively, responded favorably according to an analogue scale used in the evaluation of serial ulcer photos. Significant differences in treatment effects between the groups ($p < 0.05$) were obtained. The authors concluded that the results of this study emphatically suggest that PGE_1 infusions at individualized doses is the treatment of choice in patients with peripheral vascular disorders for whom amputations are necessary.

One limitation of the study from the point of view of atherosclerosis is that the vast majority of the patients suffered from thrombangitis obliterans, a common cause of ischemic ulcers in Japan, but less common in Europe and in the U.S. Therefore, this study does not demonstrate long-term efficacy of PGE_1 in atherosclerosis. Another disadvantage of that study was the method of administering PGE_1: long-term intraarterial infusions (2 to 6 weeks). This type of administration is hardly feasible as a routine treatment in many places.

We have recently published a small double-blind controlled study with PGE_1 given intravenously by frequent injections for 3 days on two occasions.[14] The end point was ulcer healing as documented by serial stereophotography evaluated by computerized determination of ulcer areas and volumes.[16] This method determines ulcer dimensions with great accuracy. We showed a significant short-term healing effect after PGE_1, which was not noted after placebo. One month after the second treatment, however, no difference was seen between PGE_1 and placebo-treated groups. The conclusion of that study was that PGE_1 should be studied using longer treatment periods and higher doses. Again, controlled studies are mandatory because of the considerable placebo effect.

B. PGI₂

1. Uncontrolled Observations

Szczeklik et al.[17] reported in 1979 on 5 patients with advanced arteriosclerosis obliterans of the lower limbs treated with PGI_2 in doses of 5 to 10 ng/kg/min intraarterially for 72 hr. Focal necrosis regressed completely in 3 of 5 patients. Rest pain disappeared in all patients. One puzzling finding was that muscle blood flow to the limb, as measured by xenon-133 clearance, increased significantly not only during PGI_2 infusion, but also during 6 weeks of measurement after its termination.

We also note a good healing response to PGI_2 given intravenously in 6 of 8 patients treated openly in a dose of 1 to 5 ng/kg/min.[18] The effect on pain was equal to that of PGE_1 in our experience; however, the PGI_2 infusions in contrast to those with PGE_1 were often accompanied by side effects such as flushing, headache, nausea, and vomiting. The patients also often experienced a feeling of uneasiness.

Since these two encouraging initial studies of PGI_2, taken intraarterially and intravenously, our findings have been supported by some,[19] but not all[10,20] workers in uncontrolled studies.

2. Controlled Studies

Only one published study of controlled design has so far come to our attention.[21] Belch and associates carried out a double-blind controlled trial of intravenous PGI_2 as a treatment for rest pain due to severe peripheral arterial disease in 28 patients. Patients received either a 4 day PGI_2 infusion in buffer in a dose of up to 10 ng/kg/min or placebo infusion (buffer alone). The primary end point was the absence or improvement in rest pain on day 5. Patients were followed for 6 months after treatment and the following secondary end points were measured: recurrence of pain, healing of skin lesions, and surgical intervention. Results showed that on day 5 the PGI_2-treated patients had significantly less pain and required less analgesia than controls. At 1 and 6 months the PGI_2 patients were still improved and had undergone less surgery than controls.

Facial flushing was noted in nearly all patients during PGI_2 infusion with mild headache in over half. Four PGI_2 patients experienced nausea and vomiting, requiring decrease in PGI_2 dose to 7.5 ng/kg/min in 3 of the 4 patients.

The high frequency of side effects also demonstrated in this study raises questions regarding the reliability of the results. How could the study be kept blind as the authors claimed the study to be with these side effects? This is important, as only the subjective measurement of pain was used as end point.

IV. WHAT HAS NOT BEEN SHOWN AND WHAT REMAINS TO BE DONE

A. PGE_1

To summarize, PGE_1 has proven in a well-performed controlled study to be of prolonged therapeutic benefit in the treatment of ischemic ulcers due to thrombangitis obliterans when given intraarterially. When given intravenously in a low dose to patients with ulcers due to atherosclerotic PAD it has a temporary healing effect.

It has not been demonstrated so far that intravenous treatment with PGE_1 is of lasting benefit in healing and pain relief of ulcers due to atherosclerotic PAD. Consequently, this remains to be shown before the substance could be generally used.

The optimal treatment schedule of PGE_1 dose, timing, and duration has not yet been established. We do not know if there are certain subcategories of patients that benefit more than others.

B. PGI_2

No controlled study of PGI_2 given intraarterially is available. There is one study on the effects of ischemic pain by PGI_2 given intravenously. This showed that patients given PGI_2 had significantly less pain and took fewer analgesic tablets than the controls; however, the design of the study raises doubts regarding its blindness and to what extent the conclusions are valid. Controlled studies on the effects of intravenous PGI_2 on ulcer healing still remain to be done.

C. PGE_1 and PGI_2

It cannot be stated at present which of the PGs, PGE_1 or PGI_2, is better with regard to beneficial effects in PAD. Our impression is that PGI_2 has more frequent and severe side effects such as nausea, vomiting, flushing, and feeling of uneasiness than PGE_1. To assess both the effects on PAD and side effects, however, controlled comparative studies between PGE_1 and PGI_2 must be performed.

It should also be pointed out that it is by no means certain that the two PGs will equally affect different conditions in PAD. For example, treatment with PGE_1 might influence more vasospastic peripheral symptoms as it is primarily a vasodilator, while PGI_2 might have its best effects in thrombotic complications of PAD.

D. Prostaglandin Metabolism and Future Treatment

PGs are normally synthesized in the organism from certain essential fatty acids such as linoleic acid. It has recently been shown in man that the endogenous production of PGs can be augmented by the addition of essential fatty acids. Linoleic acid infusion induced a profound increase in immunoassayable 6-oxo-PGF_2 excretion (a PGI_2 metabolite).[22] Thus, another method of "PG treatment" would be the provision of ample amounts of precursor fatty acids.

Still another way of increasing PGI_2 production is the administration of specific blockers of thromboxane synthesis, thereby shunting the metabolism of endoperoxides from the thromboxane[23] pathway to the PGI_2 pathway. Such specific thromboxane synthetase inhibitors are already at hand and are being subjected to clinical evaluation.

ACKNOWLEDGMENTS

Supported by grants from the Swedish Medical Research Council (19X-204) and Tore Nilsons fond for medicinsk forskning and Torsten Soderbergs och Ragnar Soderbergs stiftelser.

REFERENCES

1. Hughson, W. G., Mann, J. I., and Garrod, I., Intermittent claudication: prevalence and risk factors, *Br. Med. J.,* 1, 179, 1978.
2. Bevegard S. and Oro, L., Effect of prostaglandin E_1 on forearm blood flow, *Scand. J. Clin. Lab. Invest.,* 23, 347, 1969.
3. Emmons, P. R., Hampton, J. R., Harrison, M. J. G., Honour, A. J., and Mitchell, R. A., Effect of prostaglandin E_1 on platelet behaviour in vitro and in vivo, *Br. Med. J.,* 2, 468, 1967.
4. Moncada, S., Gryglewski, R., Bunting, S., and Vane, J. R., An enzyme isolated from arteries transforms prostaglandin endoperoxides to an unstable substance that inhibits platelet aggregation, *Nature (London),* 263, 663, 1976.
5. Carlson, L. A. and Eriksson, I., Femoral-artery infusion of prostaglandin E_1 in severe peripheral vascular disease, *Lancet,* 1, 155, 1973.
6. Carlson, L. A. and Olsson, A. G., Intravenous prostaglandin E_1 in severe peripheral vascular disease, *Lancet,* 2, 810, 1976.
7. Carlson, L. A. and Olsson, A. G., PGE_1 in ischaemic peripheral vascular disease, in *The Practical Applications of Prostaglandins and Their Synthesis Inhibitors,* Karim, S. M. M., Ed., MTP Press, Lancaster, England, 1979, 39.
8. Molony, B. A., The early clinical experience with the vasodilator effects of PGE_1, as reported to the sponsor by several investigators, in *Proc. 13th Int. Congr. Intern. Med.,* Helsinki, 1976, 216.
9. Gruss, J. D., Kawai, S., Karadedos, C., and Bartels, D., Preliminary results with intraaterial long-term perfusion with prostaglandin E_1 in advanced peripheral arterial occlusive disease of the lower limbs in stage IV, *Dtsch. Med. Wochenschr.,* 103, 1624, 1978.
10. Pardy, J. B., Lewis, J. D., and Eastcott, H. H. G., Preliminary experience with prostaglandin E_1 and I_2 in peripheral vascular disease, *Surgery,* 88, 826, 1980.
11. Sethi, G. K., Scott, S. M., and Takaro, T., Effect of intra-arterial infusion of PGE_1 in patients with severe ischemia of lower extremity, *J. Cardiovasc. Surg.,* 21, 185, 1980.
12. Gruss, J. D., Karadedos, C., Bartels, D. and Okta, D., Intra-arterial perfusion with prostaglandin E_1 for limb salvage in cases with severe inoperable occlusive disease, in *Hormones and Vascular Disease,* Greenhalgh, R., Ed., Pitman, New York, 1981, 177.

13. Lowe, G. D. O., Dunlop, D. J., Lawson, D., Pollock, J. G., Watt, J. K., Forbes, C. D., Prentice, C. R. M., and Drummond, M. M., Double-blind controlled clinical trial of ancrod for ischaemic rest pain of the leg, *Angiology*, 33, 46, 1982.

14. Eklund, A. E., Eriksson, G., and Olsson, A. G., A controlled study showing significant short term effect of prostaglandin E₁ in healing of ischaemic ulcers of the lower limb in man, *Prostaglandins, Leukotrienes, Med.*, 8, 265, 1982.

15. Sakaguchi, S., Kusaba, A., Mishima, Y., Kamiya, K., Nishimura, A., Furukawa, K., Shionoya, S., Kawashima, M., Katsumura, T., and Sakuma, A., A multi-center double blind study with PGE₁ (α-cyclodextrin clathrate) in patients with ischemic ulcer of the extremities, *VASA*, 7, 263, 1978.

16. Eriksson, G., Eklund, A. E., Torlegard, K., and Dauphin, E., Evaluation of leg ulcer treatment with stereophotogrammetry, *Br. J. Dermatol.*, 101, 123, 1979.

17. Szczeklik, A., Skawiński, S., Głuszko, P., Niżankowski, R., Szczeklik, J., and Gryglewski, R. J., Successful therapy of advanced arteriosclerosis obliterans with prostacyclin, *Lancet*, 1, 1111, 1979.

18. Olsson, A. G., Intravenous prostacyclin for ischaemic ulcers in peripheral artery disease, *Lancet*, 2, 1076, 1980.

19. Hossman, V., Heinen, A., Auel, H., and Fitzgerald, A., A randomized, placebo controlled trial of prostacyclin (PGI₂) in peripheral arterial disease, *Thromb. Res.*, 22, 481, 1981.

20. Vermylen, J., Chamore, D. A. F., Machin, S. J., and Verstraete, M., Prostacyclin in inoperative ischaemic rest pain, *Acta Ther.*, 6, 33, 1980.

21. Belch, J. J., McArdle, B., Pollock, J. G., Forbes, C. D., McKay, A., Lieberman, P., Lowe, G. D. O., and Prentice, C. R. M., Epoprostenol (prostacyclin) and severe arterial disease. A double-blind trial, *Lancet*, 1, 315, 1983.

22. Epstein, M., Lifschitz, M., and Rappaport, K., Augmentation of prostaglandin production by linoleic acid in man, *Clin. Sci.*, 63, 565, 1982.

23. Vermylen, J., Carreras, L. O., Van Schaeren, J., Defreyn, G., Machin, S. J., and Verstraete, M., Thromboxane synthetase inhibiton as antithrombotic strategy, *Lancet*, 1, 1073, 1981.

Chapter 14

EFFECTS OF PROSTACYCLIN DURING CARDIOPULMONARY BYPASS

F. Reinhard Matthias, Heinrich Ditter, Dieter Heinrich, and Friedrich W. Hehrlein

TABLE OF CONTENTS

I. INTRODUCTION

Treatment of patients with techniques employing extracorporeal circulation (ECC) of blood leads to considerable alterations in hemostatic balance, which is often the cause of bleeding disorders and renal, pulmonary, or cerebral dysfunction.[1-7] Improvement in operative technique and in the equipment used did not sufficiently eliminate these problems until now. A major factor in the development of hemostatic defects during hemodialysis, hemoperfusion, or cardiopulmonary bypass (CPB), other than the contact activation of clotting factors, seems to be the platelet contact with foreign surfaces.[4,8] This results in an activation of platelets with partial or complete loss of platelet functions (e.g., platelet adhesivity and aggregability) and a decrease in platelet counts, which in the case of CPB can only partially be ascribed to dilution effects by nonblood priming solutions.[9-11]

While increasing plasma levels of platelet-specific proteins from α-granules during ECC were observed by several groups,[4,8,10] few reports exist on measurements of platelet or vessel wall prostaglandin (PG) metabolism during ECC. Addonizio et al.[8,12] found a marked elevation of plasma thromboxane B_2 (TXB_2) levels during simulated ECC, indicating a stimulation of the platelet cyclooxygenase/thromboxane synthetase system, which was only partially related to the release of α-granule contents and platelet loss. Davies et al.[13] reported an increase in thromboxane plasma levels during CPB, and they assumed that this could be attributed to consecutive induction of platelet aggregation and vasoconstriction.

Considering the increasing number of surgical procedures using a cardiopulmonary bypass system, many attempts were made to prevent ECC-induced platelet activation and consumption by substances influencing platelet metabolism or platelet membrane stability. PGE_1 was reported to preserve, at least partially, platelet count and function during and after ECC.[14,15] Over the last few years, prostacyclin (PGI_2), the most potent platelet inhibitor,[16] has been used by several groups. All reports showed a preservation of platelet counts, platelet function, and granule contents during hemodialysis, hemoperfusion, and cariopulmonary bypass.[11,17-26] Formation of microaggregates during hemodialysis and hemoperfusion was greatly reduced.[18,27] When PGI_2 was used without heparin anticoagulation during hemodialysis no blood clotting was observed.[27,28] This seems to be indicative of the importance of platelets in foreign surface-induced activation of hemostatic mechanisms and clot formation.[27]

II. METHODS

A prospective, randomized, and double-blind study was conducted on 40 male patients who underwent aortocoronary bypass operations.

A. Patient Groups

Twenty patients were treated with PGI_2 in a constant dose of 8 ng/kg/min from 2 min before onset of bypass circulation until the end of cardiopulmonary bypass (the PGI_2 was kindly provided by Wellcome Ltd./Beckenham, U. K.). It was dissolved 30 min before use in a glycine buffer at pH 10.5 and diluted with the same buffer to an appropriate volume. Twenty control patients received an equivalent volume of solution buffer without PGI_2 during the same period. Groups did not differ from each other with respect to age (PGI_2-treated group 54 ± 7 years, control group 53 ± 5 years) or preoperative ejection fraction.[29]

B. Anticoagulation of Patients

A heparin bolus (200 units/kg body weight) was given to all patients 6 min before

ECC (Liquemin® , Roche). Additional heparin (100 units/kg body weight) was injected after 1 hr bypass time or when activated, clotting time (Hemochron® time) decreased to 350 sec. Heparin was neutralized by injection of protamine chloride (2 mg/kg body weight, Roche) 15 min after the end of ECC.

C. ECC

A bubble oxygenator (Spiraflo® BOS-10, Bentley Laboratories, Calif.) was used. During ECC hypothermic body temperatures (approximately 30°C) were maintained. The priming solution (2941 ± 434 mℓ in the PGI$_2$ group and 2983 ± 339 mℓ in the placebo group) was composed of 250 to 500 mℓ of erythrocyte concentrate, 500 mℓ of 5% glucose, 500 mℓ of 5% laevulose, 500 to 1000 mℓ Ringer's lactate solution, 500 to 1500 mℓ plasma protein solution, 50 mℓ of 20% human albumin, and 40 to 60 mM potassium chloride. There was no significant difference in the composition of the priming solutions between the two treatment groups. Perfusion rates, arterial blood pressures and perfusion pressures, blood loss during and after operation, bleeding times, and urine production did not differ significantly between patient groups (data not shown here; for details see Heinrich et al.[29]).

D. Blood Sampling

Blood samples were collected immediately before initiation of anesthesia (sample 1), after thoracotomy (sample 2), after administration of 200 units of heparin per kilogram and before PGI$_2$ administration (sample 3), 2 min after onset of ECC (sample 4), and every 30 min thereafter (samples 5 to 9). Further blood samples were taken after termination of ECC and 5 min after protamine application (sample 10) and finally 2 hr (sample 11) and 24 hr (sample 12) after completion of CPB. All samples were taken from an arterial canule in the radial artery.

E. Laboratory Measurements

The levels of platelet α-granule constituents β-thromboglobulin (βTG) and platelet factor 4 (PF4) in plasma were determined using commercially available radioimmunoassay kits (Amersham and Abbott, respectively). Blood samples (2.5 mℓ) were immediately transferred into precooled sampling tubes (provided with the Amersham kit) containing an anticoagulant mixture of EDTA and theophylline (final concentrations 8.5 mM and 0.95 mM, respectively) and gently mixed and cooled in a crushed ice water bath until centrifugation (4°C, 30 min, 2000 g); 0.5 mℓ plasma from each sample was stored at −20°C until the radioimmunoassay was to be performed. Normal values in our laboratory for βTG and PF4 were 35.7 ± 9.7 ng/mℓ (n = 47; range 17 to 68 ng/mℓ) and 11.5 ± 4.4 ng/mℓ (n = 47; range 2.4 to 28.0 ng/mℓ), respectively, and did not differ from reported normal values obtained by anticoagulant mixtures containing PGE$_1$.[30,31]

F. Thromboxane B$_2$ (TXB$_2$) and 6-Keto-Prostaglandin F$_{1\alpha}$ (6-Keto-PGF$_{1\alpha}$) Assays

Nine volumes of blood were collected into 1 volume of a citrate buffer (final concentration 0.01 M) containing indomethacin (final concentration 55 μM), cooled, and immediately centrifuged at 4°C for 30 min at 2000 g. Plasma was stored at −20°C and processed without extraction. We used our own modifications[21] of radioimmunological procedures described by Anhut et al.[32] and Peskar et al.[33,34] Specific antibodies were purchased from Seragen Inc. of Boston. Tritium labeled TXB$_2$ (specific activity 100 to 150 Ci/mmol) and 6-keto-PGF$_{1\alpha}$ (specific activity 100 to 150 Ci/mmol) were obtained from NEN (Dreieich, West Germany). Unlabeled standards were provided by the Upjohn Company, Kalamazoo, Mich. Blanks, binding controls, and standard curves ranging from 100 to 7.8 pg were run with each assay using charcoal-absorbed human plasma which was anticoagulated with citrate and indomethacin in the same way as unknown samples. For TXB_2, coefficients of variation at the levels of 250, 125, and 62.5 pg were 15.1, 4.8, and 11.0%, respectively. The anti-TXB_2 antibody cross-reacted with $PGF_{2\alpha}$, 0.01%; PGE_2, 0.17%; PGD_2, 1.57%; and 6-keto-$PGF_{1\alpha}$, <0.01%. For 6-keto-$PGF_{1\alpha}$ the coefficients of variation at the levels of 250, 125, and 62.5 pg were 6.8, 9.4, and 9.1%, respectively. Cross-reactivities of the antibody against $PGF_{2\alpha}$ were 0.02%; PGE_2, 0.5%; PGD_2, 0.05%; and TXB_2, <0.01%.

G. Plasma Heparin Concentrations

Plasma heparin levels were determined in citrated plasma (final citrate concentration 0.01 mmol/ℓ). For measurements of total heparin concentrations we used a commercially available kit (Coatest®, Kabi). After addition of antithrombin III (AT III) and factor Xa (FXa) in excess, the resulting residual acitivity of FXa (not inhibited by the heparin-AT III complex) was determined by liberation of para-nitroanilide (pNA) from chromogenic substrates S 2222. The concentrations of the functional active portion of heparin bound by endogenous antithrombin (AT) III in patients' plasma were determined using a test kit from Boehringer, Mannheim, West Germany. For this purpose thrombin was added in excess without addition of AT III; a part of the added thrombin was neutralized by the patients' AT III-heparin complex, and the residual activity was then measured by liberation of pNA from chromogenic substrate Chromozym TH®. Platelet counts were obtained with a Linson 431 cell counter.

H. Calculations

All parameters were adjusted for hemodilution on the basis of the preoperative hematocrit, which was measured by an electronic cell (Model 30L, YSI, Yellow Springs, Ohio). Results are shown as mean values and standard deviations. Statistical comparisons between both patient groups were made, using the two-tailed Student's t test for unpaired observations.

III. RESULTS

Platelet counts of both treatment groups are shown as percent of initial values (Figure 1). Two minutes after the onset of ECC platelets had fallen to 48 ± 19% in the placebo group and to 55 ± 22% in the PGI_2-treated group. Sixty (60) and 90 min after initiation of CPB the difference between the two patient groups became statistically significant.

A. α-Granule Contents

Before operation both patient groups had elevated plasma levels of platelet α-granule proteins βTG and PF4 (Figures 2 and 3) as compared to normal donors (placebo group: βTG 65 ± 23 ng/mℓ, PF4 30 ± 12 ng/mℓ; PGI_2-treated group: βTG 72 ± 23 ng/mℓ, PF4 34 ± 15 ng/mℓ). Plasma levels of βTG and PF4 slightly increased during thoracotomy and vessel cannulation for ECC. Administration of heparin caused an additional (about 3-fold) increase in PF4 values. After onset of cardiopulmonary bypass βTG and PF4 levels were markedly increased. Maximal mean plasma βTG values were 1926 ng/mℓ (placebo group) and 1178 ng/mℓ (PGI_2-treated group). Mean PF4 values reached up to 1245 ng/mℓ (control group) and 837 ng/mℓ (PGI_2-treated group), respectively. One hour after onset of CPB until the end of bypass, PGI_2-treated patients had significantly ($p < 0.01$) lower plasma levels of both α-granule proteins than patients of the control group.

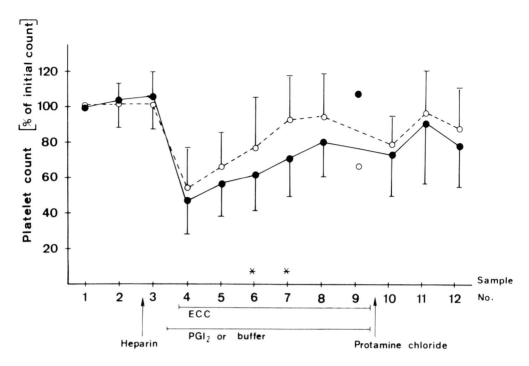

FIGURE 1.   Changes in platelet counts during extracorporeal circulation (ECC) in man in percent of initial values. Mean values ± standard deviations are depicted of PGI₂-treated patients (N = 20; O---O) and of placebo control-patients (N = 20; ●——●). In two patients the ECC lasted longer than 150 min (blood sample 9; circles without standard deviation). Significant differences between treatment groups are indicated (*p<0.05; **p<0.01; ***p<0.0001).

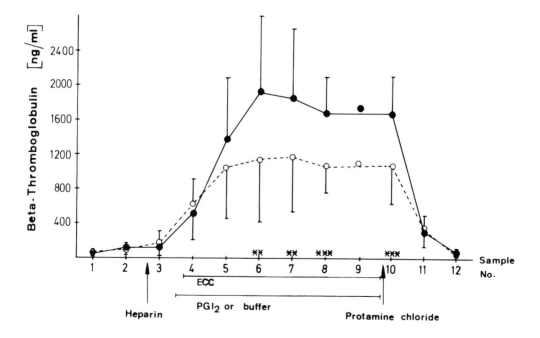

FIGURE 2.   Plasma levels of β-TG during ECC (for further details, see Figure 1).

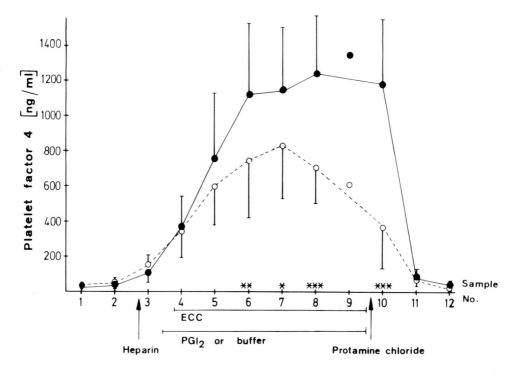

FIGURE 3.   Plasma levels of PF4 during ECC (for further details, see Figure 1).

B. TXB₂

Plasma TXB₂ levels (Figure 4) rose from normal preoperative values up to about 600 pg/ml at the end of ECC. There were no significant differences between patient groups except at 2 hr after the end of ECC, when PGI₂-treated patients showed higher levels than the control patients. Plasma TXB₂ levels increased rather slowly during ECC and did not show as pronounced changes in plasma levels as platelet α-granule proteins after onset and following termination of ECC.

6-Keto-PGF$_{1\alpha}$ plasma levels (Figure 5) of the control patients showed a continuous increase during the bypass period from normal values before ECC up to 1176 pg/ml 2 hr after onset of ECC. In the PGI₂-treated group, PGI₂ infusion resulted in a sharp increase in circulating levels of its oxidation product, reaching a constant level after ½ hr (about 2100 pg/ml). Plasma levels of both groups differed significantly during CPB ($p < 0.01$) including the measurement immediately after bypass ($p < 0.05$).

C. Heparin Plasma Levels

After the injection of a heparin bolus (200 units/kg body weight) and the following reinjections, plasma levels of total heparin (AT III-bound and -unbound; Figure 6) rose to a nearly constant level of about 3 units/ml. After protamine chloride neutralization, preoperative values were determined. Initial peaks of active heparin (AT III-bound; Figure 7) 2 min after heparinization reached 0.9 units/ml, followed by rather constant levels of 0.6 units/ml during the further course of CPB. Both methods of heparin measurement showed no differences between the two patient groups.

IV. DISCUSSION

During extracorporeal circulation, blood, plasma, and blood cells come into contact with foreign surfaces such as plastic cannulae, membranes, filters, and air interfaces.

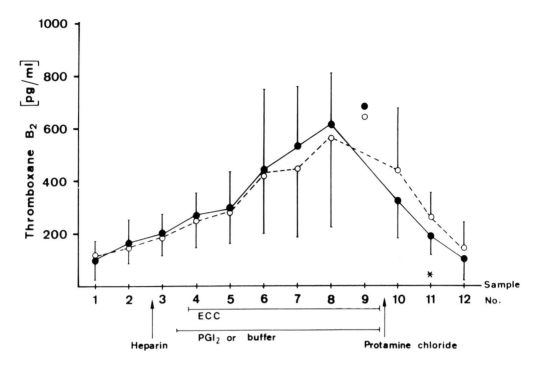

FIGURE 4. TXB₂-plasma levels during ECC (for further details, see Figure 1).

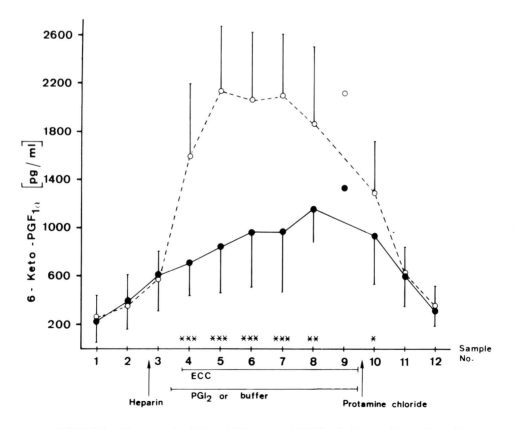

FIGURE 5. Plasma levels of 6-keto-PGF₁ₐ during ECC (for further details, see Figure 1).

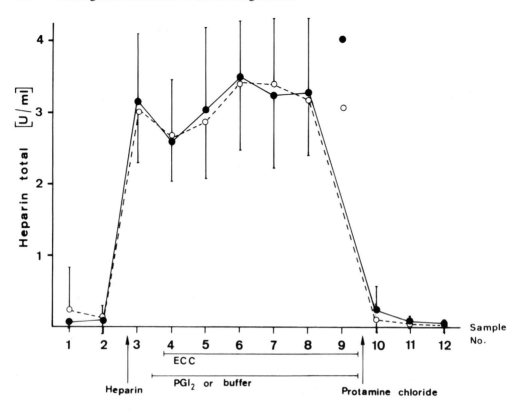

FIGURE 6.   Total amount of measurable heparin (AT III-bound and unbound) in plasma during ECC (for further details, see Figure 1).

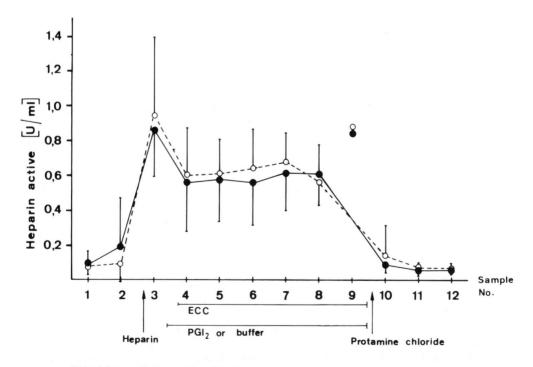

FIGURE 7.   AT III-bound heparin levels during ECC (for further details see Figure 1).

The resulting changes in the hemostatic mechanism are characterized by an activation of platelets resulting in a marked reduction of circulating platelets and, subsequently, platelet dysfunction.[6,10,19,24]

α-Granule release can be regarded as an indication of platelet activation.[35-37] The preoperatively elevated plasma levels of βTG and PF4 in our patients may be attributed to the presence of coronary artery disease.[10,35,37] Our results show that the main increase of βTG and PF4 plasma levels occurred during the first hour of ECC. At the same time platelet counts fell to about 50% of initial values. It can be concluded from this and from other observations that platelet activation is most pronounced during the first minutes of CPB.[4,14] After about 1 hr a level is reached at which release reactions and elimination of platelet granule contents counterbalance each other. Following the termination of ECC and protamine chloride injection (sample no. 10) no further release from platelets occurred. The more rapid decrease in plasma values of PF4 compared to βTG after termination of CPB is explained by the different half-life of these platelet-specific proteins.[30]

Divergent results were reported concerning the release of platelet-dense granule contents during ECC. Beurling-Harbury and Galvani[39] found that platelet contents of releasable ADP and ATP were decreased after ECC. Harker et al.,[10] however, did not see a decrease of platelet ADP and ATP content and found an unchanged number of dense granules after ECC.

It seems likely that release of dense granule contents needs a stronger platelet stimulation than release of α-granules.[36] ECC-induced partial platelet activation is accompanied by an impaired platelet function, which could be shown by measurements of platelet adhesivity or aggregability.[2-6,9] Additional formation of platelet microaggregates within extracorporeal systems was found, which can lead to a microembolization syndrome with consecutive organ dysfunction.[15,18,27,40] Heparinization cannot prevent platelet activation, decrease in platelet counts, and platelet dysfunction during and after cardiopulmonary bypass.[2,4,6,20,23] On the other hand, many experimental and clinical studies have shown that PGE$_1$ and PGI$_2$ could reduce platelet activation in various extracorporeal circulation systems.[9,11,18,19,22,24,41-43] The endogenous platelet inhibitor PGI$_2$ has a short half-life in a physiological milieu and its effects are rapidly reversible. Therefore, it seems to be the most favorable substance for preservation of platelets during ECC if it is given in addition to heparin.[9,26] Our results show that platelets of PGI$_2$-treated patients release significantly less βTG and PF4 than those of untreated patients. Platelet loss was reduced and platelet counts returned earlier toward preoperative values. This effect could be reached by a relatively small dose of PGI$_2$ (8 ng/kg/min) which had no distinct cardiovascular effects, nor led to additional prolongation of bleeding times.[29] Perhaps a higher dose or an earlier start of PGI$_2$-infusion before onset of bypass might have had even more distinct platelet preserving effects. Radegran and Papaconstantinou[42] reported a persisting preservation of platelet counts after infusion of 50 ng/kg/min PGI$_2$, while 2 to 20 ng/kg/min had no effect in their system.

In order to evaluate the possible concomitant activation of platelet PG metabolism, we measured the plasma levels of TXB$_2$. Changes in the TXB$_2$ plasma concentrations did not follow the course of initial rapid platelet loss and increases in α-granule contents in the plasma during the first phase of CPB.

Only a smaller portion of activated and releasing platelets seemed to simultaneously undergo an activation of the cyclooxygenase-thromboxane synthetase. Our results are in agreement with those reported by Addonizio et al.,[8,12] who found slowly increasing plasma TXB$_2$ values until the end of simulated ECC and did not see a correlation with the release of PF4. They also reported that inhibition of cyclooxygenase by acetylsalicylic acid could not prevent but only attenuate platelet loss and platelet release reactions during simulated ECC. Davies et al.[13] found the highest levels of plasma TXB_2 (800 ng/mℓ) during the first 20 min of bypass, but could not confirm a correlation between increase in TXB_2 and loss of platelet counts. Therefore, it can be assumed that platelet activation and adhesion during the first period of bypass leads to a partial release reaction, but is not necessarily dependent on the stimulation of the platelet PG system. Our results show that PGI_2 infusion had only a slight effect on thromboxane formation, and plasma levels of treated patients during ECC did not differ significantly from those of untreated patients. These results are comparable to those reported by Walker et al.,[43] who also did not observe lower TXB_2-levels using PGI_2 (20 ng/kg/min) during CPB. Further investigations with higher doses of PGI_2 are needed to clarify whether the prevention of thromboxane formation is possible and whether a reduction of this strongly proaggregatory and vasoconstrictive substance has additional beneficial effect for patients.

To our knowledge, 6-keto-PGF_{1a} plasma levels in patients on PGI_2 treatment during ECC have not been reported until now. As could be expected our results show a rapid increase in 6-keto-PGF_{1a} concentration with onset of PGI_2 infusion to about 2.1 ng/mℓ; however, control patients, receiving the glycine buffer only, also had elevated plasma levels of the PGI_2 oxidation product (up to 1.2 ng/mℓ at the end of ECC). Ylikorkala et al.[44] recently reported similar data on plasma levels of 6-keto-PGF_{1a} in seven patients under CPB. We presume that this increase is caused by stimulation of PGI_2 synthesis by the vessel endothelial system, which could be induced by mechanical irritation during operation and CPB. Possibly, the augmented production of endogenous PGI_2 is able to attenuate platelet activation during ECC.

Different results were reported concerning the influence of PGI_2 infusions on the requirement of heparin for anticoagulation. Attempts to replace heparin completely by PGI_2 infusion during cardiopulmonary bypass in dogs failed because extensive blood coagulation occurred in the oxygenators.[20,23] During hemodialysis or hemoperfusion, however, other groups could demonstrate that PGI_2 was able to replace heparin,[28,45] or could at least reduce the dose needed for adequate anticoagulation.[18,26] This effect can be explained by the PGI_2-induced inhibition of platelet activation and the concomitant reduction of plasma antiheparin activity which is achieved by lowering the PF4 liberation from platelets into plasma.[26] Consequently, PGI_2-treated patients should have more active heparin forming complexes with AT III. Turney et al.[26] reported a significant increase in thrombin clotting time and higher heparin levels using PGI_2 (5 ng/kg/min) during hemodialysis in humans. Bunting et al.[18] also observed a prolongation of thrombin clotting times during charcoal hemoperfusion of greyhounds when PGI_2 (50 ng/kg/min) was given in addition to heparin anticoagulation. Gimson et al.,[22] however, could not find significant differences in plasma heparin levels between PGI_2-treated (16 ng/kg/min) and untreated patients undergoing charcoal hemoperfusion. Longmore[24] and Bunting et al.[19] observed in patients during CPB a more prolonged Hemochron® time under PGI_1 treatment (10 ng/kg/min before CPB, 20 ng/kg/min during CPB). The plasma heparin concentrations measured by Bunting et al.[19] did notdiffer significantly in the PGI_2-treated and the untreated groups. We, too, failed to see significant differences in heparin plasma levels — neither in the total amount nor in the active AT III-bound heparin — between the two groups. The latter may partly depend on the fall of plasma AT III during ECC;[29] therefore, we could not confirm the heparin-saving effect, at least for the low PGI_2 concentrations used in this study.

V. SUMMARY

A double-blind randomized study was conducted on 40 male patients requiring aortocoronary bypass operations. Twenty patients received PGI_2 in a constant dose of 8 ng/kg/min from 2 min before until the end of ECC. Compared to the placebo-treated patients (n = 20), PGI_2 treatment was able to reduce the ECC-induced release of platelet α-granule proteins, β-thromboglobulin (βTG: 1178 ng/mℓ vs. 1926 ng/mℓ), and platelet factor 4 (PF4: 837 ng/mℓ vs. 1245 ng/mℓ) into plasma. The decrease in platelet counts during ECC was less pronounced in PGI_2-treated patients. Administration of PGI_2 had no effect on the increase in TXB_2 plasma levels, which amounted to 0.6 ng/mℓ at the end of ECC. PGI_2-treatment of patients resulted in elevated plasma concentrations of 6-keto-$PGF_{1\alpha}$ (2.1 ng/mℓ) throughout the infusion of PGI_2. 6-Keto-$PGF_{1\alpha}$ plasma levels increased up to 1.2 ng/mℓ in control group patients, indicating a stimulation of endogenous PGI_2-formation during ECC.

ACKNOWLEDGMENTS

The authors wish to acknowledge the help of Dr. J. O'Grady, Wellcome Research Laboratories, Beckenham, U.K., who supplied the prostacyclin. They also acknowledge the expert technical assistance of Mrs. D. Reitz, Mrs. M. Weizsaecker, Mr. J. Simon, and Mr. D. Söhngen.

REFERENCES

1. Bachmann, F., McKenna, R., Cole, E. R., and Najafi, H., The hemostatic mechanism after open heart surgery. I. Studies on plasma coagulation factors and fibrinolysis in 512 patients after extracorporeal circulation, *J. Thorac. Cardiovasc. Surg.*, 70, 76, 1975.
2. Bick, R. L., Alterations of hemostasis associated with cardiopulmonary bypass: pathophysiology, prevention, diagnosis and management, *Semin. Thromb. Hemostas.*, 3, 59, 1976.
3. Heiden, D., Mielke, C. H., Rodvien, R., and Hill, J. D., Platelets, hemostasis and thromboembolism during treatment of acute respiratory insufficiency with extracorporeal membrane oxygenation, *J. Thorac. Cardiovasc. Surg.*, 70, 644, 1975.
4. Hennessy, V. L., Hicks, R. E., Niewiarkowski, S., Edmunds, L. H., and Colman, R. W., Function of human platelet during extracorporeal circulation, *Am. J. Physiol.*, 232, H622, 1977.
5. Kalter, J. D., Saul, C. M., Wetstein, L., Soriano, C., and Reiss, R. F., Cardiopulmonary bypass. Associated hemostatic abnormalities, *J. Thorac. Cardiovasc. Surg.*, 77, 427, 1979.
6. McKenna, R., Bachmann, F., Whittaker, B., Gilson, J. R., and Weinberg, M., The hemostatic mechanism after open heart surgery. II. Frequency of abnormal platelet functions during and after extracorporeal circulation, *J. Thorac. Cardiovasc. Surg.*, 70, 298, 1975.
7. Weston, M. J., Hanid, A., Rubin, M. H., Langley, P. G., Mellon, P. J., and Williams, R., Biocompatibility of coated and uncoated charcoal during haemoperfusion in healthy dogs, *Eur. J. Clin. Invest.*, 7, 401, 1977.
8. Addonizio, V. P., Smith, J. B., Strauss, J. F., Colman, R. S., and Edmunds, L. J., Thromboxane synthesis and platelet secretion during cardiopulmonary bypass with bubble oxygenator, *J. Thorac. Cardiovasc. Surg.*, 79, 91, 1980.
9. Coppe, D., Wonders, T., Snider, M., and Salzman, E. W., Preservation of platelet number and function during extracorporeal membrane oxygenation by regional infusion of prostaglandin, in *Prostacyclin*, Vane, J. R. and Bergstrom, S., Eds., Raven Press, New York, 1979, 371.
10. Harker, L. A., Malpass, T. W., Branson, H. E., Hessel, E. A., II, and Slichter, S. J., Mechanism of abnormal bleeding in patients undergoing cardiopulmonary bypass: acquired transient platelet dysfunction associated with selective alpha-granule release, *Blood*, 56, 824, 1980.
11. Longmore, D. B., Hoyle, P. M., Gregory, A., Bennett, G. J., Smith, M. A., Osivand, T., and Jones, W. A., Prostacyclin administration during cardiopulmonary bypass in man, *Lancet*, 1, 800, 1981.
12. Addonizio, V. P., Smith, J. B., Guiod, L. R., Strauss, J. F., Colman, R. W., and Edmunds, L. H., Thromboxane synthesis and platelet protein release during simulated extracorporeal circulation, *Blood*, 54, 371, 1979.
13. Davies, G. C., Mowschenson, P. M., and Salzman, E. W., Thromboxane B_2 and fibrinopeptide A levels in platelet consumption and thrombosis, *Surg. Forum*, 29, 471, 1978.

14. Addonizio, V. P., Strauss, J. F., Colman, P. W., and Edmunds, L. H., Effects of prostaglandin E_1 on platelet loss during in vivo and in vitro extracorporeal circulation with a bubble oxygenator, *J. Thorac. Cardiovasc. Surg.*, 77, 119, 1979.

15. Stibbe, J., Ong, G. L., ten Hoor, F., Nauta, J., Van der Plas, P. M., Vergroesen, A. J., de Jong, D., and Krenning-Douma, E., Influence of prostaglandin E_1 on platelet decrease in the heart-lung machine, *Haemostasis*, 2, 294, 1973.

16. Tateson, J. E., Moncada, S., and Vane, J. R., Effects of prostacyclin (PGX) on cyclic AMP concentration in human platelets, *Prostaglandins*, 13, 389, 1977.

17. Bennett, J. G., Longmore, D. B., and O'Grady, J., Use of prostacyclin in cardiopulmonary bypass in man, in *Clinical Pharmacology of Prostacyclin*, Lewis, P. J. and O'Grady, J., Eds., Raven Press, New York, 1981, 201.

18. Bunting, S., Moncada, S., Vane, J. R., Woods, H. F., and Weston, M. J., Prostacyclin improves hemocompatibility during charcoal hemoperfusion, in *Prostacyclin*, Vane, J. R. and Bergstrom, S., Eds., Raven Press, New York, 1979, 361.

19. Bunting, S., O'Grady, J., Fabiani, J. N., Terrier, E., Moncada, S., Vane, J. R., and Dubost, C. H., Cardiopulmonary bypass in man: effects of prostacyclin, in *Clinical Pharmacology of Prostacyclin*, Lewis, P. J. and O'Grady, J., Eds., Raven Press, New York, 1981, 181.

20. Coppe, D., Sobel, M., Seamans, L., Levine, F., and Salzman, E., Preservation of platelet function and number by prostacyclin during cardiopulmonary bypass, *J. Thorac. Cardiovasc. Surg.*, 81, 274, 1981.

21. Ditter, H., Heinrich, D., Matthias, F. R., Sellmann-Richter, R., Wagner, W. L., and Hehrlein, F. W., Effect of prostacyclin during cardiopulmonry bypass in men on plasma levels of β-thromboglobulin, platelet factor 4, thromboxane B_2, 6-keto-prostaglandin F_{1a} and heparin, *Thromb. Res.*, 32, 393, 1983.

22. Gimson, A. E. S., Hughes, R. D., Mellon, P. J., Woods, H. F., Langley, P. G., Canalese, J., Williams, R., and Weston, M. J., Prostacyclin to prevent platelet activation during charcoal haemoperfusion in fulminant hepatic failure, *Lancet*, 1, 173, 1980.

23. Koshal, A., Krausz, M. M., Utsunomiya, T., Hechtman, H. B., Collins, J. J., and Cohn, L. H., Preservation of platelets and their function in prolonged cardiopulmonary bypass using prostacyclin, *Circulation*, 64, 1124, 1981.

24. Longmore, D. B., Experience with prostacyclin in cardiopulmonary bypass in dog and man, *Philos. Trans. R. Soc. London Ser. B*, 294, 399, 1981.

25. Matthias, F. R., Ditter, H., Heinrich, D., Simon, J., Söhngen, D., Schleussner, E., and Walter, P., Effect of prostacyclin (PGI_2) on the release of β-thromboglobulin (β-TG) and platelet factor 4 (PF4) during extracorporeal circulation (ECC), *Thromb. Haemost.*, 46, 316, 1981.

26. Turney, J. H., Fewell, M. R., Williams, L. C., Parsons, V., and Weston, M. J., Platelet protection and heparin sparing with prostacyclin during regular dialysis therapy, *Lancet*, 1, 219, 1980.

27. Woods, H. F., Weston, M. J., Bunting, S., Moncada, S., and Vane, J. R., The use of prostacyclin (PGI_2) during charcoal hemoperfusion, *Thromb. Haemost.*, 42, 131, 1979.

28. Zusman, R. M., Rubin, R. W., Cato, A. E., Coccheto, D. M., Crow, J. W., and Tolkoff-Rubin, N., Hemodialysis using prostacyclin instead of heparin as the sole antithrombotic agent, *N. Engl. J. Med.*, 304, 934, 1981.

29. Heinrich, D., Schleussner, E., Wagner, W. L., Sellmann-Richter, R., and Hehrlein, F. W., Prostacyclin in aorto-coronary bypass surgery. A double-blind, placebo-controlled study, *Thromb. Res.*, 32, 409, 1983.

30. Dawes, J., Smith, R. C., and Pepper, D. S., The release, distribution and clearance of human β-thromboglobulin and platelet factor 4, *Thromb. Res.*, 12, 851, 1978.

31. Ludlam, C. A., Evidence for the platelet specifity of β-thromboglobulin and studies on its plasma concentrations in healthy individuals, *Br. J. Haematol.*, 41, 271, 1979.

32. Anhut, H., Bernauer, W., and Peskar, B. A., Radioimmunological determination of thromboxane release in cardiac anaphylaxis, *Eur. J. Pharmacol.*, 44, 85, 1977.

33. Peskar, B. A., Anhut, H., Kroner, E. E., and Peskar, B. M., Development, specifity and some applications to radioimmunoassays for prostaglandins and related compounds, in *Advances in Pharmacology and Therapeutics*, Vol. 7, *Biochemical Clinical Pharmacology*, Tillement, J. P., Ed., Oxford, New York, 1979, 275.

34. Peskar, B. A., Steffens, Ch., and Peskar, B. M., Radioimmunoassay of 6-keto-prostaglandin F_{1a} in biological material, in *Radioimmunoassay of Drugs and Hormones in Cardiovascular Medicine*, Albertini, A., DaPrada, M., and Peskar, B. A., Eds., Elsevier/North Holland, Amsterdam, 1979, 239.

35. Files, J. C., Malpass, T. W., Yee, E. K., Ritchie, J. L., and Harker, J. A., Studies of human platelet α-granule release in vivo, *Blood*, 58, 607, 1981.

36. Kaplan, K. L., Nossel, H. L., Drillings, M., and Lesznik, G., Radioimmunoassay of platelet factor 4 and β-thromboglobulin: development and application to studies of platelet release in relation to fibrinopeptide A generation, *Br. J. Haematol.*, 39, 129, 1978.

37. Zahavi, J. and Dakkar, V. V., β-thromboglobulin — a specific marker of in-vivo platelet release reaction, *Thromb. Haemost.,* 44, 23, 1980.
38. Ellis, J. B., Kreutz, L. S., and Levine, S. P., Increased plasma platelet factor 4 (PF4) in patients with coronary artery disease, *Circulation,* 57/58(Suppl. 2), 116, 1978.
39. Beurling-Harbury, C. and Galvani, C. A., Acquired decrease in platelet secretory ADP associated with increased post-operative bleeding in post-cardiopulmonary bypass patients and in patients with severe valvular heart disease, *Blood,* 52, 13, 1978.
40. Longmore, D. B., Gueirrara, D., Bennett, G., Smith, M., Bunting, S., Reed, P., Moncada, S., Read, N. G., and Vane, J. R., Prostacyclin: a solution to some problems of extracorporeal circulation (experiments in greyhounds), *Lancet,* 1, 1002, 1979.
41. Malpass, T. W., Hanson, S. R., Savage, B., Hessel, E. A., and Harker, L. A., Prevention of acquired transient defect in platelet plug formation by infused prostacyclin, *Blood,* 57, 736, 1981.
42. Radegran, K. and Papaconstantinou, C., Prostacyclin infusion during cardiopulmonary bypass in man, *Thromb. Res.,* 19, 267, 1980.
43. Walker, I. D., Davidson, J. F., Faichney, A., Wheatley, D. J., and Davidson, K. G., A double blind study of prostacyclin in cardiopulmonary bypass surgery, *Br. J. Haematol.,* 49, 415, 1981.
44. Ylikorkala, O., Saarela, E., and Viinikka, L., Increased prostacyclin and thromboxane production in man during cardiopulmonary bypass, *J. Thorac. Cardiovasc. Surg.,* 82, 245, 1981.
45. Woods, H. F., Ash, G., Weston, M. J., Bunting, S., Moncada, S., and Vane, J. R., Prostacyclin can replace heparin in hemodialysis in dogs, *Lancet,* 2, 1075, 1978.

Chapter 15

CEREBRAL INFARCTION: BIOCHEMICAL CHANGES, DEFICIT IN BRAIN FUNCTION, AND NEW TRENDS IN THERAPY

Marie-Gilberte Borzeix and Jean Cahn

TABLE OF CONTENTS

I. INTRODUCTION

Clinically, the general and rather static concept of cerebral infarction was of a permanent arterial occlusion. Spontaneous reperfusion of the artery was, for many years, considered a rare event. Recent advances in this field showed that two types of infarcts occur in the acute phase: the first one is a permanent occlusion resulting in complete ischemia which ends in tissue necrosis; the second one corresponds to a transient occlusion which is removed allowing the reperfusion of the previously ischemic area.[1,2] Experimental models reproduce these clinical situations.

In the first part of this chapter, various types of experimental models leading to brain infarction will be briefly reviewed. An exhaustive review has been published recently in the *Journal of Cerebral Blood Flow and Metabolism.* In the second part, the consequences of both cerebral embolization and transient oligemia will be discussed more precisely as well as some therapeutic procedures for ameliorating brain function. In the third part, new trends in the treatment of cerebral infarction will be discussed through experimental findings. The common feature of the pathophysiological situations related to cerebral infarction is that the blood supply to the brain is reduced, and consequently the oxygen and metabolite delivery. The difference consists in the extent, the duration, and the localization of the cerebral insult. It may be global (complete, incomplete, or diffuse), regional, transient, or long-lasting. The consequences for the brain function are directly related to all these events.

II. DIFFERENT MODELS LEADING TO BRAIN INFARCTION

A. Complete Cerebral Ischemia

This can be obtained using the four-vessel occlusion model in rats,[3] rabbits,[4] cats and monkeys,[5-7] by cardiac arrest,[8] by an increased CSF pressure in the dog,[9] and others. For a complete review see Reference 10.

Very rapidly after ischemia is induced, the EEG flattens and disappears; the energy charge of the nucleotides pool declines and reaches a minimum value within about 5 to 7 min.[11] Saturated and unsaturated fatty acids gradually accumulate in the free fatty acid (FFA) pool of the brain — mostly stearic, arachidonic, and palmitic acids. This increase in FFA, which reaches approximately 11 times the basal value over a 30-min period of complete ischemia, results from a disintegration of membrane phospholipids.[12] Membranes are depolarized, and as shown by Symon,[13] Astrup,[14] and Branston et al.[15] a reduction in local blood flow below 10 mℓ/100 g/min produces a massive efflux of K^+ from the cellular compartment and a great rise in extracellular K^+ concentration. As these authors showed, there are different thresholds of blood flow leading to membrane failure and to subsequent tissue infarction.[16] The important event which rapidly follows the efflux of potassium is a dramatic rise in intracellular calcium, the accumulation of which in cells rapidly ends in cell death as defined by Farber,[17] Schanne et al.,[18] and Hass.[19] In parallel, lactic acidosis occurs, the degree of which is dependent on the preischemic store of glucose and glycogen. Whether the animals are normally fed, hypo-, or hyperglycemic,[20,21] markedly influences the clinical restitution following ischemia.

As Hossmann[10] outlined, complete ischemia must be limited in duration in order to be reversible and many events occur during recirculation. Only animals presenting a reactive hyperemia have a chance to recover,[22] but this hyperemic period is generally followed by secondary hypoperfusion during which cerebral blood flow (CBF) remains below the pre-ischemic values. In contrast, the postischemic metabolism increases[23,24] (postischemic hypermetabolism), a phenomenon which has been also described by Cahn et al.[25] in the course of a posthypocapnic period in the dog. Peroxidative processes to FFA take place during reperfusion which may cause additional damage during the postischemic phase. Free radicals, mainly superoxides and hydroperoxides, are thus damaging membrane phospholipids.[26-29]

B. Regional Cerebral Ischemia

This results from the occlusion of a cerebral vessel, most often the middle cerebral artery in rats, cats, or monkeys. The severity of the brain insult is a function of the duration of ischemia and of the importance of the surrounding anastomotic circulation. Many years ago, Symon[30] described a zone of moderate energy imbalance surrounding the area of infarction that he termed the "ischemic penumbra". For a review, see Reference 10.

C. Cerebral Oligemia

The combination of bilateral carotid artery ligation for 1 hr with a mild drop (to about 7.9 to 9.3 kPa) in blood pressure obtained by injecting (s.c.) 1 mg per rat of sodium nitroprusside, results in cerebral infarction. Outcome can be assessed in terms of vasospasm, reactive hyperemia associated or not with brain hemorrhages, brain edema, intracellular accumulation of calcium, changes in the activity of the membrane Na^+/K^+ATPase, and changes of the blood/brain barrier (BBB) permeability to serum proteins. All of these events end in a failure of the brain function, i.e., in the ability of a rat to aquire learning and conditioning.[31] Oligemia may also be induced by blood withdrawal.[32,33]

D. Cerebral Microembolization

A permanent microembolization of the cerebral circulation can be obtained by the intravascular injection (generally into an internal carotid artery) of solid microspheres.[34-37] According to Hossmann,[10] if this technique gives rise to very reproducible results, it does not correspond to what occurs in human pathology. Unstable and transient cerebral microembolism may be obtained by the intraarterial injection of fat droplets, gas bubbles,[38] or atheromatous material.[39] It can also be induced by disseminated platelet aggregates due to ADP,[40] arachidonic acid,[41,42] or by a fragment of clot obtained from autologous blood.[43,44]

III. NEW FINDINGS IN TRANSIENT CEREBRAL OLIGEMIA, IN TIAs, OR IN IRREVERSIBLE CEREBRAL MICROEMBOLISM — DEFICIT IN BRAIN FUNCTIONS AND NEW TRENDS IN THERAPY

A. Transient Cerebral Oligemia in the Rat

This experimental model has been studied during the acute phase (from the time of carotid artery ligation to hour 5 following clipping-off) as well as during the subacute period of evolution (until day 3 postligation).[31] In the course of the 60 min of oligemia, behavioral manifestations occur, such as piloerection in all cases, severe hypotonia marked by ventral decubitus in 93% of cases, and occasional clono-tonic discharges in 19% of rats. Following clipping-off, after 3 hr, the first event noted is the occurrence of clonic discharges. As during the period of oligemia, these occur in 20% of rats, but not necessarily the same rats. From this moment, a marked lateralization is observed as well as a protrusion of the eyeballs. After removal of the brain, it is seen that exophthalmus corresponds to the more injured cerebral hemisphere, which exhibits vasospasm and sometimes brain hemorrhages (Figure 1). The more severe brain insult slightly predominates in the right hemisphere (60% of cases). Over a period of 6 days, the mortality rate is about 40%.

Two major facts are characteristic of the postoligemic period. First, such a brain insult is mainly related to the tremendous rise in intracellular Ca^{++}. Second, the severity of the lesion increases with time, at least until day 3 (Table 1). Brain edema marked by

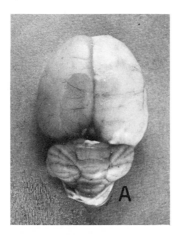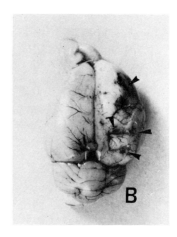

FIGURE 1.   Brains of postoligemic rats removed 72 hr after clipping-off. Vasospasm predominates in the right hemisphere (case A) and several hemorrhages (arrows) are present in case B.

a mild increase in water content develops in parallel with a K^+ efflux which induces a membrane depolarization. The CBF threshold described by Astrup et al.[16] from which K^+ leaves the cell, immediately followed by Ca^{++} entry, is confirmed by the highly significant correlation plotted in Figure 2. Similarly, and as has been discussed by Hass[19] recalling the work of Farber's group,[17,18] the tremendous intracellular accumulation of Ca^{++} exerts a detergent effect upon membranes and inhibits oxidative phosphorylation.[45] The damaging effect of Ca^{++} upon membranes is reflected by the significant increase in the cerebral FFA pool, which seems to be due more to a splitting of membrane phospholipids than of cholesterol, since the amount of cerebral cholesterol remains unchanged. Finally, the alteration of the integrity of the membrane layers ends in a slowing of the activity of the $Na^+/K^+ATPase$[46] (Table 1). Directly connected with the above changes in cerebral biochemistry are the very important disturbances of brain function revealed by learning and conditioning tests. A simple one-trial learning procedure (passive avoidance test) derived from that described many years ago by Burešova et al.,[47] was used. Conditioning to sound in a shuttle-box was used as an active avoidance learning test.

In Burešova's test, a naive rat is placed in an apparatus consisting of a large lighted compartment (about 40×40 cm) connected by a small opening to a small dark one (10 $\times$ 10 cm) with an electrified grid floor. The rats are allowed to explore this new environment for 3 min. Very rapidly (11 sec) they discover the small, dark compartment, enter it, and remain there for about 160 sec. At the end of the 3-min exploratory period, the opening between the two compartments is closed and each rat receives, in the small compartment, intermittent electrical foot shocks for 30 sec. It remains in this small dark box for 90 sec and finally it is allowed to enter the large lighted compartment and kept there for 2 min. After 24 hr none of the control rats will reenter the small compartment. There is retention of the punishment (Table 2). By contrast, 75% of the postoligemic rats reenter the small compartment 48 hr after having been injured (punishment took place 24 hr after oligemia). The difference between the two groups is highly significant and may be related to the markedly increased intracerebral Ca^{++} concentration (Table 2).

We defined normal active avoidance learning as the ability to exhibit 10 consecutive escape responses in a shuttle-box by 80 to 90% of healthy young (9 weeks old) rats. In a second session performed 24 hr later, the performance of controls improved as the number of trials fell from 37 to only 17. When similarly aged rats are first submitted to a transient oligemia as described above, only 1 rat out of 9 is able to acquire such conditioning. The difference between the two groups is highly significant and may also be related to the increase in intracerebral Ca^{++} content (Table 3).

B. From TIAs To Irreversible Cerebral Microembolism In The Rat

As reported by Fieschi et al.[40] using ADP, or Furlow and Bass[41] using arachidonate, it is possible to reproduce TIAs experimentally by injecting pro-aggregatory agents into the internal carotid artery of heparinized animals.

The most important phenomenon following the injection of arachidonate is a reactive hyperemia concomitant with the occurrence of an immediate BBB breakdown and with a marked and widespread cerebral edema.[42] The edematous reaction usually involves not only the frontal part of the injected hemisphere, but also spreads down to posterior structures and often reaches the opposite side, realizing a diaschisis as noted by Lavy et al.[48] in human beings. The mortality is high in the first 3 hr following embolization (about 80%) and must be directly related to the severity and extent of the edematous reaction, which also depends on the dose of arachidonate. Animals surviving 24 hr exhibit no neurological deficit or cerebral biochemical disturbances. All the events occurring in the course of this cerebral microembolization have been described by Cahn et al.[49]

Furlow and Bass[41] reported (1976) the prophylactic value of aspirin in this animal model of platelet-mediated stroke. Their conclusion was that although aspirin is known to inhibit the arachidonic acid cascade through the cyclooxygenase pathway, it offered little protection against arachidonate-induced stroke. As reported above, many events result from stroke. The disease, being related to so many phenomena, its prevention as well as its treatment, must also be diverse. It may be thought that a more direct antagonist to the effect of arachidonate would be prostacyclin (PGI$_2$). To test this hypothesis, a new chemically stable carbacyclin derivative, ZK 36374 (Schering) was continuously infused either immediately or from the 30th minute following the intracarotid injection of arachidonate, to the 90th minute, when the rats were sacrificed. The goal of this study was to determine the extent of the BBB breakdown by measuring the intracerebral extravasation of Evans Blue. Results were recently reported at the 5th International Conference on Prostaglandins.[50] The most effective dose was 0.5 μg/kg/min of ZK 36374, but a therapeutic effect only occurred when the perfusion started long after the onset of stroke. This suggests that the vasodilating effect of the PGI$_2$-analogue aided the reactive hyperemia of the disease. However, BBB breakdown is a transient phenomenon and more prolonged disturbances affect the cerebral biochemistry, notably brain edema and intracerebral accumulation of Ca^{++} (Table 4). Since stroke generates an increase in the intracerebral content of arachidonic acid, the use of indomethacin as a pretreatment against the deleterious effect of this FFA was tested. As shown in Table 4, three oral administrations of indomethacin did not result in any significant reduction of brain edema, but caused a more pronounced Ca^{++} entry into the brain. This detrimental pathophysiological effect of indomethacin was mentioned by Harris et al.,[51] who noted an increased brain water accumulation after focal cerebral ischemia in primates. There are many hypotheses for this, among which that of Volpi et al.[52] is the most attractive. Volpi proposed that indomethacin not only inhibits the formation of products of the cyclooxygenase pathway, but also stimulates the lipoxygenase route of arachidonic acid metabolism, a product of which may be involved in the above deleterious effect.

Since arachidonate is transformed into free radicals through peroxidative mechanisms, the protective effect of free radical scavengers was also tested. Superoxide radicals are destroyed by superoxide dismutase (SOD). SOD was injected intravenously to

Table 1

CEREBRAL BIOCHEMICAL DISTURBANCES RELATED TO TRANSIENT OLIGEMIA IN YOUNG SD RATS

Series	Time of sacrifice[a]	N	H₂O (%)	Cerebral content			FFA (mmol/kg wet weight)	Membrane Na/K/ATPase (µmol/Pi/ mg/protein/hr)
				K⁺	Ca⁺⁺	Cholesterol		
				(mmol/kg dry weight)				
Controls	—	36	78.7 ± 0.05	499 ± 3.5	4.4 ± 0.20	198 ± 2.9	3.18 ± 0.068	4.72 ± 0.118
Oligemic rats	+15 min	5	79.8 ± 0.22	411 ± 11.7[b]	8.2 ± 1.8	165 ± 7.9[b]	—	—
	+5 hr	4	81.8 ± 0.20[b]	378 ± 23.8[b]	9.5 ± 2.02	222 ± 8.4[b]	—	—
	+24 hr	12	80.0 ± 0.54	400 ± 14.2[b]	10.4 ± 1.71[b]	205 ± 3.7	—	—
	+72 hr	11	80.1 ± 0.37[b]	366 ± 12.6[b]	28.2 ± 3.20[b]	200 ± 6.6	—	—
	+72 hr	6	—	—	—	—	5.97 ± 0.963[b]	—
	+72 hr	6	—	—	—	—	—	3.72 ± 0.287[b]

Note: N = Number of rats per series.

[a] Post clipping-off.

[b] $p \leq 0.05$ according to Student's t test or to Cochran's t test vs. controls.

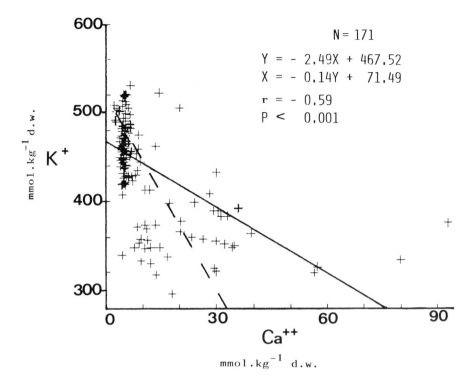

FIGURE 2.   Correlation between intracerebral Ca^{++} and K$^+$ content.

avoid free radical damage to the brain. But as Michelson[53] recalled recently, in some circumstances, SOD may be good and superoxides bad, as well as the converse. Under our experimental conditions, at doses ranging from 0.25 to 2 mg for free SOD, and doses ranging from 0.125 to 0.5 mg for liposomal SOD, a similar impairment of the disease was observed. Contrary to these results, a prophylactic intravenous injection of reduced glutathione, at a relatively high dose, improved the situation by reducing brain edema. The primary role of glutathione in brain reamination was described many years ago by Cahn et al.[54,55] This suggested that Ubiquinone 50 (coenzyme Q10) be tested as a free radical scavenger.[49-56] CoQ10 markedly reduced the water and Na$^+$ contents of the brain and limited the accumulation of Ca^{++} (Table 4). An alpha blocker such as dihydroergotoxine (DHET) may also be used as it is thought to reduce any spasm related to sympathetic stimulation. Brain edema was reduced, but the Ca^{++} influx into the cerebral tissue was unchanged (Table 4). All these results were obtained in young rats, about 8 to 10 weeks old. In old (28 to 32 months) or adult (15 to 24 months) rats, both the disease and its prevention and treatment may be different. Aging causes spontaneous changes in the brain biochemistry[57] and in the cerebral function, i.e., in the plasticity of the brain. Aging is marked by a reduction of the water content of the brain and by an accumulation of Ca^{++} ions. These changes are small but statistically significant. There is also an increase in the plasma thiobarbituric reactive material (TBAR) mainly malonedialdehyde (MDA).[57] This means that with aging, spontaneous peroxidation of lipids occurs, leading progressively to free radical reactions. This results in the accumulation of cerebral lipofuscin pigments described long ago by histologists. The severity of the brain insult due to arachidonate was quite similar to that described in the young rats. Under these conditions, an α-1 blocker such as nicergoline was able to completely suppress the biochemical brain injury even when it was injected after the intracarotid injection of sodium arachidonate. By contrast,

Table 2

PERFORMANCE OF RATS IN BUREŠOVA'S TEST RELATED TO BRAIN BIOCHEMICAL CHANGES

Series	N	No. rats entering small compartment			Latency (sec) to enter small compartment			Time spent in small compartment			H_2O (%)	Cerebral content K^+ (mmol/kg dry weight)	Cerebral content Ca^{++} (mmol/kg dry weight)
		Before	+48 hr	+72 hr	Before	+48 hr	+72 hr	Before	+48 hr	+72 hr			
Healthy control rats	36	—	—	—	—	—	—	—	—	—	78.7 ± 0.05	499 ± 3.5	4.4 ± 0.20
Buresova control rats	10	10	0	0	11 ± 4.9	180 ± 0	180 ± 0	167 ± 5.5	0 ± 0	0 ± 0	78.2 ± 0.16[a]	454 ± 5.6[a]	4.9 ± 0.13
Buresova oligemic rats	12	12	9[a]	7[a]	11 ± 2.7	115 ± 19.2[a]	103 ± 23.3[a]	166 ± 3.5	41 ± 17.4[a]	55 ± 21.5[a]	78.8 ± 0.38	399 ± 12.9[a]	19.1 ± 4.4[a]

Note: N = number of rats per series.

[a] $p \leqslant 0.05$ according to Chi square test (no. of rats) or according to Student's *t* test or Cochran's *t* test (other parameters).

Table 3

PERFORMANCE OF RATS IN THE SHUTTLE-BOX TEST RELATED TO BRAIN BIOCHEMICAL CHANGES

Series	N	No. conditioned rats	No. trials nec. to acquire learning		Cerebral content		
			+48 hr	+72 hr	H_2O (%)	K^+ mmol/kg dry weight	Ca^{++} mmol/kg dry weight
Healthy control rats	36	—	—	—	78.7 ± 0.05	499 ± 3.5	4.4 ± 0.20
Shuttle-box control rats	10	8	37 ± 3.5	17 ± 3.4	78.1 ± 0.11[a]	461 ± 4.6[a]	5.3 ± 0.35[a]
Shuttle-box oligemic rats	9	1[a]	37	21	78.4 ± 0.39	401 ± 15.3[a]	14.4 ± 4.2[a]

Note: N = number of rats per series.

[a] $p \leqslant 0.05$ according to Chi square test (no. of rats) or according to Student's *t* test or Cochran's *t* test (other parameters).

Table 4

PROPHYLACTIC EFFECT OF DRUGS UPON ARACHIDONATE-INDUCED STROKE IN YOUNG RATS (9 WEEKS)

Series		N	Dose	Route of admin.	Cerebral content			
					H_2O (%)	Na^+	K^+ (mmol/kg dry weight)	Ca^{++}
Controls		35	—	—	78.8 ± 0.05	230 ± 2.0	499 ± 3.5	4.4 ± 0.23
Arachidonate controls,		35	—	—	81.1 ± 0.22[a]	358 ± 15.3[a]	408 ± 9.7[a]	7.6 ± 0.64[a]
Anti-inflammatory	Indomethacin	10	5	mg/kg, p.o.	80.4 ± 0.45	328 ± 21.8	450 ± 14.5[b]	10.4 ± 1.64[b]
		3	2	mg, i.v.	81.7	436	372	11.9
		3	1	mg, i.v.	88.2	474	354	13.6
Free radical scaven-gers	Free SOD	3	0.5	mg, i.v.	80.3	329	447	6.5
		3	0.25	mg, i.v.	81.2	413	373	31.2
		3	0.5	mg, i.v.	81.8	429	364	8.4
	Liposomal SOD	3	0.25	mg, i.v.	81.2	374	402	10.5
		10	0.125	mg, i.v.	80.5 ± 0.40	358 ± 14.6	342 ± 8.1[b]	7.4 ± 0.59
	Reduced glutathione	3	100	mg, i.v.	78.7	222	470	5.6
	Co Q 10	10	10	mg/kg, i.p.	79.0 ± 0.20[b]	211 ± 4.6[b]	456 ± 3.7[b]	5.9 ± 2.0
Alpha blocker	DHET	10	0.5	mg/kg, i.v.	79.9 ± 0.51[b]	288 ± 29.7[b]	454 ± 15.7[b]	9.7 ± 0.91

Note: N = number of rats per series.

[a,b] $p \leqslant 0.05$ according to Student's *t* test or to Cochran's *t* test; footnote a: vs. controls, footnote b: vs. arachidonate controls.

Table 5
TREATMENT OF ARACHIDONATE-INDUCED STROKE IN ADULT RATS
(18 MONTHS)

Series		N	Dose (mg/ kg, i.v.)	Cerebral content			
				H_2O (%)	Na^+	K^+	Ca^{++}
					(mmol/kg dry weight)		
Controls		10	—	76.3 ± 0.27	209 ± 19	397 ± 6.7	5.3 ± 0.29
Arachidonate controls		10	—	78.1 ± 0.41^a	265 ± 14.5^a	352 ± 13.7^a	9.5 ± 1.28^a
Alpha 1 blocker	Nicergoline	10	2	76.2 ± 0.29^b	208 ± 5.8^b	390 ± 6.5^b	6.2 ± 0.67^b
Ca^{++} entry blockers	Nicardipine	10	1	78.3 ± 0.83	306 ± 36.8	336 ± 20.4	5.7 ± 0.36^b

Note: N = number of rats per series.

[a,b] $p \leqslant 0.05$ according to Student's *t* test or to Cochran's *t* test; footnote a: vs. controls, footnote b: vs. arachidonate controls.

with a Ca^{++} channel blocker such as nicardipine the Ca^{++} content of the brain returned to normal, but there was no improvement in the other parameters (Table 5).

IV. DISCUSSION

Given the different models of experimental cerebral infarction mentioned above, the problem arises as to what extent they correspond to the clinical situation and whether they can provide information concerning therapy.

The most investigated situation is cerebral ischemia, whether global or regional, and this corresponds to what happens during and after a large cerebral vessel occlusion or a cardiac arrest. The main clinical problem is the eradication of postischemic edema, which is the common feature of these conditions associated with hyper- or hypometabolism and hypoperfusion of the brain.

Microembolization of the brain ranging from TIAs (ADP or arachidonate-induced) to permanent microembolism by small blood clot emboli are relevant to the clinical situation.[10] Drugs that interfere with arachidonic acid metabolism may prevent injury in models related to platelet aggregation, but have no effect or increase injury when used therapeutically.[51] Chronic cerebrovascular insufficiency is a most difficult condition to reproduce experimentally and, from a clinical point of view, one of the most important therapeutic problems. The model described above of postoligemia seems to reproduce the major part of this condition since there is progressive cerebral biochemical failure and a parallel circulatory insufficiency as shown by increasing partial vasospasm with time. Finally, the most interesting aspect of this model is that concomitantly with the biochemical and hemodynamic changes, there is a progressive functional disturbance illustrated by the inability of the rats to acquire learning or conditioning. This situation closely resembles what occurs during aging, i.e., that CBF slightly but gradually declines, calcium ions tend to accumulate in brain tissue, and most importantly, brain function progressively declines. Thus, about 90% of young rats (9 weeks old) easily acquire shuttle-box learning as do 80% of 8-month-old rats. From the age of 12 months, this learning rate falls to 55%.[58] As outlined elsewhere,[59] the etiology of ischemia-induced cerebral injury is polymorphic, so the therapy of these brain insults must necessarily also be diverse. The same major events are always present:

1.   Brain edema — Depending on whether it is cytotoxic or vasogenic, either glycerol or steroids will be more efficient.
2.   Intracerebral accumulation of Ca^{++} ions — This stimulates phospholipase A_2-induced lipolysis. The increased cerebral pool of FFA comes directly from membrane phospholipids. It is obvious that Ca^{++} entry blockers are able to impede this damaging effect, but as shown in Table 5, they are without effect on edema.
3.   Since arachidonic acid is one of the more important FFA released during ischemia, its peroxidation gives rise to end products such as TXA_2, PGI_2, or leukotrienes. Inhibitors or cyclooxygenase and/or lipoxygenase and inhibitors of TXA_2 synthetase may be useful in acting against platelet aggregation, edema, and vasospasm.
4.   The free radical-induced membrane damage can be treated by free radical scavengers such as CoQ10, reduced glutathione, or even alpha-tocopherol or ascorbic acid. SOD and glutathione peroxidase are ineffective in this situation, but it is well known that many drugs can be antioxidants at one range of doses and become prooxidants at larger doses. The problem is similar for inhibitors of cyclooxygenase (e.g., aspirin), the effect of which may be reveresed depending on the dose given.

These views on postischemic therapy are close to those of Hallenbeck and Furlow,[9] who proposed combined treatment with heparin, indomethacin, and PGI_2 to prevent impairment of postischemic brain reperfusion. Finally, it must be stressed that the future for postischemic cerebral therapy will necessarily be polymorphic and that no single drug will effectively treat brain ischemia of all etiology.

ACKNOWLEDGMENT

We gratefully acknowledge the technical assistance of the scientific staff of SIR International.

REFERENCES

1. Olsen, T. S., Larsen, B., Skriver, E. B., Herning, M., Enevoldsen, E., and Lassen, N. A., Focal cerebral hyperhemia in acute stroke. Incidence, pathophysiology and clinical significance, *Stroke,* 12, 598, 1981.
2. Olsen, T. S. and Lassen, N. A., Dynamic changes of regional cerebral blood flow in the acute state of cerebral infarction: therapeutical consequences, *J. Cereb. Blood Flow Metab.,* 2(Suppl. 1), S35, 1982.
3. Pulsinelli, W. A. and Brierley, J. B., A new method of bilateral hemispheric ischemia in the unanesthetized rat, *Stroke,* 10, 267, 1979.
4. Kolata, R. J., Survival of rabbits after prolonged cerebral ischemia, *Stroke,* 10, 272, 1979.
5. Hossmann, K. A. and Kleihues, P., Reversibility of ischemic brain damage, *Arch. Neurol.,* 29, 375, 1973.
6. Hossmann, K. A., Total ischemia of the brain, in *Brain and Heart Infarct,* Zülch, K. J., Kaufmann, W., Hossmann, K. A., and Hossmann, V., Eds., Springer-Verlag, Berlin, 1977, 107.
7. Hossmann, K. A., Matzuoka, Y., Blöink, M., Fitzgerald, G., and Hossmann, V., Treatment of experimental infarction of the cat brain, in *Drugs and Methods in CVD,* Cahn, J., Ed., Pergamon Press, Oxford, 1981, 427.
8. Hirsch, H. and Schneider, M., Uberlebens-, Erholungs- und Wiederbelebungszeit des Gehirns bei Normo- und Hypothermie, in *Handbuch der Neurochirurgie,* Grundlagen II, I, 2, Olivecrona, H. and Tonnis, W., Eds., Springer-Verlag, Berlin, 1968, 509.
9. Hallenbeck, J. M. and Furlow, T. W., Jr., Prostaglandin I_2 and indomethacin prevent impairment of post-ischemic brain reperfusion in the dog, *Stroke,* 10, 629, 1979.

10. Hossmann, K. A., Review: treatment of experimental cerebral ischemia, *J. Cereb. Blood Flow Metab.,* 2, 275, 1982.
11. Siesjo, B. K., Current views on Ca⁺⁺ and lipid metabolism in ischemia, paper presented at 3rd Int. Beaune Conf., Beaune, France, October 15 to 16, 1982.
12. Yoshida, S., Inoh, S., Asano, T., Sano, K., Kubota, M., Shimazaki, H., and Ueta, N., Effect of transient ischemia on free fatty acids and phospholipids in the gerbil brain. Lipid peroxidation as a possible cause of post-ischemic injury, *J. Neurosurg.,* 53, 323, 1980.
13. Symon, L., Investigations into the biochemistry of ischaemic brain, in *Energy Transduction and Neurotransmission,* Benzi, G., Giuffrida Stella, A. M., Bachelard, H. S., and Agnoli, A., Eds., Fondazione Internazionale Menarini, Milan, 1982, 117.
14. Astrup, J., Energy-requiring cell functions in the ischemic brain. Their critical supply and possible inhibition in protective therapy, *J. Neurosurg.,* 56, 482, 1982.
15. Branston, N. M., Strong, A. J., and Symon, L., Extracellular potassium activity, evoked potential and tissue blood flow. Relationships during progressive ischemia in baboon cerebral cortex, *J. Neurol. Sci.,* 32, 305, 1977.
16. Astrup, J., Symon, L., and Branston, N. M., Cortical evoked potential and extracellular K⁺ and H⁺ at critical levels of brain ischemia, *Stroke,* 8, 51, 1977.
17. Farber, J. L., Mini-review: the role of calcium in cell-death, *Life Sci.,* 29, 1289, 1981.
18. Schanne, F. A. X., Kane, A. B., Young, E. E., and Farber, J. L., Calcium dependance of toxic cell death: a final common pathway, *Science,* 260, 700, 1979.
19. Hass, W. K., Beyond cerebral blood flow, metabolism and ischemic thresholds: an examination of the role of calcium in the initiation of cerebral infarction, in *Cerebral Vascular Disease,* Vol. 3, Meyer, J. S., Lechner, H., Reivich, M., Ott, E. O., and Aranibar, A., Eds., Excerpta Medica, Amsterdam, 1981, 3.
20. Siemkowicz, E. and Hansen, A. J., Clinical restitution following cerebral ischemia in hypo-, normo- and hyperglycemic rats, *Acta Neurol. Scand.,* 58, 1, 1978.
21. Siemkowicz, E. and Hansen, A. J., Brain extracellular ion composition and EEG activity following 10 minutes ischemia in normo- and hyperglycemic rats, *Stroke,* 12, 236, 1981.
22. Hossmann, K. A. and Kleihues, P., Reversibility of ischemic brain damage, *Arch. Neurol.,* 29, 375, 1973.
23. Hossmann, K. A., Sakaki, S., and Kimoto, K., Cerebral uptake of glucose and oxygen in the cat brain after prolonged ischemia, *Stroke,* 7, 301, 1976.
24. Nemoto, E. M., Hossmann, K. A., and Cooper, H. K., Post-ischemic hypermetabolism in cat brain, *Stroke,* 12, 666, 1981.
25. Cahn, J., Herold, M., and Borzeix, M. G., Introduction à la pathopharmacologie des substances vaso-actives cérébrales, in *Actualites de Chimie Thérapeutique: 4ème Série,* Société de Chimie Thérapeutique, Paris, 1976, 65.
26. Demopoulos, H. B., Flamm, E. S., Seligman, M. L., Power, R., Pietronigro, D., and Ransohoff, J., Molecular pathology of lipids in CNS membranes, in *Oxygen and Physiological Function,* Jöbsis, F. F., Ed., Professional Information Library, Dallas, 1977, 491.
27. Demopoulos, H. B., Flamm, E. S., Seligman, M. L., Mitamura, J. A., and Ransohoff, J., Membrane perturbations in central nervous system injury: theoretical basis for free radical damage and a review of the experimental data, in *Neural Trauma,* Popp, A. J., Ed., Raven Press, New York, 1979, 63.
28. Demopoulos, H. B., Flamm, E. S., Pietronigro, D. D., and Seligman, M. L., The free radical pathology and the microcirculation in the major central nervous system disorders, *Acta Physiol. Scand.,* 492(Suppl.), 91, 1980.
29. Flamm, E. S., Demopoulos, H. B., Seligman, M. L., Poser, R. G., and Ransohoff, J., Free radicals in cerebral ischemia, *Stroke,* 9, 445, 1978.
30. Symon, L., The relationship between CBF, evoked potential and the clinical features in cerebral ischemia, in *Drugs and Methods in CVD,* Cahn, J., Ed., Pergamon Press, Oxford, 1981, 397.
31. Borzeix, M. G., Charles, P., and Souil, J. M., Unpublished data.
32. Mossakowski, M. J., Cerebral circulation disturbances in various hypoxic conditions, in *Advances in Neurology,* Vol. 20, Cervos-Navarro, J., Betz, E., Ebhardt, G., Ferszt, R., and Wüllenweber, R., Eds., Raven Press, New York, 1978, 161.
33. Borzeix, M. G., Labos, M., Hartl, C., and Billeau, P., Vincamine effect on EEG disturbances induced by a transitory hypovolemic hypotension, in *Pathophysiology and Pharmacotherapy of Cerebrovascular Disorders,* Betz, E., Grote, J., Heuser, D., and Wüllenweber, R., Eds., Verlag Gerhard Witzstrock, Baden-Baden, 1980, 321.
34. Kogure, K., Busto, R., Reinmuth, O., and Scheinberg, P., Energy metabolites, water content, and catecholamine changes in a model of cerebral embolic infarction, *Neurology,* 23, 438, 1973.
35. Bralet, A. M., Beley, A., Beley, P., Bralet, J., Brain edema and blood brain barrier permeability following quantitative cerebral microembolism, *Stroke,* 10, 34, 1979.
36. Rapin, J. R., Modèle d'ischémie cérébrale chez le rat. Captation et phosphorylation du déoxyglucose, in *Barrière Hémoencéphalique et Souffrance Cérébrale,* Excerpta Medica, Amsterdam, 1981, 78.

37. Le Poncin-Lafitte, M., Modèle d'ischémie cérébrale chez le rat. Etude d'une activité fonctionnelle, in *Barrière Hémoencéphalique et Souffrance Cérébrale,* Excerpta Medica, Amsterdam, 1981, 87.

38. Meldrum, B. S., Papy, J. J., and Vigouroux, R. A., Intracarotid air embolism in the baboon: effects on cerebral blood flow and the electroencephalogram, *Brain Res.,* 25, 301, 1971.

39. Jeynes, B. J. and Warren, B. A., Cerebral atheroembolism. An animal model, *Stroke,* 13, 312, 1982.

40. Fieschi, C., Battistini, N., Volante, F., Zanette, E., and Passero, S., Animal model of TIA: an experimental study with intracarotid ADP infusion in rabbits, *Stroke,* 6, 617, 1975.

41. Furlow, T.W., Jr. and Bass, N.H., Arachidonate-induced cerebrovascular occlusion in the rat, *Neurology,* 26, 297, 1976.

42. Cahn, J., Borzeix, M. G., Akimjak, J. P., Dupont, J. M., and Lemas, C., Nonspecific breakdown of the BBB in rats. Comparative study between cerebral infarctions due to sodium lactate, or sodium arachidonate and mechanical opening of BBB by rapid infusion of blood into the internal carotid artery, in *Cerebral Vascular Disease 3,* Meyer, J. S., Lechner, H., Reivich, M., Ott, E. O., and Aranibar, A., Eds., Excerpta Medica, Amsterdam, 1981, 223.

43. Cahn, J. and Borzeix, M. G., Experimental models related to acute brain ischemia in the dog, *J. Cereb. Blood Flow Metab.,* in press.

44. Kudo, M., Aoyama, A., Ichimori, S., and Fukunaga, N., An animal model of cerebral infarction. Homologous blood clot emboli in rats, *Stroke,* 13, 505, 1982.

45. Ferrari, R., Di Lisa, F., Raddino, R., and Visioli, O., Effects of myocardial calcium overloading during ischaemia and reperfusion on ATP synthesis, in *Calcium Modulators,* Godfraind, T., Albertini, A., and Paoletti, R., Eds., Elsevier Biomedical Press, Amsterdam, 1982, 99.

46. Rigoulet, M., Guerin, F., Cohadon, F., and Vandendreissche, M., Unilateral brain injury in the rabbit. Reversible and irreversible damage to the membranal ATPase, *J. Neurochem.,* 32, 535, 1979.

47. Burešova, O., Bureš, J., Bohdanecky, Z., and Weiss, T., Effect of atropine on learning, extinction, retention and retrieval in rats, *Psychopharmacologia,* 5, 255, 1964.

48. Lavy, S., Melamed, E., and Portnoy, Z., Cerebral blood flow response in non affected hemisphere of patients with acute cerebral infarction, in *Cerebral Function, Metabolism and Circulation,* Ingvar, D. H. and Lassen, N. A., Eds., Munksgaard, Copenhagen, 1977, 246.

49. Cahn, J., Borzeix, M. G., Anignard, J., Akimjak, J. P., and Dupont, J. M., Possible use of Coenzyme Q10 in acute cerebral disease, in *Biomedical and Clinical Aspects of Coenzyme Q,* Vol. 3, Folkers, K. and Yamamura, Y., Eds., Elsevier/North-Holland, Amsterdam, 1981, 385.

50. Borzeix, M. G. and Cahn, J., Effect of ZK 36374 (PGI$_2$ analog) on Na arachidonate-induced cerebral infarct in hypertensive rats, in *Proc. 5th Int. Conf. Prostaglandins,* Fondazione Giovanni Lorenzini, Milan, 1982, 800.

51. Harris, R. J., Bayhan, M., Branston, N. M., Watson, A., and Symon, L., Modulation of the pathophysiology of primate focal cerebral ischaemia by indomethacin, *Stroke,* 13, 17, 1982.

52. Volpi, M., Naccache, P. H., and Sha'afi, R. I., Arachidonate metabolite (s) increase the permeability of the plasma membrane of the neutrophil membranes to calcium, *Biochem. Biophys. Res. Comm.,* 92, 1231, 1980.

53. Michelson, A. M., Inflammatory aspects of free radicals, paper presented at 3rd Int. Beaune Conf., Beaune, France, October 15 to 16, 1982.

54. Cahn, J. and Herold, M., Importance des groupes sulfhydryles en biologie. Physiopathologie des derives sulfhydryles, *Agressologie,* 1, 157, 1960.

55. Cahn, J. and Herold, M., Importance du glutathion reduit dans le metabolisme du cerveau, *C. R. Seances Soc. Biol. Paris,* 154, 304, 1960.

56. Cahn, J., Herold, M., Kabacoff, O., Helbecque, C., Barre, N., and Tassart, O., Action de l'Ubiquinone 50 sur le systeme cardio-vasculaire et le comportement psychomoteur chez le chien et le rat, *Agressologie,* 2, 221, 1961.

57. Cahn, J. and Borzeix, M. G., Aging and hypertension as risk factors for the brain related to freeradical damages to cell membranes. Curative effect of ergot alkaloids in case of a multiple cerebral infarct, in *Aging,* Vol. 23, Agnoli, A., Ed., Raven Press, New York, 1983, 413.

58. Borzeix, M. G. and Charles, P., Unpublished data.

59. Cahn, J., Borzeix, M. G., Akimjak, J. P., Anignard, J., Labos, M., and Lebeau, M., Revue sur certains antagonistes des la peroxydation des lipides membranaires par les radicaux libres dans la therapeutique des accidents vasculaires cerebraux aigus d'origine ischemique, *Agressologie,* 23, 21, 1982.

Chapter 16

HYPERTENSION

Peter S. Chan and Peter Cervoni

TABLE OF CONTENTS

I. INTRODUCTION

The etiology of 90% of all human hypertension cases is unknown. The level of arterial blood pressure at any given time is determined by the balance of the vasopressor and vasodepressor systems operating in various organs and tissues of the body. The major vasopressor systems identified to date consist of the adrenergic nervous system, the renin-angiotensin-aldosterone system, the thromboxane (TX) and prostaglandin (PG) $F_{2\alpha}$ system, and the vasopressin system. The major vasodepressor systems that have been identified are the parasympathetic nervous system, the kallikrein-kinin system, the PGE_2 and PGI_2 systems, and the renal neutral-lipids system. The CNS can exert either a vasopressor or vasodepressor influence, depending on the level of homoeostasis.

The overactivity of the vasopressor systems with normal vasodepressor systems will, no doubt, cause hypertension. In the past 50 years of hypertension research, the emphasis has been on the etiology and modulation of the overactivity of these vasopressor systems; however, normal vasopressor systems with underactivity or deficiency of the vasodepressor systems to oppose the vasopressor effect will theoretically lead to hypertension. This latter mechanism, particularly the PG system, has been proposed mainly by Lee and associates[1-14] and McGiff and associates[15-23] as a working hypothesis in the last two decades. Many review articles are available on this subject.[1-33]

This chapter will focus on the available evidence and examine the contribution of PGs in the regulation of blood pressure and their role in the etiology of hypertension.

II. BIOSYNTHESIS AND METABOLISM OF PROSTAGLANDINS

PGs of various types are synthesized by all tissues studied.[24,25] Arachidonic acid, the common precursor for the major PGs, is derived from food or formed from linoleic acid from the diet, and is stored in the membrane phospholipids of cells. It is released by the actions of the phospholipases. Once released, depending on the tissue, arachidonic acid is metabolized via two important pathways, the cyclooxygenase pathway and the lipoxygenase pathway. The latter pathway, which is responsible for the formation of leukotrienes, is outside the scope of this chapter and will not be discussed; however, agents that inhibit the actions of the phospholipases, such as the steroidal anti-inflammatory drugs and mepacrine, will block both pathways.

Arachidonic acid is catalyzed by cyclooxygenase to form the endoperoxides. The endoperoxides, PGG_2 and PGH_2 are common precursors for the major PGs and TXs. Prostacyclin (PGI_2, epoprostenol) and TXA_2 are formed from the endoperoxides by the action of PGI_2 synthetase (synthase) and TX synthetase, respectively. PGE_2, PGD_2, and $PGF_{2\alpha}$ are formed by isomerases or reductases. It is now generally accepted that PGA_2 does not occur naturally in the body in any significant amount and probably is an artifact resulting from rearrangement of PGE_2 during isolation procedures.[35]

Cyclooxygenase activity is inhibited by indomethacin, meclofenamate, aspirin, and other nonsteroidal anti-inflammatory (NSAI) agents. TX synthetase activity is inhibited by imidazole, 1-benzylimidazole, dazoxiben-HCl (UK 37248-01), CGS-13080,[36] and OKY-1581, etc., while PGI_2 synthetase is inhibited by 15-hydroperoxy arachidonic acid (15-HPAA), other lipid peroxides, β-thromboglobulin, low-density lipoprotein (LDL), and tranylcypromine, etc.[32,37-40] Both TXA_2 and PGI_2 are unstable in aqueous solution with a half-life of a fraction of a minute to several minutes and are metabolized to TXB_2 and 6-keto-$PGF_{1\alpha}$, respectively.[34] In blood, PGI_2 binding to albumin has a half-life of 3 min. 6-Keto-PGE_1 can be formed from PGI_2 by 9-hydroxy-PG dehydrogenase. It has similar biological effects and can, therefore, serve as an extension of the effects of PGI_2[40-49] because 6-keto-PGE_1 has a much longer half-life. Initially, it was reported that 6-keto-PGE$_1$ could be formed from 6-keto-PGF$_{1\alpha}$ in some tissues, but the fact that infusion of large amounts of 6-keto-PGF$_{1\alpha}$ and PGI$_2$ in animals and man did not result in formation of a significant amount of 6-keto-PGE$_1$ casts some doubt on the importance of the transformation from 6-keto-PGF$_{1\alpha}$ in vivo.[49,50] Furthermore, 6-keto-PGE$_1$ was not detected in patients with Bartter's syndrome who were reported to have high levels of 6-keto-PGF$_{1\alpha}$. PGE$_2$, PGD$_2$, and PGF$_{2\alpha}$ are mainly inactivated by 15-hydroxy PG dehydrogenase. In a normal diet, the intake of dihomo-γ-linoleic acid and eicosapentaenoic acid (EPA), the precursors of the PGs of the 1 and 3 series, respectively, is low, and therefore significant levels of the PGs of the 1 and 3 series such as PGE$_1$ and PGI$_3$ are not formed and exert little influence in biological systems. PGs are not stored in any cells or organs, but are formed in cells at the site of action on demand by stimuli. Therefore, the levels of PGs in tissues and blood are very low.

III. PROSTAGLANDINS AND REGULATION OF BLOOD PRESSURE

PGE$_2$ and PGI$_2$ (epoprostenol) are the major vasodepressor PGs, while PGF$_{2\alpha}$ and TXA$_2$ are the major vasopressor PGs. Vasodepressor PGs exert their effects (1) by direct vasodilation of the blood vessels in counteracting the vasopressor systems, (2) by increasing renal blood flow and by inducing diuresis and natriuresis in the kidney, (3) by attenuating the hypertensive effects of the renin-angiotensin system, and (4) by amplifying the hypotensive effects of the kallikrein-kinin system. PGE$_2$ has also been shown to attenuate transmission in the adrenergic nervous system by decreasing norepinephrine release.[51-52]

PGs appear to be critically involved in human hypertension in the regulation of renin release, vascular resistance, renal blood flow, and by counteracting the pressor response to vasopressor hormones. Therefore, deficiency in PG formation may contribute to the increase in vascular resistance and increased responsiveness to vasopressor agents such as norepinephrine and angiotensin II. Patients with essential hypertension show a decrease in responsiveness to increased plasma renin activity (PRA) stimulated by furosemide.[53] This suggests that the kidneys of patients with essential hypertension produce less PGE$_2$. Indeed, impairment in renal production and a decrease in the excretion of PGE$_2$ has been reported in patients with essential hypertension.[54-56] In addition, it was reported that the urinary ratio of PGF$_{2\alpha}$:PGE$_2$ was increased under basal conditions and after stimulation with furosemide.[57] High salt intake shifted the ratio of PGF$_{2\alpha}$:PGE$_2$ in urine from 1 to 4.[58] In spontaneously hypertensive rats[59,60] and in salt plus indomethacin-induced hypertension in rats,[61] the production of PGF$_{2\alpha}$ was increased.[59-61]

In conscious human subjects, indomethacin has been shown to increase total peripheral resistance and renal resistance. The contribution of the PG system in maintaining the relaxation of the vasculature depends on the vasoconstrictor influence. The greater the vasoconstrictor influence, the greater the response of the PG system. Therefore, the end result of PG systhesis blockade varies widely.[62]

Indomethacin causes sodium retention, which has been proposed to be the mechanism by which it blocks the antihypertensive effect of propranolol.[63]

If the PGs synthesized locally in blood vessels are important in the regulation of blood pressure by counteracting the vasopressor systems, then the removal of this PG system should increase blood pressure or aggravate the existing hypertension. Indeed, significant increases in blood pressure in normotensive and hypertensive subjects have been observed after acute[64,65] or after 4 days of treatment with high doses in indomethacin.[66] Indomethacin and meclofenamate also increase the blood pressure in anesthetized rabbits, dogs, and other species after acute administration.[67-71] Subchronic dosing

(14 days) with indomethacin elevates the blood pressure of rabbits;[72] however, this was not observed routinely in other conscious animals or humans.[32,65,73,74]

Long-term heavy users of NSAI drugs such as aspirin and indomethacin, etc., which are potent cyclooxygenase inhibitors, have not been reported to develop hypertension in association with their use. In addition, other studies using indomethacin at lower doses and/or for a shorter treatment period did not demonstrate an increase in blood pressure.[32,75] It has been estimated that the production of PGs has to be inhibited more than 80% for an increase in blood pressure to occur.[19] It appears that there is a basal efflux of renal PGs which cannot be suppressed even by high doses of indomethacin. This may explain why attempts to produce hypertension by inhibition of PG production have failed in many species.

At least five different forms of experimental hypertension, namely, deoxycorticosterone (DOCA) hypertension, post-salt hypertension, Goldblatt hypertension, post-Goldblatt hypertension, and Okamoto-Kyoto spontaneous hypertension are characterized by reduced lipid granules (rich in arachidonic acid) in the renal papilla of the kidney. This suggests that a possible reduction in PG synthesis may lead to hypertension.[76-80]

On the other hand, in many forms of hypertension in animals, such as spontaneous hypertension, renal hypertension, and DOCA-salt hypertension, increased capability of PG synthesis was observed in many tissues.[81,82] The increase in PG synthesis is interpreted as a protective or defensive mechanism in an attempt to counteract the effects of the vasopressor systems.

It has been shown that the administration of epinephrine, norepinephrine, angiotensin II, and stimulation of the adrenergic nervous system leads to release of the PGs, primarily PGE_2 and PGI_2, which in turn counteracts the vasoconstricting effects of the stimuli.[83] Therefore, the PG system attenuates the reactivity of the blood vessels, and the deficiency in the production of PGs may lead to hypertension.

Even though production of TXA_2 in blood vessels, lungs, kidneys, and other tissues as compared to PGI_2 is small in absolute amounts, the level of biological activities (concentration × potency) may be in comparable ranges. Whether TXA_2 synthesis is increased in hypertension is not well studied; therefore, the significance of TXA_2 as a vasoconstrictor in hypertension may be underestimated at present.[84]

A. Circulating Prostaglandins

1. Direct Vasodilatation

PGI_2 was discovered in 1976 and it is the major PG in all vascular tissues studied to date,[85-88] except perhaps the umbilical blood vessels where PGE_2 appears to be dominant as reported in one study. Prostacyclin is 4 to 8 times more potent that PGE_2 as a hypotensive agent when given intravenously. It is also the most potent endogenous inhibitor of platelet aggregation known, being 40 times more potent than PGE_1 and has been shown to inhibit thrombus formation in vivo. Whether there is any significant consequence of the antithrombotic effects of PGI_2 on blood pressure regulation is unknown. PGI_2 dilates all vascular beds studied. Armstrong et al.[89] proposed that PGI_2, not PGE_2, synthesized locally in the arterioles throughout the body, is the PG vasodepressor system responsible for counteracting other vasopressor systems. A decrease in PGI_2 synthesis may, therefore, contribute to hypertension.

Many agents have been reported to stimulate the synthesis and release of PGI_2 in vitro or in vivo. These agents are angiotensin II,[90-93] bradykinin, A23187 (a calcium ionophore),[94-95] nafazatrom (Bay g 6575),[96-98] vitamins C and E, nitroglycerin,[99] dipyridamole,[100-102] nicotinic acid, catecholamines, isoproterenol, suloctidil, dazoxiben HCl (UK 37248-01), thrombin,[95-103] trypsin,[95] bendrofluazide,[104] high density lipoprotein (HDL),[105] and other agents.[86,106-109] Dazoxiben HCl, a TX synthetase inhibitor, has been reported to increase PGI_2 in vivo and ex vivo probably by shifting the PG endoperoxides from the platelets to other tissues for the synthesis of PGI_2.

Many agents that have been reported to stimulate the formation of PGI_2 or increase its concentration in the circulation probably will also increase the formation and release of PGE_2, although this has not been studied in detail. Theoretically, an agent which can selectively stimulate the synthesis and release of PGI_2 and PGE_2 to a significant level, but not that of TXA_2 formation may be useful as an antihypertensive agent. However, the known agents do not have the desired activity, potency, and profile; therefore, the testing of such a hypothesis is not possible at present.

Agents that inhibit the activity of 15-hydroxy-PG dehydrogenase should also be useful clinically, particularly if used in combination with stimulators of PGI_2 and PGE_2 release. Furosemide, nafazatrom, theophylline, sulfasalazine, ethacrynic acid, probenecid, and xylocaine, etc. are known to inhibit this enzyme.[110,111]

PGI_2 does not block the effects of angiotensin on the microcirculation[112] and does not block the release of norepinephrine from the nerve terminals.[113] Besides spontaneous degradation in water, PGI_2 is also metabolized by 15-hydroxy-PG dehydrogenase. Over 85% of the PGI_2 that passes through the circulation of the lungs remains intact, not because of its resistance to the enzyme for degradation but probably because of its poor penetration into sites of catabolism.[114] In fact, PGI_2 is released from the pulmonary vascular bed into the general circulation.[115,116] For this reason, PGI_2 was proposed as a circulatory hormone acting as a systemic antihypertensive principle;[117,118] however, under normal conditions, the amount of PGI_2 found in the blood may be too small to have any significant antihypertensive effect.[25,119-121]

Intravenous injections or infusions of PGE_2 decrease arterial blood pressure in all species studied.[122,123] When blood pressure is raised by the infusion of norepinephrine, simultaneous infusion of PGE_2 still produces lowering of arterial blood pressure in all species tested. PGE_2 is synthesized in the body at a rate of about ten times that of PGI_2.[124-126] Since the discovery of PGI_2 the research of PGE_2 has temporarily been deemphasized. The relative importance and contribution on PGE_2 in the control of blood pressure has yet to be determined.

2. Administration of Prostaglandins and Their Precursors

PGI_2 produces peripheral vasodilation and blood pressure lowering.[85-88,127,128] Even though the existence of PGA as a naturally occurring PG has been questioned,[129,130] the intravenous administration of PGA_1 and PGA_2 infusion produces hypotension in hypertensive patients.[131-138] PGE_1 and PGE_2 have also been reported to decrease the elevated blood pressure in humans.[122,139,140]

PGs of the A and E series, at high intravenous doses, have been demonstrated to lower the blood pressure in animals with spontaneous, renovascular, and renoprival hypertension. PGE_1 and PGE_2 produce natriuresis, diuresis, and lower arterial blood pressure mainly by decreasing the peripheral resistance in all species studied.[122,123] The blood flows through various vascular beds are increased. Intravenous infusions of prostaglandins PGE_1, PGE_2, PGI_2, PGA, and PGD produce natriuresis and diuresis.[132,141,142]

Intravenous administration of arachidonic acid, the precursor of PGs, lowers the blood pressure in various species.[143] A synthetic PGE_2 analogue, 16(R)-methyl-13,14-dihydro-PGE_2 methyl ester given orally produces antihypertensive effects in hypertensive patients.[144] Another synthetic PGE_2 analogue CL 115,347, (±)-15-deoxy-16-hydroxy-16-vinyl PGE_2 methyl ester, produces very impressive antihypertensive effects with a long duration of action in rats, cats, dogs, and monkeys following oral or transdermal administration.[145-150] The 16-methylene PGE_1 methyl ester and other PGE_1 analogues[151] have been reported to exert potent antihypertensive activity. Many synthetic stable PGI_2 analogues have also been reported to produce potent hypotensive effects.[152-155]

Lowering of blood pressure has been reported in patients and normotensive subjects as well as in animals after treatment with linoleic acid, the precursor of arachidonic acid.[156-161] Deprivation of linoleic acid in the diet leads to hypertension.[160-162] In spontaneously hypertensive rats, linoleic acid supplemented diets not only increase PG synthesis, but also proportionately increase the production of PGE_2, rather than $PGF_{2\alpha}$ in the kidney, leading to a favorable ratio for decreasing the blood pressure.[162,164] Linoleic acid also delays the onset of salt-induced hypertension in Dahl S rats.[165]

B. Prostaglandins in the Kidney

The role of the PGs in the regulation of blood pressure through the kidney mainly reside in (1) its direct effect in inducing saluretic and diuretic effects, (2) increasing renal blood flow, (3) its amplification of the kinin system, and (4) its attenuation of the hypertensive effects of the renin-angiotensin-aldosterone system.[14,15,166,167] PGI_2, PGE_2, and $PGF_{2\alpha}$ are the major PGs synthesized by the kidney.[14] PGE_2 is the main PG of the renal medulla and papilla, while $PGF_{2\alpha}$ is mostly synthesized in the outer renal medulla. PGI_2 is mainly produced in the renal vasculature and the renal cortex.[14] This observation forms the basis for the suggestion that PGI_2 may play a more important role in the release of renin and in decreasing renal vascular resistance rather that PGE_2.

PGE_2 causes vasodilation, diuresis, and inhibition of the release of norepinephrine from nerve endings, while $PGF_{2\alpha}$ causes vasoconstriction and augmentation of the adrenergic nervous system. PGI_2 produces vasodilation and release of renin. The latter action may counteract part of its vasodilator action. $PGF_{2\alpha}$ can be formed in the kidney from PGE_2 by the action of PGE-9-ketoreductase.[141] The balance between PGE_2 and $PGF_{2\alpha}$ may determine the feedback for the control of arterial blood pressure. PGE_2 is synthesized in the interstitial and collecting tubular cells of the renal medulla and it is mainly metabolized in the renal cortex.[168] PGE_2 produces natriuresis in animals and humans, probably secondary to renal vasodilation. Bradykinin and angiotensin II release PGE_2 from the kidneys.

1. Water and Sodium Excretion

Arachidonic acid by virtue of its conversion to PGs increases renal blood flow with a concomitant natriuresis. Indomethacin inhibits both effects.[169,170] The diuretics, furosemide, bumetanide, and ethacrynic acid increase PGE_2 production, renal blood flow, and natriuresis. Indomethacin also blocks such effects.[14,171] Infusions of exogenous PGs types E and A cause diuresis and natriuresis in animals and man.[132,141,142] PGE_2 has been shown to inhibit sodium reabsorption in the isolated collecting ducts;[172,173] however, other investigators have not been able to reproduce this effect.[174] There is overwhelming evidence to show that inhibition of PG synthesis by NSAI agents leads to water and sodium retention in man. PGE_2 exerts its renal effects by renal vasodilation, anti-antidiuretic hormone (ADH), and effects on sodium reabsorption.[14,167,171]

Indomethacin has been shown to suppress the diuretic and natriuretic effects of diuretics with diversified structures such as hydrochlorothiazide, furosemide, MK-196, and MK-447.[175,176] This suggests that the actions of many diuretics are mediated by PGs.

2. Renal Vasodilatation

Increase in renal vascular resistance has been recognized as an important initiating factor in the pathogenesis of human hypertension.[177] Renal blood flow depends on renal PGs in situations under stress such as in sodium deprivation, laparotomy, and infusion of angiotensin II, but not in conscious, normotensive, and salt-repleted animals.[14,15,167,171,178] In stress situations, infusion of arachidonic acid, PGA_2, PGD_2, PGE_2, and PGI_2 decrease renal vascular resistance, while inhibition of the PG system decreases renal blood flow and increases renal vascular resistance.[14,167,171] Since PGE_2 opposes the renal vasoconstricting effects of angiotensin II, the impairment in the synthesis and release of intrarenal PGE_2 will leave the effects of the renin-angiotensin system unopposed. This may lead to the initiation of hypertension.

3. Interaction with the Kallikrein-Kinin System

Bradykinin is a potent vasodilator formed by kallikrein and degraded by kininase II. It is 10 times as active as histamine. The kidney has a very high kininase II activity in the proximal tubule. Kallikrein excretion is increased in patients with aldosteronism and decreased following treatment with an antagonist of aldosterone, spironolactone.[179] It is possible that the release of kallikrein may be regulated by the mineralocorticoids.[30] Bradykinin is known to release PGs in the kidney by activation of phospholipase A_2.[180,181] Kinins are reported to increase the activity of PGE-9-ketoreductase, which catalyzes the formation of $PGF_{2\alpha}$ from PGE_2.[182] It has been suggested that the vasodepressor effect of bradykinin is mediated by PGE_2 and the vasoconstrictor effect, particularly in the veins, is mediated by $PGF_{2\alpha}$[183] and norepinephrine.

PGE_1 and PGE_2 antagonize the effects of ADH in stimulating water transport in vitro in the toad bladder and in the isolated renal collecting duct;[184-186] therefore, at least part of the renal vasodilator action, diuresis, and natriuresis of bradykinin is mediated by PGE_2.[187] Both bradykinin and PGE_2 attenuate the renal vasoconstrictor effect of norepinephrine or stimulation of the sympathetic nervous system.[187,188] The attenuation was reversed by the inhibition of PG synthesis, implying that PGE_2 mediates the action of bradykinin in the regulation of renal blood flow.[189] Stimulation of the production or inhibition of the degradation of the kinins produces diuresis, natriuresis, and an increase in PGE_2 excretion. Therefore, PGE_2 amplifies the action of the kinin system by increasing urinary sodium excretion and by attenuating the reactivity of the renal vasculature to adrenergic stimulation in an attempt to protect the circulation in the kidney.

4. Interaction with the Renin-Angiotensin-Aldosterone System

Angiotensin II infusion causes an initial decrease in renal blood flow, but also causes the release of PGE_2 in the kidney. The PGE_2 released in the kidney was found to counteract the vasoconstrictor and antidiuretic effects of the infused angiotensin II and to return the renal blood flow and urine flow to the control level despite the continued infusion of angiotensin II. When the synthesis of PGs is inhibited by indomethacin, the renal blood flow and diuresis are drastically reduced by angiotensin II infusion, and the return to normal phase is not observed,[17] implying that PGs are responsible for returning the renal blood flow and urine flow to the normal level.

On the other hand, arachidonic acid, endoperoxides, PGE_2, PGA_1, PGE_1, and PGI_2 are potent stimulators of the release of renin,[14,30] which in turn produces angiotensin II and aldosterone, while $PGF_{2\alpha}$ inhibits renin release.[30] Renal nerve stimulation, ischemia, low sodium diet, and diuretics increase PG production in the kidney. This increase may be mediated through the renin-angiotensin system because renin production is increased. Therefore, the mechanism by which PGs release renin and the end product of renin, angiotensin II (which in turn releases PGs) serves as a positive feedback between the two systems. The initiation and the significance of this positive feedback is poorly understood.

Indomethacin decreases the basal levels of PRA and inhibits the renin release induced by orthostasis, renal hypertension, low sodium intake, furosemide, and other diuretics, indicating that PGs may play a role in the release of renin in many situations.[14,62,187,190-192] Furthermore, indomethacin was shown to lower basal PRA in normotensive and hypertensive humans and rabbits. Thus, indomethacin attenuates the angiotensin pressor system in addition to the removal of the PG system by inhibition of cyclooxygenase.

Urinary excretion of PGE_2 decreases while that of $PGF_{2\alpha}$ is normal in patients with essential hypertension.[30,32] Captopril is an angiotensin converting enzyme and kininase II inhibitor and, therefore, a bradykinin potentiator. Captopril has been shown to increase urinary excretion of PGE_2 200% over the control.[30,32] Another study on captopril reported the increase of kinin, but not that of PGE_2 excretion. The increase of $PGF_{2\alpha}$ excretion was not statistically significant; however, captopril did not alter the plasma levels of PGs. Endogenous PGs may be responsible for the blood pressure lowering effects of captopril in low renin hypertensive patients, since the effects were reversed by indomethacin.[30]

Other preliminary reports suggest that part of the antihypertensive effect of hydralazine, angiotensin converting enzyme inhibitors, β-adrenoceptor blockers, and diuretics may be mediated by endogenous PGs.[193,194]

IV. CONCLUSIONS

The evidence available at present shows that the vasodepressor PGs, PGI_2 and PGE_2, are powerful regulators of arterial blood pressure by counteracting the vasopressor influences in blood vessels and kidney, locally as well as systemically. The reactivity of blood vessels, peripheral resistance, and the renal functions are intimately modulated by the PG systems, which serve a protective role when they are challenged in situations such as hypertension and ischemia. Whether a deficiency in PG production leads to hypertension requires more study. Considering the available evidence, it appears that without the operation of the PG vasodepressor system to oppose the effects of the vasoconstrictor hormones, the existing hypertension is likely to become more severe. PGI_2 and PGE_2 are among the most potent vasodepressors known, and they possess desirable mechanisms for lowering arterial blood pressure. The next generation of new antihypertensives may evolve from this system. Several synthetic PGs are under clinical trials for the treatment of essential hypertension. Whether these synthetic PGs can serve as replacements of the "missing hormone" (i.e., deficiency of endogenous PGs) remains to be seen. They may become valuable additions to the armamentarium for hypertension therapy.

Even though the synthesis of the vasodepressor PGs in many tissues is reported to increase in some forms of hypertension, the increase without other stimuli is obviously not high enough to overcome the prevailing vasopressor mechanisms and to normalize the elevated arterial blood pressure. Therefore, stimulators of PG synthesis are needed to further elevate the vasodepressor PG synthesis. However, the present known stimulators of endogenous PGI_2 and PGE_2 release do not have the required potency, profiles, and duration of action. Better compounds have yet to be discovered. Thus, manipulation in the stimulation of production and inhibition of the degradation of PGI_2 and PGE_2 or inhibition of TXA_2 and $PGF_{2\alpha}$ formation by chemical agents appear to offer novel approaches to new, desirable antihypertensive agents.

REFERENCES

1. Lee, J. B., Antihypertensive activity of the kidney — the renomedullary prostaglandins, *N. Engl. J. Med.*, 277, 1073, 1967.
2. Lee, J. B., Hypertension, natriuresis and the renal prostaglandins, *Ann. Intern. Med.*, 70, 1033, 1969.
3. Lee, J. B., Renal homeostasis and the hypertensive state: a unifying hypothesis, in *The Prostaglandins*, Ramwell, P. W., Ed., Plenum Press, New York, 1973, 133.
4. Lee, J. B., The antihypertensive function of the kidney, in *Perspective Prostaglandins*, Lee, J. B., Ed., Medcom Press, New York, 1973, 48.
5. Vance, V. K. and Lee, J. B., Hypertension and human renal prostaglandins, *Med. Ann.*, 42, 419, 1973.
6. Lee, J. B., Cardiovascular-renal effects of prostaglandins. Antihypertensive, natriuretic renal endocrine function, *Arch. Intern. Med.*, 133, 56, 1974.
7. Lee, J. B., Renal prostaglandins and the antihypertensive endocrine function, *Med. Clin. North Am.*, 59, 713, 1975.
8. Lee, J. B. and Attallah, A. A., Renal prostaglandins, *Nephron*, 15, 352, 1975.
9. Lee, J. B., Prostaglandins and blood pressure control, *Am. J. Med.*, 61, 681, 1976.
10. Lee, J. B., The renal prostaglandins and blood pressure regulation, in *Advances in Prostaglandins and Thromboxane Research*, Vol. 2, Samuelson, B. et al., Eds., Raven Press, New York, 1976, 573.
11. Lee, J. B. and Mookerjee Basab, B. K., The renal prostaglandins as etiologic factor in human essential hypertension: fact or fantasy? *Cardiovasc. Med.*, 1, 302, 1976.
12. Lee, J. B., Prostaglandins, neutral lipids, renal interstitial cells and hypertension, in *Hypertension: Physiopathological Treatment*, Genest, J., Koiw, E., and Kuchel, O., Eds., McGraw-Hill, New York, 1977, 373.
13. Carr, A. A. and Lee, J. B., Prostaglandins and blood pressure regulation, *Renal Prostaglandins*, 1, 121, 1978.
14. Attallah, A. A. and Lee, J. B., Prostaglandins, renal function, and blood pressure regulation, in *Prostaglandins*, Lee, J. B., Ed., Elsevier, New York, 1982, 251.
15. McGiff, J. C. and Nasjletti, A., Renal prostaglandins and the regulation of blood pressure, in *Prostaglandins and Cyclic AMP: Biological Actions and Clinical Applications*, Kahn, R. and Lands, W. E. M., Eds., Academic Press, New York, 1973, 119.
16. Vane, J. R. and McGiff, J. C., Possible contributions of endogenous prostaglandins to control of blood pressure, *Circ. Res.*, 36, 68, 1975.
17. McGiff, J. C. and Vane, J. R., Prostaglandins and the regulation of blood pressure, *Kidney Int.*, 8, S-262, 1975.
18. McGiff, J. C., Prostaglandins as regulators of blood pressure, *Hosp. Prac.*, 10, 101, 1975.
19. McGiff, J. C. and Quilley, J., Prostaglandins, kinins and regulation of blood pressure, *Clin. Exp. Hypertension*, 2, 729, 1980.
20. McGiff, J. C. and Quilley, J., Prostaglandins, hypertension and the cardiovascular system, in *Prostaglandins and Cardiovascular Disease*, Hegyeli, R. J., Ed., Raven Press, New York, 1981, 101.
21. McGiff, J. C., Prostaglandins and blood pressure control, in *Biochemical Regulation of Blood Pressure*, Soffer, R. L., Ed., John Wiley & Sons, New York, 1981, 360.
22. McGiff, J. C., Prostaglandins and hypertension, in *Prostaglandins, Platelets, Lipids: New Developments in Atherosclerosis*, Conn, H. L., DeFelice, and Kuo, P. T., Eds., Elsevier/North Holland, New York, 1981, 49.
23. McGiff, J. C. and Spokas, E. G., Regulation of blood pressure by prostaglandin-kinin interactions, in *Frontiers in Hypertension Research*, Laragh, J. H., Bühler, F. R., and Seldin, D. W., Eds., Springer-Verlag, New York, 1981, 105.
24. Frölich, J. C., Gill, J. R., McGiff, J. C., Needleman, P., and Nies, A. S., Prostaglandins, in *Subgroup Report of the Hypertension Task Force*, DHEW Publ. No. 79-1629, U.S. Government Printing Office, Washington, D.C., 1979, 3.
25. Frölich, J. C. and Rosenkranz, B., Role of prostaglandins in the regulation of blood pressure, in *Cardiovascular Pharmacology of the Prostaglandins*, Herman, A. G., Vanhoutte, P. M., Denolin, H., and Goossens, A., Eds., Raven Press, New York, 1982, 259.
26. Nasjletti, A. and Malik, K. U., Interactions between prostaglandins and vasoconstrictor hormones: contribution to blood pressure regulation, *Fed. Proc. Fed. Am. Soc. Exp. Biol.*, 41, 2394, 1982.
27. Wennmalm, Å., Participation of prostaglandins in the regulation of peripheral vascular resistance, in *Advances in Prostaglandin, Thromboxane, Leukotriene Research (Prostaglandins and the Cardiovascular System)*, Vol. 10, Oates, J. A., Ed., Raven Press, New York, 1982, 303.
28. Sullivan, J. M., Prostaglandins and regulation of blood pressure: clinical implications, *Pharmacol. Ther.*, 15, 447, 1982.
29. McGiff, J. C., Prostaglandins, prostacyclin, and thromboxanes, *Ann. Rev. Pharmacol. Toxicol.*, 21, 479, 1981.

30. Abe, K., The kinins and prostaglandins in hypertension, *Clin. Endocrinol. Metab.*, 3(3), 577, 1981.
31. Pace-Asciak, C. R., Prostacyclin and hypertension, *Mater. Med. Polona*, 3, 181, 1980.
32. Hornych, A., Role of prostaglandins in control of blood pressure, in *Prostaglandin Synthetase Inhibitors: New Clinical Applications,* Alan R. Liss, New York, 1980, 231.
33. Hornych, A., Prostaglandins and high blood pressure, *Contrib. Nephrol.*, 12, 54, 1978.
34. Samuelsson, B., Prostaglandins, thromboxanes, and leukotrienes: formation and biological roles, *Harvey Lect.*, 75, 1, 1981.
35. Frölich, J. C., Sweetman, B. J., Carr, K., Hollifield, J. W., and Oates, J. A., Assessment of the levels of PGA_2 in human plasma by gas chromatography-mass spectrometry, *Prostaglandins*, 10, 185, 1975.
36. Cohen, D. S., Povalski, H. J., Rinehart, R. R., Barclay, B. W., VanOrsdell, D., Tsai, C., and Sakane, Y., Thromboxane A_2 (TXA_2) synthetase inhibition causes endoperoxide shunting towards PGI_2 and PGE_2 synthesis in canine whole blood, *Fed. Proc. Fed. Am. Soc. Exp. Biol.*, 42, 640, 1983.
37. Salmon, J. A., Inhibition of arachidonic acid metabolism, in *Cardiovascular Pharmacology of Prostaglandins,* Herman, A. G., Vanhoutte, P. M., Denolin, H., and Goossens, A., Eds., Raven Press, New York, 1982, 7.
38. Cross, P. E., Antithrombotic agents, in *Annual Reports of Medical Chemistry,* Vol. 17, Hess, H.-J., Ed., Academic Press, New York, 1982, 79.
39. Vermylen, J. and Carreras, L. O., Pharmacological manipulation of prostacyclin release and activity, in *5-Hydroxytryptamine in Peripheral Reactions,* DeClerck, F. and Vanhoutte, P. M., Eds., Raven Press, New York, 1982, 107.
40. McGiff, J. C., Spokas, E. G., and Wong, P. Y-K., 6-KetoPGE$_1$, a stable and biologically active metabolite of prostacyclin, in *Cardiovascular Pharmacology of the Prostaglandins,* Herman, A. G., Vanhoutte, P. M., Denolin, H., and Goossens, A., Eds., Raven Press, New York, 1982, 149.
41. Wong, P. Y-K., Lee, W. H., and McGiff, J. C., Metabolism of prostacyclin (PGI_2) by the 9-hydroxyprostaglandin dehydrogenase (9-OH-PGDH) in human platelets, *Circulation*, 60, 269, 1979.
42. Wong, P. Y-K., Lee, W. H., Reiss, R. F., and McGiff, J. C., 6-Keto-prostaglandin E_1 inhibits the aggregation of human platelets, *Euro. J. Pharmacol.*, 60, 245, 1979.
43. Wong, P. Y-K., Lee, W. H., Chao, P. H. W., Reiss, R. F., and McGiff, J. C., Metabolism of prostacyclin by 9-hydroxyprostaglandin dehydrogenase in human platelets—formation of a potent inhibitor of platelet aggregation and enzyme purification, *J. Biol. Chem.*, 255, 9021, 1980.
44. Wong, P. Y-K., Malik, K. U., Desiderio, D. M., McGiff, J. C., and Sun, F. F., Hepatic metabolism of prostacyclin (PGI_2) in the rabbit—Formation of a potent novel inhibitor of platelet aggregation, *Biochem. Biophys. Res. Comm.*, 93, 486, 1980.
45. Wong, P. Y-K., Lee, W. H., Reiss, R. F., and McGiff, J. C., Metabolism of prostacyclin (PGI_2) by purified 9-hydroxy-prostaglandin dehydrogenase (9-OH-PGDH) of rabbit liver and human platelets, *Fed. Proc.*, 39, 392, 1980.
46. Quilley, C. P., Wong, P. Y-K., and McGiff, J. C., Hypotensive and renovascular actions of 6-keto-prostaglandin E_1, a metabolite of prostacyclin, *Euro. J. Pharmacol.*, 57, 273, 1979.
47. Quilley, C. P., McGiff, J. C., Lee, W. H., Sun, F. F., Wong, P. Y-K., 6-Keto PGE$_1$—A possible metabolite of prostacyclin having platelet anti-aggregatory effects, *Hypertension*, 2, 524, 1980.
48. VanDam, J., Fitzpatrick, T. M., Friedman, L. S., Ramwell, P. W., Rose, J. C., and Kot, P. A., Cardiovascular responses to 6-keto-prostaglandin E_1 in the dog, *Proc. Soc. Exp. Biol. Med.*, 166, 76, 1981.
49. Rosenkranz, B., Fischer, C., Reimann, I., Weimer, K. E., Beck, G., and Frölich, J. C., Identification of the major metabolite of prostacyclin and 6-keto-prostaglandin $F_{1\alpha}$ in man, *Biochem. Biophys. Acta*, 619, 207, 1980.
50. Jackson, E. K., Goodman, R. P., Fitzgerald, G. A., Oates, J. A., and Branch, R. A., Assessment of the extent to which exogenous prostaglandin I_2 is converted to 6-keto-prostaglandin E_1 in human subjects, *J. Pharmacol. Exp. Ther.*, 221, 183, 1982.
51. Hedqvist, P., Autonomic neurotransmission, in *The Prostaglandins,* Vol. 1, Ramwell, P. W., Ed., Plenum Press, New York, 1973, 101.
52. Malik, K. U., Prostaglandins — modulation of adrenergic nervous system, *Fed. Proc. Fed. Am. Soc. Exp. Biol.*, 37, 203, 1978.
53. Rumpf, K. W., Frenzel, S., Lowetz, H. D., and Scheler, F., The effect of indomethacin on plasma renin activity in man under normal conditions and after stimulation of the renin-angiotensin system, *Prostaglandins*, 10, 641, 1975.
54. Tan, S. Y., Sweet, P., and Mulrow, P. J., Impaired renal production of prostaglandin E_2: a newly identified lesion in human essential hypertension, *Prostaglandins*, 15, 139, 1978.
55. Abe, K., Yasujima, M., Irokawa, N., Seino, M., Chiba, S., Sakurai, Y., Sato, M., Imai, Y., Saito, K., Ito, T., Hasuyama, T., Otsuka, Y., and Yoshinasa, K., The role of intrarenal vasoactive substances in the pathogenesis of essential hypertension, *Clin. Sci. Mol. Med.*, 55, 363S, 1978.

56. Weber, P. C., Siess, W., and Scherer, B., Possible significance of renal prostaglandins in essential hypertension, *Clin. Exp. Hypertension,* 2, 741, 1980.
57. Weber, P. C., Scherer, B., Heed, E., Siess, W., and Stoffel, H., Urinary prostaglandins and kallikrein in essential hypertension, *Clin. Sci.,* 57, 259S, 1979.
58. Weber, P. C., Larsson, C., and Scherer, B., Prostaglandin E_2-9-ketoreductase as a mediator of salt intake-related prostaglandin-renin interaction, *Nature (London),* 226, 65, 1977.
59. Ahnfelt-Ronne, I. and Arrigoni-Martelli, E., Increased $PGF_{2\alpha}$ synthesis in renal papilla of spontaneously hypertensive rats, *Biochem. Pharmacol.,* 27, 2363, 1978.
60. Taube, C., Block, H. U., and Förster, W., Antihypertensive drugs alter the production and the ratio of prostaglandins E and F in the organs of spontaneously hypertensive rats, *Acta Biol. Med.,* 41, 477, 1982.
61. Nekrasova, A. A., Sokolova, R. N., Levitskaya, Y., Speranakaya, N. V., Kulagina, V. P., and Leghonkaya, N. P., Prostaglandins of blood vessels and vessel reactivity in rats receiving sodium chloride and indomethacin, in *Advances in Prostaglandin and Thromboxane Research,* Vol. 7, Samuelsson, B. et al., Eds., Raven Press, New York, 1980, 1139.
62. Weber, P. C., Siess, W., Scherer, B., Briggs, J. P., and Schnermann, J., Prostaglandins and the renal circulation, in *Cardiovascular Pharmacology of the Prostaglandins,* Herman, A. G., Vanhoutte, P. M., and Goossens, A., Eds., Raven Press, New York, 1982, 267.
63. Frölich, J. C., Prostaglandins: role in renin regulation and mediation of antihypertensive drug effects, *Arch. Int. Pharmacodyn. Ther.,* Suppl., 213, 1980.
64. Wennmalm, Å., Hypertensive effect of the prostaglandin synthesis inhibitor, indomethacin, *IRCS Libr. Compend.,* 2, 1099, 1974.
65. Ylitalo, P., Pitkäjärvi, T., Metsä-Ketelä, T., and Vapaatalo, H., The effect of inhibition of prostaglandin synthesis on plasma renin activity and blood pressure in essential hypertension, *Prostaglandins Med.,* 1, 479, 1978.
66. Patak, R. V., Mookerjee, B. K., Bentzel, C. J., Hysert, P. E., Babeu, M., and Lee, J. B., Antagonism of the effect of furosemide by indomethacin in normal hypertensive man, *Prostaglandins,* 10, 649, 1975.
67. Larsson, C. and Änggård, E., Arachidonic acid lowers and indomethacin increases the blood pressure of the rabbit, *J. Pharm. Pharmacol.,* 25, 653, 1973.
68. Lonigro, A. J., Itskovitz, H. D., Crowshaw, K., and McGiff, J. C., Dependency of renal blood flow on prostaglandin synthesis in the dog, *Circ. Res.,* 32, 712, 1973.
69. Yun, J., Kelly, G., Bartter, F. C., and Smith, H., Jr., Role of prostaglandins in the control of renin secretion in the dog, *Circ. Res.,* 40, 459, 1977.
70. Romero, J. C. and Strong, C. G., The effect of indomethacin blockade of prostaglandin synthesis on blood pressure of normal rabbits and rabbits with renovascular hypertension, *Circ. Res.,* 40, 35, 1977.
71. Scholkens, B. A. and Steinbach, R., Increase of experimental hypertension following inhibition of prostaglandin biosynthesis, *Arch. Int. Pharmacodyn. Ther.,* 214, 328, 1975.
72. Colina-Chourio, J., McGiff, J. C., and Nasjletti, A., Effect of indomethacin on blood pressure in the normotensive unanesthetized rabbit: possible relation to prostaglandin synthesis inhibition, *Clin. Sci.,* 57, 359, 1979.
73. Muirhead, E. E., Brooks, B., and Brosius, W. L., Indomethacin and blood pressure control, *J. Lab. Clin. Med.,* 88, 578, 1977.
74. Frölich, J. C., Hollifield, J. W., Dormois, J. C., Frölich, B. L., Seyberth, H., Michelakis, A. M., and Oates, J. A., Suppression of plasma renin activity by indomethacin in man, *Circ. Res.,* 39, 447, 1976.
75. Negus, P., Tannen, R. L., and Dunn, M., Indomethacin potentiates the vasoconstrictor actions of angiotensin II in normal man, *Prostaglandins,* 12, 175, 1976.
76. Tobian, L., Ishii, M., and Duke, M., Relationship of cytoplasmic granules in renal papillary interstitial cells to "postsalt" hypertension, *J. Lab. Clin. Med.,* 73, 309, 1969.
77. Tobian, L. and Ishii, M., Interstitial cell granules and solutes in renal papilla in post-Goldblatt hypertension, *Am. J. Physiol.,* 217, 1699, 1969.
78. Ishii, M. and Tobian, L., Interstitial cell granules in renal papilla and the solute composition of renal tissue in rats with Goldblatt hypertension, *J. Lab. Clin. Med.,* 74, 1, 1969.
79. Muehrcke, R. C., Mandal, A. K., and Volini, F., A pathophysiological review of the renal medullary interstitial cells and their relationship to hypertension, *Circ. Res.,* 27(Suppl. 1), 109, 1970.
80. Muehrcke, R. C., Mandal, A. K., Epstein, M., and Volini, F. I., Cytoplasmic granularity of the renal medullary interstitial cells in experimental hypertension, *J. Lab. Clin. Med.,* 73, 299, 1969.
81. Rioux, F., Quirion, R., and Regoli, D., The role of prostaglandins in hypertension. I. The release of prostaglandins by aorta strips of renal, DOCA-salt and spontaneously hypertensive rats, *Can. J. Physiol. Pharmacol.,* 55, 1330, 1977.

82. Limas, C. and Limas, C. J., Enhanced renomedullary prostaglandin synthesis in spontaneously hypertensive rats: role of a phospholipase A_2, *Am. J. Physiol.*, 233, H87, 1977.

83. Weber, P. C., Siess, W., Lorenz, R., and Scherer, B., The role of prostaglandins in essential hypertension, *Int. J. Obesity*, 5(Suppl. 1), 125, 1981.

84. Ally, A. I. and Horrobin, D. F., Thromboxane A_2 in blood vessel walls and its physiological significance: relevance to thrombosis and hypertension, *Prostaglandins Med.*, 4, 431, 1980.

85. Moncada, S., Prostacyclin and arterial wall biology, *Arteriosclerosis*, 2, 193, 1982.

86. Moncada, S., Biological importance of prostacyclin, *Br. J. Pharmacol.*, 76, 3, 1982.

87. Vane, J. R., Clinical potential of prostacyclin, in *Advances in Prostaglandin, Thromboxane and Leukotriene Research*, Vol. 11, Samuelsson, B. et al., Eds., Raven Press, New York, 1983, 449.

88. Higgs, E. A. and Moncada, S., Prostacyclin — physiology and clinical uses, *Gen. Pharmacol.*, 14, 7, 1983.

89. Armstrong, J. M., Dusting, G. J., Moncada, S., and Vane, J. R., Cardiovascular actions of prostacyclin (PGI$_2$), a metabolite of arachidonic acid which is synthetized by blood vessels, *Circ. Res.*, 43(Suppl 1), 112, 1978.

90. Danon, A., Chang, L. C., Sweetman, S. J., Nies, A. S., and Oates, J. A., Synthesis of prostaglandins by the rat renal papilla in vivo; mechanism of stimulation by angiotensin II, *Biochem. Biophys. Acta*, 388, 71, 1975.

91. Dusting, G. J. and Mullane, K. M., Stimulation by angiotensin of prostacyclin biosynthesis in rats and dogs, *Clin. Exp. Pharmacol. Physiol.*, 7, 545, 1980.

92. Gryglewski, R. J., Spławinski, J., and Korbut, R., Endogenous mechanisms that regulate prostacyclin release, in *Advances in Prostaglandin and Thromboxane Research*, Vol. 7, Samuelsson, B., Ramwell, P. W., and Paoletti, R., Eds., Raven Press, New York, 1980, 777.

93. Gryglewski, R., Prostacyclin experimental and clinical approach, in *Advances in Prostaglandin, Thromboxane and Leukotriene Research*, Vol. 11, Samuelsson, B. et al., Eds., Raven Press, New York, 1983, 457.

94. Knapp, H. R., Oelz, O., Roberts, L. J., Sweetman, B. J., Oates, J. A., and Reed, P. W., Ionophores stimulate prostaglandin and thromboxane biosynthesis, *Proc. Natl. Acad. Sci. U.S.A.*, 74, 4251, 1977.

95. Weksler, B. B., Ley, C. W., and Jaffe, E. A., Stimulation of endothelial cell prostacyclin production by thrombin, trypsin and the ionophore A23187, *J. Clin. Invest.*, 62, 923, 1978.

96. Honn, K. V., Busse, W. D., and Sloane, B. F., Prostacyclin and thromboxanes: implication for their role in tumor cell metastasis, *Biochem. Pharmacol.*, 32, 1, 1983.

97. Carreras, L. O., Chamone, D. A. F., Klercks, P., and Vermylen, J., Decreased vascular prostacyclin (PGI$_2$) in diabetic rats. Stimulation of PGI$_2$ release in normal and diabetic rats by the antithrombotic compound Bay g 6575, *Thromb. Res.*, 19, 663, 1980.

98. Vermylen, J., Chamone, D. A. F., and Verstaete, M., Stimulation of prostacyclin release from vessel wall by Bay g 6575, an antithrombotic compound, *Lancet*, 1, 518, 1979.

99. Levin, R. I., Jaffe, E. A., Weksler, B. B., and Tack-Goldman, K., Nitroglycerin stimulates synthesis of prostacyclin by cultured human endothelial cells, *J. Clin. Invest.*, 67, 762, 1981.

100. Blass, K. E., Block, H. U., Förster, W., and Pönicke, K., Dipyridamole: a potent stimulator of prostacyclin (PGI$_2$) biosynthesis, *Br. J. Pharmacol.*, 68, 71, 1980.

101. Van deVelde, V., Beetens, J., and Herman, A. G., Interactions of dipyridamole with prostacyclin biosynthesis, *Acta Ther.*, 6(Suppl.), 15, 1980.

102. Neri Serneri, G. G., Masotti, G., Poggesi, L., Galanti, G., and Morettini, A., Enhanced prostacyclin production by dipyridamole in man. *Eur. J. Clin. Pharmacol.*, 21, 9, 1981.

103. Hong, S. L., Effect of bradykinin and thrombin on prostacyclin synthesis in endothelial cells from calf and pig aorta and human umbilical cord vein, *Thromb. Res.*, 18, 787, 1980.

104. Webster, J., Dollery, C. T., and Hensby, C. N., Circulating prostacyclin concentrations may be increased by bendrofluazide in patients with essential hypertension, *Clin. Sci.*, 59, 125S, 1980.

105. Fleisher, L. N., Tall, A. R., Witte, L. D., and Cannon, P. J., Effects of high-density lipoprotein and the apoprotein of high-density lipoprotein on prostacyclin synthesis by endothelial cells, in *Advances in Prostacyclin, Thromboxane and Leukotriene Research*, Vol. 11, Samuelsson, B. et al., Eds., Raven Press, New York, 1983, 475.

106. Vermylen, J. and Carreras, L. O., Pharmacological manipulation of prostacyclin release and acitvity, in *5-Hydroxytryptamine in Peripheral Reactions*, DeClerck, F. and Vanhoutte, P. M., Eds., Raven Press, New York, 1982, 107.

107. Förster, W., Effect of various agents on prostaglandin biosynthesis and the anti-aggregatory effect, *Acta Med. Scand.*, 642(Suppl.), 35, 1980.

108. Mullane, K. M. and Moncada, S., Prostacyclin release and the modulation of some vasoactive hormones, *Prostaglandins*, 20, 25, 1980.

109. Kirstein, A., Cardiac prostacyclin release: stimulation by hypoxia and various agents, *Scand. J. Haematol.*, 23(Suppl. 34), 105, 1979.

110. Hansen, H. S., 15-Hydroxyprostaglandin dehydrogenase: a review, *Prostaglandins*, 12, 647, 1976.
111. Iijima, Y., Kawakita, N., and Yamazaki, M., Inhibition of 15-hydroxy prostaglandin dehydrogenase by antiallergic agents, *Biochem. Biophys. Res. Comm.*, 93, 912, 1980.
112. Messina, E. J. and Kaley, G., Microcirculatory response to PGI_2 and PGE_2 in the rat cremaster muscle, in *Advances in Prostaglandin and Thromboxane Research*, Samuelsson, B., Ramwell, P. W., and Paoletti, R., Raven Press, New York, 1980, 719.
113. Hedqvist, P., Actions of prostacyclin (PGI_2) on adrenergic neuroeffector transmission in the rabbit kidney, *Prostaglandins*, 17, 249, 1979.
114. Mullane, K. M., Moncada, S., and Vane, J. R., Formation and disappearance of prostacyclin in the circulation, in *Prostacyclin*, Vane, J. R. and Bergstrom, S., Eds., Raven Press, New York, 1979, 221.
115. Gryglewski, R. J., Is the lung an endocrine organ that secretes prostacyclin? in *Prostacyclin*, Vane, J. R. and Bergstrom, S., Eds., Raven Press, New York, 1979, 275.
116. Gryglewski, R., Korbut, R., and Ocetkiewicz, A., Generation of prostacyclin by lungs in vivo and its release into the arterial circulation, *Nature (London)*, 273, 765, 1978.
117. Moncada, S., Korbut, R., Bunting, S., and Vane, J. R., Prostacyclin is a circulatory hormone, *Nature (London)*, 273, 767, 1978.
118. Gryglewski, R. J., Prostacyclin as a circulating hormone, *Biochem. Pharmacol.*, 28, 3161, 1979.
119. Pace-Asciak, C. R., Carrara, M. C., Levine, L., and Nicolaou, K. C., PGI_2-specific antibodies administered in vivo suggest against a role for endogenous PGI_2 as a circulating vasodepressor hormone in the normotensive and spontaneously hypertensive rat, *Prostaglandins*, 20, 1053, 1980.
120. Pace-Asciak, C. R., Carrara, M. C., and Levine, L., PGI_2 is not a circulating vasodepressor hormone, *Prog. Lipid Res.*, 20, 113, 1981.
121. Christ-Hazelhof, E. and Nugteren, D. H., Prostacyclin is not a circulating hormone, *Prostaglandins*, 22, 739, 1981.
122. Karim, S. M. and Somers, K., Cardiovascular and renal actions of prostaglandins, in *The Prostaglandins, Progress in Research*, Karim, S. M., Ed., Wiley Interscience, New York, 1972, 165.
123. Nakano, J., Prostaglandins: cardiovascular actions, in *The Prostaglandins*, Ramwell, P. W., Ed., Plenum Press, New York, 1973, 239.
124. Samuelsson, B., Roundtable discussion of analytical methods, in *Advances in the Biosciences*, Bergstrom, S. and Bernhard, S., Eds., Pergamon Press, Oxford, 1973, 121.
125. Samuelsson, B., Quantitative aspects on prostaglandin synthesis in man, in *Advances in the Biosciences*, Bergstrom, S. and Bernhard, S., Eds., Pergamon Press, Oxford, 1973, 7.
126. Rosenkranz, B., Fischer, C., Reimann, I., Weiner, K. E., Beck, G., and Frölich, J. C., Identification of the major metabolite of prostaglandin and 6-ketoprostaglandin $F_{1\alpha}$ in man, *Biochem. Biophys. Acta*, 619, 207, 1980.
127. Vane, J. R., Prostacyclin: a hormone with a therapeutic potential, *J. Endocrinol.*, 95, 3P, 1982.
128. Sutter, D. M. and Weeks, J. R., An antihypertensive effect of prostacyclin, in *Advances in Prostaglandin and Thromboxane Research*, Vol. 7, Samuelsson, B. et al., Eds., Raven Press, New York, 1980, 789.
129. Frölich, J. C., Gas chromatography-mass spectrometry of prostaglandins, in *The Prostaglandins*, Vol. 3, Ramwell, P., Ed., Plenum Press, New York, 1976, 1.
130. Granström, E., Metabolism of prostaglandins, in *Prostaglandins and Thromboxane*, Berti, F., Samuelsson, B., and Velo, G. P., Eds., Plenum Press, New York, 1977, 75.
131. Lee, J. B., Chemical and physiological properties of renal prostaglandins: the antihypertensive effects of medullin in essential human hypertension, in *Nobel Symposium 2: Prostaglandins*, Bergstrom, S. and Samuelsson, B., Eds., Almqvist & Wiksell, Stockholm, 1967, 197.
132. Lee, J. B., McGiff, J. C., Kannegiesser, H., Aykent, Y. Y., Mudd, J. G., and Frawley, T. F., Prostaglandin A_1: antihypertensive and renal effects, *Ann. Intern. Med.*, 74, 703, 1971.
133. Christlieb, A. R., Dobrzinsky, S. J., Lyons, C. J., and Hickler, R. B., Short term PGA_1 infusions in patients with essential hypertension, *Clin. Res.*, 17, 234, 1969.
134. Westura, E. E., Kannegiesser, H., O'Tool, J. B., and Lee, J. B., Antihypertensive effects of prostaglandin A_1 in essential hypertension, *Circ. Res.*, 27(Suppl. 1), I131, 1970.
135. Krakoff, L. R., DeGuia, D., Vlachakis, N., Stricker, J., and Goldstein, M., Effect of sodium balance on arterial blood pressure and renal responses to prostaglandin A_1 in man, *Circ. Res.*, 33, 539, 1973.
136. Carr, A. A., Effect of PGA_1 on renin and aldosterone in man, *Prostaglandins*, 3, 621, 1973.
137. Hornych, A., Safar, M., Weiss, Y., Menard, J., Corvol, P., Bariety, J., and Milliez, P., in *Euro. J. Clin. Invest.*, 6, 314, 1976.
138. Krakoff, L. R., Vlachakis, N. D., and DeGuia, D., Effect of prostaglandin A_1 infusion in hypertensive patients with renal artery stenosis, *Prostaglandins*, 14, 1153, 1977.
139. Bergstrom, S., Düner, H., von Euler, U. S., Pernow, B., and Sjövall, J., Observations on the effects of infusion of prostaglandin E in man, *Acta Physiol. Scand.*, 45, 145, 1959.

140. Bergstrom, S., Carlson, L. A., Ekelund, L. G., and Orö, L., Cardiovascular and metabolic response to infusions of prostaglandin E_1 to simultaneous infusions of noradrenaline and prostaglandin E_1 in man, *Acta Physiol. Scand.*, 64, 332, 1965.

141. Dunn, M. J. and Hood, V. L., Prostaglandins and the kidney, *Am. J. Physiol.*, 233, F169, 1977.

142. Flamenbaum, W. and Kleinman, J. G., Prostaglandins and renal function, or "A trip down the rabbit hole", in *The Prostaglandins*, Vol. 3, Ramwell, P. W., Ed., Plenum Press, New York, 1977, 267.

143. Kot, P. A. and Fitzpatrick, T. M., Cardiovascular actions of prostaglandin precursors and elected prostanoic compounds, in *Prostaglandins*, Lee, J. B., Ed., Elsevier, New York, 1982, 177.

144. Shimada, Y., Okamoto, T., Inoue, T., Ohtsuka, Y., Morii, H., and Wada, M., Antihypertensive effect of prostaglandin E_2 analogue by oral administration, *Osada City Med. J.*, 21, 71, 1975.

145. Cervoni, P., Chan, P. S., Lai, F. M., and Birnbaum, J. E., CL 115,347 (DHV-PGE₂ ME): a new orally and topically active prostaglandin antihypertensive agent, *Fed. Proc. Fed. Am. Soc. Exp. Biol.*, 42, 157, 1983.

146. Chan, P. S., Scully, P. A., Accomando, R. C., and Cervoni, P., Mechanism of action of a new prostaglandin antihypertensive, CL 115,347 (15-deoxy-16-hydroxy-16-vinyl-prostaglandin E_2 methyl ester), *Fed. Proc. Fed. Am. Soc. Exp. Biol.*, 41, 1647, 1982.

147. Chan, P. S., Emma, J. E., Cervoni, P., Quirk, G., and Stubbs, C. S., The diuretic effects of (±) 15 deoxy-16-hydroxy-16-vinyl-prostaglandin E_2 methyl ester (CL 115,347) and its metabolite CL 115,129 in dogs, *Fed. Proc. Fed. Am. Soc. Exp. Biol.*, 42, 1133, 1983.

148. Chan, P. S., Cervoni, P., Lai, F., Ronsberg, M., and Stubbs, C. S., Further studies on CL 115,347 (15-deoxy-16-hydroxy-16-vinyl-prostaglandin E_2 methyl ester), a new prostaglandin antihypertensive, *Pharmacologist*, 24, 138, 1982.

149. Birnbaum, J. E., Chan, P. S., Cervoni, P., Dessy, F., and Van Humbeeck, L., Cutaneous erythema and blood pressure lowering effects of topically applied 16-vinylprostaglandins, *Prostaglandins*, 23, 185, 1982.

150. Birnbaum, J. E., Cervoni, P., Chan, P. S., Chen, S.-M. L., Floyd, M. B., Grudzinskas, C. V., Weiss, M. J., and Dessey, F., Prostaglandins and congeners. XXIX. (16RS)-(±)-15 deoxy-16hydroxy-16-vinyl-prostaglandin E_2, an orally and transdermally active hypotensive agent of prolonged duration, *J. Med. Chem.*, 25, 492, 1982.

151. Schaaf, T. K., Johnson, M. R., Eggler, J. F., Bindra, J. S., Constantine, J. W., and Hess, H. J., Hypotensive prostaglandin structure activity relationships: 11-desoxy-16-aryl-ω-tetranor prostaglandins, in *Advances in Prostaglandin, Thromboxane and Leukotriene Research*, Vol. 11, Samuelsson, B. et al., Eds., Raven Press, New York, 1983, 313.

152. Aristoff, P. A., Harrison, A. W., Aiken, J. W., Gorman, R. R., and Pike, J. E., Synthesis and structure-activity relationship of novel stable prostacyclin analogs, in *Advances in Prostaglandin, Thromboxane and Leukotriene Research*, Vol. 11, Samuelsson, B., Paoletti, R., and Ramwell, P., Eds., Raven Press, New York, 1983, 267.

153. Bartmann, W., Beck, G., Knolle, J., Rupp, R. H., Schölkens, B. A., and Werthmann, U., Synthesis of stable prostacyclin analogs, in *Advances in Prostaglandin, Thromboxane and Leukotriene Research*, Vol. 11, Samuelsson, B., Paoletti, R., and Ramwell, P., Eds., Raven Press, New York, 1983, 287.

154. Haslanger, M. F., Sprague, P. W., Snitman, D., Vu, T., Harris, D. N., Greenberg, R., and Powell, J., Novel 7-oxabicyclo(2.2.1.) heptane prostacyclin agonists, in *Advances in Prostaglandin, Thromboxane and Leukotriene Research*, Vol. 11, Samuelsson, B. et al., Eds., Raven Press, New York, 1983, 293.

155. Skuballa, W. and Vorbrüggen, H., Synthesis of cipoprost (ZK 36374): a chemically stable and biologically potent prostacyclin analog, in *Advances in Prostaglandin, Thromboxane and Leukotriene Research*, Vol. 11, Samuelsson, B. et al., Eds., Raven Press, New York, 1983, 299.

156. Comberg, H. U., Heyden, S., Hames, C. G., Vergroesen, A. J., and Fleischman, A. I., Hypotensive effect of dietary prostaglandin precursors in hypertensive man, *Prostaglandins*, 15, 193, 1978.

157. Rao, R. H., Rao, U. B., and Srikantia, S. G., Effect of polyunsaturate-rich vegetable oils on blood pressure in essential hypertension, *Clin. Exp. Hypertension*, 3, 27, 1981.

158. Hoffmann, P. and Förster, W., Influence of dietary linoleic acid content on blood pressure regulation in salt-loaded rats (with special reference to the prostaglandin system), *Adv. Lipid Res.*, 18, 203, 1981.

159. Iacono, J. M., Judd, J. T., Marshall, M. W., Canary, J. J., Dougherty, R. M., Mackin, J. F., and Weinland, B. T., The role of dietary essential fatty acids and prostaglandins in reducing blood pressure, *Prog. Lipid Res.*, 20, 349, 1981.

160. Triebe, G., Block, H. U., and Förster, W., On the blood pressure response of salt-loaded rats under different content of linoleic acid in the food, *Acta Biol. Med. Ger.*, 35, 1223, 1976.

161. Düsing, R., Scherhag, R., Glänzer, K., Budde, U., and Kramer, H. J., Effect of changes in dietary prostaglandin precursor fatty acids on arterial blood pressure and vascular prostacyclin synthesis, in *Advances in Prostaglandin, Thromboxane and Leukotriene Research,* Vol. 12, Samuelsson, B. et al., Eds., Raven Press, New York, 1983, 209.

162. Rosenthal, J., Simone, P. G., and Silbergleit, A., Effect of prostaglandin deficiency of natriuresis, diuresis and blood pressure, *Prostaglandins,* 5, 435, 1974.

163. Schoene, N. W., Reeves, V. B., and Ferreti, A., Effect of dietary linoleic acid on the biosynthesis of PGE$_2$ and PGF$_{2o}$ in kidney medullae in spontaneously hypertensive rats, in *Advances in Prostaglandin and Thromboxane Research,* Vol. 8, Samuelsson, B. et al., Eds., Raven Press, New York, 1980, 1791.

164. Dusting, G. J., Davies, W., Drysdale, T., and Doyle, A. E., Increased conversion of arachidonic acid to vasodilators prostanoids in spontaneously hypertensive rats, *Clin. Exp. Pharmacol. Physiol.,* 8, 435, 1981.

165. Tobian, L., Ganguli, M., Johnson, M. A., and Iwai, J., Influence of renal prostaglandins and dietary linoleate on hypertension in Dahl S rats, *Hypertension,* 4, II-149, 1982.

166. Weber, P. C., Renal prostaglandins, kidney function and essential hypertension, *Contrib. Nephrol.,* 23, 83, 1980.

167. Frölich, J. C. and Fejes-Toth, G., Renal prostaglandins, *Klin. Wochenschr.,* 60, 1155, 1982.

168. Larsson, C. and Änggård, E., Regional differences in the formation and metabolism of prostaglandins in the rabbit kidney, *Eur. J. Pharmacol.,* 21, 30, 1976.

169. Tannenbaum, J., Spławinski, J. A., Oates, J. A., and Nies, A. S., Enhanced renal prostaglandin production in the dog. I. Effects on renal function, *Circ. Res.,* 36, 197, 1975.

170. Larsson, C., Weber, P., and Änggård, E., Stimulation and inhibition of renal PG biosynthesis: effects on renal blood flow and on plasma renin activity, *Acta Biol. Med. Ger.,* 35, 1195, 1976.

171. Gerber, J. G., Anderson, R. J., Schrier, R. W., and Nies, A. S., Prostaglandins and the regulation of renal circulation and function, in *Prostaglandins and the Cardiovascular System,* Oates, J. A., Ed., Raven Press, New York, 1982, 227.

172. Stokes, J. B. and Kokko, J. P., Inhibition of sodium transport by prostaglandin E$_2$ across the isolated perfused rabbit collecting tubule, *J. Clin. Invest.,* 59, 1099, 1977.

173. Iino, Y. and Imai, M., Effects of prostaglandins on Na transport in isolated collecting tubules, *Pfluegers Arch.,* 373, 125, 1978.

174. Fine, L. G. and Trizna, W., Influence of prostaglandins on sodium transport of isolated medullary nephron segments, *Am. J. Physiol.,* 232, F383, 1977.

175. Scriabine, A., Watson, L. S., Fanelli, G. M., Jr., Shum, W. K., Blaine, E. H., Russo, H. F., and Bohidar, N. R., Studies on the interaction of indomethacin with various diuretics, in *Prostaglandins in Cardiovascular and Renal Function,* Scriabine, A. et al., Eds., Spectrum Publishers, New York, 1980, 471.

176. Attallah, A., Interaction of prostaglandins with diuretics, *Prostaglandins,* 18, 369, 1979.

177. Tobian, L. and O'Donnell, M., Renal prostaglandins in relation to sodium regulation and hypertension, *Fed. Proc. Fed. Am. Soc. Exp. Biol.,* 35, 2388, 1976.

178. Terragno, N. A., Tarragno, D. A., and McGiff, J. C., Contribution of prostaglandins to renal circulation in conscious, anesthetized and laparotomized dogs, *Circ. Res.,* 40, 590, 1977.

179. Kaizu, T. and Margolius, H. S., Studies on rat renal cortical cell kallikrein. I. Separation and measurement, *Biochem. Biophys. Acta,* 411, 305, 1975.

180. McGiff, J. C., Terragno, N. A., Malik, K. U., and Lonigro, A. J., Release of a prostaglandin E-like substance from canine kidney by bradykinin, *Circ. Res.,* 31, 36, 1972.

181. Zusman, R. M. and Keiser, H. R., Prostaglandin E$_2$ biosynthesis by rabbit renomedullary interstitial cells in tissue culture. Mechanism of stimulation by angiotensin II, bradykinin and arginine vasopressin, *J. Biol. Chem.,* 252, 2069, 1977.

182. Wong, P. Y.-K., Terragno, D. A., Terragno, N. A., and McGiff, J. C., Dual aspects of bradykinin on prostaglandin metabolism: relationship to the dissimilar vascular action of kinins, *Prostaglandins,* 13, 1113, 1977.

183. Bobbin, R. P. and Guth, P. S., Venoconstrictive action of bradykinin, *J. Pharmacol. Exp. Ther.,* 160, 11, 1968.

184. Ozer, A. and Shapr, G. W. G., Effects of prostaglandins and their inhibitors on osmotic water flow in the toad bladder, *Am. J. Physiol.,* 222, 674, 1972.

185. Lipson, L. C. and Sharp, G., Effect of prostaglandin E$_1$ on sodium transport and osmotic water flow in the toad bladder, *Am. J. Physiol.,* 220, 1046, 1971.

186. Grantham, J. J. and Orloff, J., Effect of prostaglandin E$_1$ on the permeability response of the isolated collecting tubule to vasopressin, adenosine, 3′,5′-monophosphate and theophylline, *J. Clin. Invest.,* 47, 1154, 1968.

187. Nasjletti, A. and Malik, K. U., Interaction of kinins and renal prostaglandins, in *Frontiers in Hypertension Research,* Laragh, J. H., Bühler, F. R., and Seldin, D. W., Eds., Springer-Verlag, New York, 1981, 119.

188. Blasingham, M. C. and Nasjletti, A., Contribution of renal prostaglandins to the natriuretic action of bradykinin in the dogs, *Am. J. Physiol.,* 237, F182, 1979.

189. Nasjletti, A. and Mailk, K. U., Interrelationships among prostaglandins and vasoactive substances, *Med. Clin. North Am.,* 65, 881, 1981.

190. Yun, J. C. H., Kelly, G. D., Bartter, F. C., and Smith, G. W., II, Role of prostaglandins in the control of renin secretion in the dog, *Life Sci.,* 23, 945, 1978.

191. Jackson, E. K., Branch, R. A., and Oates, J. A., Participation of prostaglandins in the control of renin release, in *Prostaglandins and the Cardiovascular System,* Oates, J. A., Ed., Raven Press, New York, 1982, 255.

192. Gerber, J. G., Keller, R. T., and Nies, J. A., Prostaglandins and renin release, *Circ. Res.,* 44, 796, 1979.

193. Frölich, J. C., Robertson, D., Kitajima, W., Rosenkranz, B., and Reimann, I., Prostaglandins in human hypertension: relationships to renin, sodium and antihypertensive drug action, in *Frontiers in Hypertension Research,* Laragh, J. H., Bühler, F. R., and Seldin, D. W., Eds., Springer-Verlag, New York, 1981, 114.

194. Mullane, K. M., Moncada, S., and Vane, J. R., Prostacyclin release induced by bradykinin may contribute to the antihypertensive action of angiotensin-converting enzyme inhibition, in *Advances in Prostaglandin and Thromboxane Research,* Vol. 7, Samuelsson, B. et al., Eds., Raven Press, New York, 1980, 1159.

Chapter 17

ARACHIDONIC ACID METABOLITES AND CONTROL OF AIRWAY SMOOTH MUSCLE

Satoshi Kitamura

TABLE OF CONTENTS

I. MAJOR METABOLIC PATHWAYS IN THE CONVERSION OF ARACHIDONIC ACID IN THE HUMAN

Arachidonic acid, the precursor of all bisenoic prostaglandins (PGs), is the most common fatty acid present in cellular phospholipids and can be obtained directly from the food or by desaturation and chain elongation from dietary linoleic acid. Figure 1 depicts the pathways involved in arachidonate metabolism, i.e., arachidonate cascade. Release of arachidonic acid from cell membrane-bound phospholipids, the rate-limiting step in PG, thromboxane (TX), and leukotriene biosynthesis is catalyzed by the enzyme phospholipase A_2,[1] and possibly other specific lipases.[2] Molecular oxygen is enzymatically added to arachidonate by the action of fatty acid cyclooxygenase which yields a pair of unstable endoperoxide intermediates, PGG_2 and PGH_2.[3] Each PG has a half-life of 4 to 6 min at $37°C$.[4] These endoperoxides are further metabolized and synthesized by isomerases, reductases, and synthetases to PGD_2, PGE_2, $PGF_{2\alpha}$, PGI_2, TXA_2, and HHT (12-hydroxy-5-8-10-heptadecatrienoic acid). Furthermore, PGE_2 can be transformed to $PGF_{2\alpha}$ by the action of 9-ketoreductase.[5] Degradation of PGs and TXA_2, occurring by both enzymatic and nonenzymatic processes, yields a series of products that generally have little or no biologic activity. The first step in the enzymatic degradation of PGE_2, $PGF_{2\alpha}$, and PGI_2 is catalyzed by 15-hydroxy-PG dehydrogenase.[6] Subsequent degradation involves various enzymes including 13-reductase and 9-hydroxydehydrogenase. Thus, PGE_2 and $PGF_{2\alpha}$ are metabolized and finally excreted in urine as 7α-hydroxy-5,11-diketotetranorprosta-1,16-dioic acid (PGE_2-MUM) and 5α, 7α-dihydroxy-11-ketotetranorprosta-1,16-dioic acid ($PGF_{2\alpha}$-MUM), respectively. PGI_2 (prostacyclin), with a half-life in blood at $37°C$ of about 3 min, is metabolized by nonenzymatic conversion to 6-keto $PGF_{1\alpha}$[7] and then undergoes enzymatic degradation.[8] TXA_2, which has a half-life of about 30 sec at $37°C$,[4] spontaneously reduces to physiologically inactive TXB_2 and thereafter may undergo further metabolism before excretion.[9] Leukotrienes are synthesized from arachidonic acid by the action of lipoxygenase. In the past few years investigators in Sweden, the U.S., and the U.K. have established that the activity which comprises SRS-A is almost entirely attributable to leukotrienes C_4, D_4, and E_4 (LTC_4, LTD_4, and LTE_4).

II. ACTIONS OF PRIMARY PROSTAGLANDINS ON THE AIRWAY SMOOTH MUSCLE

It is well known that PGs of the E series have potent inhibitory actions on smooth muscle of the respiratory tract. Contraction of the smooth muscle in response to acetylcholine, histamine, barium ions, and serotonin are all inhibited by PGE_1. Isolated human bronchial smooth muscle is also relaxed by PGE_1.[10] Both PGE_1 and PGE_2 relaxed isolated human bronchial muscle although PGE_1 appeared to be slightly more potent. $PGF_{2\alpha}$ can either relax or contract respiratory smooth muscle depending on the species investigated. Thus, on the cat tracheal preparation $PGF_{2\alpha}$ has a relaxant effect, but is about 30 times less active that PGE_2,[11] whereas on guinea pig and human preparations $PGF_{2\alpha}$ causes the muscle to contract.[12] Dawson et al.[13] reported that 15-oxo-$PGF_{2\alpha}$, the first product of $PGF_{2\alpha}$ metabolism in many tissues, is more active than $PGF_{2\alpha}$ in contracting guinea pig tracheal and human bronchial strips. On the other hand, 15-oxo-$PGF_{2\alpha}$ and 13,14-dihydro-15-oxo-$PGF_{2\alpha}$ exhibit much lower bronchoconstrictor activity than $PGF_{2\alpha}$ in pentobarbitone anesthetized dogs. $PGF_{2\alpha}$ given by aerosol to man is a powerful bronchoconstrictor. Moreover, some asthmatic patients are as much as 8000 times more sensitive than normals to the bronchoconstrictor action of $PGF_{2\alpha}$,[14] whereas the sensitivity to another bronchoconstrictor agent, histamine, is increased in asthmatics only by a factor of 10. Therefore, following the administration

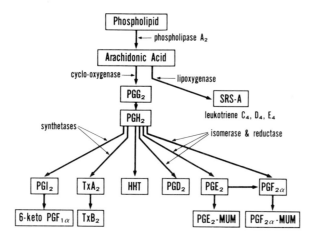

FIGURE 1.   Major metabolic pathways in the conversion of arachidonic acid.

of $PGF_{2\alpha}$ severe bronchospasm is produced with signs and symptoms closely resembling an asthmatic attack. Although PGA_1 is 30 times less active than PGE_1 as an inhibitor of the contractions of the tracheal muscle, its effect is of longer duation.[15]

III. COMPARISON OF THE EFFECTS OF PGD_2 AND $PGF_{2\alpha}$ ON GUINEA PIG TRACHEAL STRIPS[16]

A. Materials and Methods

Male Hartley strain guinea pigs weighing about 200 g were used as the experimental animals. Guinea pig trachea (GPT) was removed immediately after the animal was killed by a blow on the head and was cut spirally into a segment 1.0 to 1.5 mm in width and 3 to 4 cm in length, and one end of tracheal strip was attached to the notch in the bottom of a bioassay glass funnel the diameter of which was 4.6 cm, depth of 10 cm, and the diameter of outlet was 1-cm wide, enough to have a constant outflow. GPT had a preload of 0.5 g as a counterbalance. Krebs-Henseleit solution saturated with oxygen and carbon dioxide (95:5, v/v) in the reservoir was superfused by a pump at a flow rate of 20 mℓ/min and temperature was adjusted to 37°C through water bath to reach GPT. Chemical agents were infused at the rate of 0.97 mℓ/min within 60 sec by a slow-speed infusion pump (Harvard Apparatus, U.S.). Responses of GPT induced by chemical agents were detected by an isotonic transducer (ME Commercial, Japan) and displayed on a polyrecorder. Figure 2 shows the tissue bioassay system.[17] The grade of response was expressed as the contraction index (C.I.) measuring the area (cm²) enclosed by response curve and the base line, using a planimeter. The response curve above and below the base line means contraction and relaxation and is shown by a positive and a negative sign, respectively.

B. Results and Discussion

Figure 3 shows dose-response curves of PGD_2 and $PGF_{2\alpha}$. It is obvious from this figure that both PGD_2 and $PGF_{2\alpha}$ contracted guinea pig tracheal strips dose-dependently, and that the former showed significantly larger contractile responses than the latter at the dose of 350 ng/mℓ and 500 ng/mℓ. Figure 4 shows effects of PGD_2 and $PGF_{2\alpha}$ on guinea pig tracheal strips after increasing their tonus with continuous infusion of neostigmine bromide (500 ng/mℓ). $PGF_{2\alpha}$ shows relaxation responses, and such responses became less dominant by increasing the dose, while PGD_2 shows contractile responses dose dependently. These results suggest that PGD_2 may play a very impor-

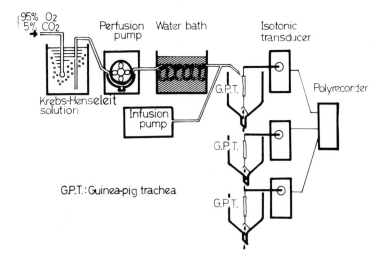

FIGURE 2.   Tissue bioassay system.

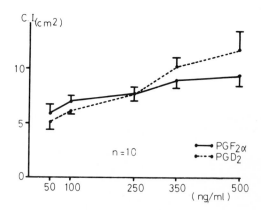

FIGURE 3.   Effects of PGD_2 and $PGF_{2\alpha}$ on guinea pig tracheal strips.

tant role in pathological conditions such as bronchial asthma in which the tonus of tracheobronchial smooth muscle is markedly elevated.

IV. EFFECTS OF PROSTAGLANDINS E_1, E_2, D_2, $F_{2\alpha}$, AND I_2 ON THE CANINE AIRWAY AND PULMONARY VASCULAR BED[18] IN VIVO

The cardiovascular actions of PGE_1, PGE_2, PGD_2, $PGF_{2\alpha}$, and PGI_2 have been extensively investigated. In most peripheral vascular beds E-type PGs are potent vasodilators, whereas $PGF_{2\alpha}$ is a weak vasoconstrictor. The present investigation was conducted to compare the effects of PGE_1, PGE_2, PGD_2, $PGF_{2\alpha}$, and PGI_2 on the canine airway and pulmonary vascular bed. Thirty-two (32) mongrel dogs, weighing between 18 and 28 kg, were anesthetized with intravenous adminstration of 25 mg/kg of sodium pentobarbital. Each dog was subjected to cannulation of the trachea for artificial ventilation with a volume type Harvard respirator, catheterization of left pulmonary artery and vein for measurement of systemic blood pressure (P_{SYST}), and for drop infusion or drug infusion such as heparin Na (100 units/kg) or succinyl choline chloride (2%, 0.2 mℓ/kg/hr), respectively. The left hemithorax was opened under artificial

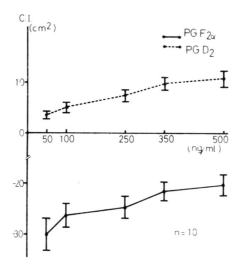

FIGURE 4.   Effects of PGD$_2$ and PGF$_{2\alpha}$ on guinea pig tracheal strips with continuous infusion of neostigmine bromide.

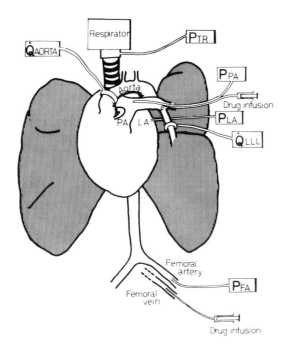

FIGURE 5.   Schema of the experimental arrangement.

respiration and catheters were inserted into the pulmonary artery trunk and left atrium for measurement of pulmonary artery pressure (P$_{PA}$) and left atrium pressure (P$_{LA}$), respectively. The noncannulating electromagnetic flow probes were placed around the ascending aorta and pulmonary artery of the left lower lobe for measurement of cardiac output ($\dot{Q}_{AORTA}$) and blood flow to the left lower lobe ($\dot{Q}_{LLL}$), respectively. Tracheal pressure (P$_{TR}$) was measured at the orifice of tracheal cannula using pressure transducer. Various PGs were injected into the left pulmonary artery through a polyethylene

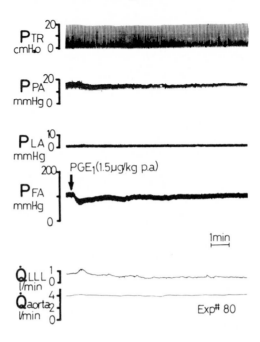

FIGURE 6.   A typical record of various parameters changed by an injection of PGE$_1$ into the pulmonary artery to left lower lobe in an anesthetized dog.

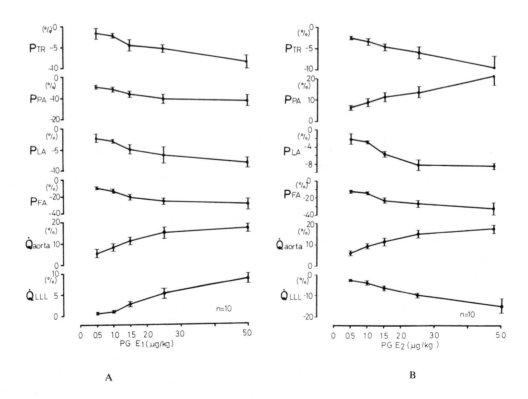

A   B

FIGURE 7.   The effect of injections of different doses of (A) PGE$_1$ and (B) PGE$_2$ into the pulmonary artery of left lower lobe in anesthetized dogs.

catheter using a Harvard low speed infusion pump. P_{TR}, P_{PA}, P_{LA}, P_{SYST}, $\dot{Q}_{AORTA}$, and $\dot{Q}_{LLL}$ were recorded and displayed on an electric polyrecorder (Nihon Kohden, Japan), Figure 5 shows a schema of the experimental arrangement. Figure 6 is a typical record of various parameters changed by an injection of PGE_1 into the pulmonary artery of left lower lobe in an anesthetized dog. Injection of PGE_1 induced a slight decrease of P_{TR} and P_{LA}, a marked decrease of P_{PA} and P_{FA}, and a transient increase of $\dot{Q}_{LLL}$ and $\dot{Q}_{AORTA}$.

Figure 7 is the summary of experimental data from 10 dogs having percent change of P_{TR}, P_{PA}, P_{LA}, P_{FA}, $\dot{Q}_{AORTA}$, and $\dot{Q}_{LLL}$ on the ordinate, and the dose ($\mu g/kg$) of PGE_1 (Figure 7A) and PGE_2 (Figure 7B) on the abscissa. It is obvious from this figure that P_{TR}, P_{LA}, and P_{FA} decreased and $\dot{Q}_{AORTA}$ increased dose-dependently with injection of PGE_1 and PGE_2 into the left pulmonary artery, while PGE_1 caused a decrease and PGE_2 an increase in P_{PA}, and PGE_1 caused an increase and PGE_2 a decrease in $\dot{Q}_{LLL}$. In the same way, P_{TR}, P_{PA}, and P_{FA} increased, P_{LA} and $\dot{Q}_{AORTA}$ decreased dose dependently with injection of $PGF_{2\alpha}$, while P_{TR} and P_{PA} increased and $\dot{Q}_{LLL}$ decreased dose dependently with injection of PGD_2 into the left pulmonary artery. P_{PA}, P_{LA}, and P_{FA} decreased and $\dot{Q}_{AORTA}$ and $\dot{Q}_{LLL}$ increased dose dependently with injection of PGI_2 into the left pulmonary artery. The above results suggest that these PGs may act on the pulmonary vascular, tracheobronchial, and pulmonary lymphatic systems, ameliorating the ventilation perfusion ratio and modulating the pulmonary circulation.

V. COMPARISON OF RESPONSES TO PGD_2, $PGF_{2\alpha}$, AND TXB_2 IN VARIOUS PARTS OF TRACHEOBRONCHIAL TREE[19]

Bronchoactive agents can exert their effects locally on the smooth muscle of the terminal bronchioles and alveolar ducts, as well as reflexively on the trachea. Nevertheless, most studies involving the action of drugs on respiratory smooth muscle utilize the isolated mammalian trachea as the test organ. Thus, unless large and small airways of the tracheobronchial tree are pharmacologically identical, results obtained with this tissue might be misleading.

The present investigation was conducted to compare the effects of various bronchoactive agents in guinea pig tracheal, 1st order bronchial (main bronchus), and 2nd bronchial (lobar bronchus) strips. Male Hartley strain guinea pigs, weighing 250 to 300 g, were sacrificed. Guinea pig tracheal, 1st bronchial, and 2nd bronchial strips were suspended in bioassay glass funnels, superfused with Krebs-Henseleit solution at 37°C, and saturated with oxygen and carbon dioxide (95:5, v/v) as previously described.[17] Contraction of tissues was detected by an isotonic transducer and displayed on a polyrecorder. From the dose-response curves of agents we determined the ED_{50}. ED_{50} of acetylcholine was markedly low in trachea compared with 1st and 2nd bronchi, suggesting that the trachea is most responsive to acetylcholine. ED_{50} of neostigmine bromide, serotonin, and histamine were lowest in trachea, although they were also low in 1st and 2nd bronchi, suggesting that all of the trachea and 1st and 2nd bronchi are responsive to these agents.

Figure 8A shows ED_{50} of PGD_2 in different parts of the tracheobronchial tree. Mean values and standard deviation (SD) of ED_{50} in trachea and 1st and 2nd bronchi were 4.91 ± 0.45, 8.68 ± 0.90, and 11.73 ± 1.48 $\mu g/m\ell$, respectively. Figure 8B shows ED_{50} of $PGF_{2\alpha}$ in different parts of the tracheobronchial tree. Mean values and SD of ED_{50} in trachea and 1st and 2nd bronchi were 8.76 ± 0.97, 10.63 ± 1.37, and 12.64 ± 1.64 $\mu g/m\ell$, respectively. In the same way, Figure 8C shows ED_{50} of TXB_2 in different parts of the tracheobronchial tree. Mean values and SD of ED_{50} in trachea and 1st and 2nd bronchi were 17.67 ± 1.76, 20.56 ± 2.11, and 24.23 ± 3.21 $\mu g/m\ell$, respectively. Above results may suggest that all of the trachea and 1st and 2nd bronchi are responsive to

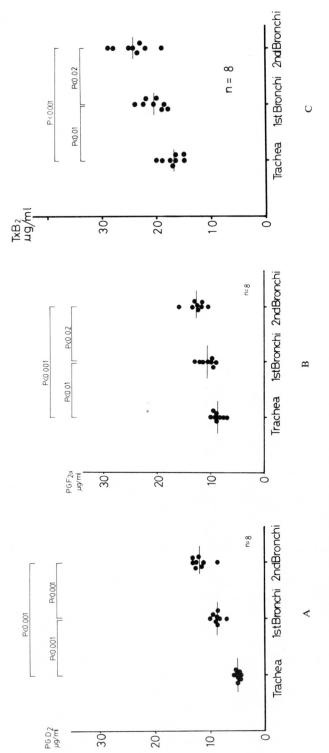

FIGURE 8.   ED$_{50}$ of (A) PGD$_2$, (B) PGF$_{2\alpha}$, and (C) TXB$_2$ in different parts of the tracheobronchial tree.

PGD_2 and $PGF_{2\alpha}$, and that the trachea is most sensitive to these agents. Although ED_{50} of TXB_2 was lowest in trachea, all of ED_{50} in trachea and 1st and 2nd bronchi were higher compared to those of other agents, suggesting that trachea and 1st and 2nd bronchi are less responsive to TXB_2.

VI. EFFECT OF 6-KETO $PGF_{1\alpha}$, THE MAIN METABOLITE OF PROSTACYCLIN, ON GUINEA PIG TRACHEAL STRIPS[20]

PGI_2 induces slight relaxation in tracheal smooth muscle and marked relaxation in arterial smooth muscle. In addition, PGI_2 has a powerful anticoagulant action. PGI_2 is unstable and has a half-life of 3 min in blood at 37°C.[21] It has recently been reported that PGI_2 has an extended stability in plasma and in blood[22] and that this may be associated with binding to albumin or with metabolism to 6-oxo-PGE_1.[23] The biotransformation of PGI_2 in the human circulation is not yet fully understood, and the assumption that 6-oxo-$PGF_{1\alpha}$ (6-keto $PGF_{1\alpha}$) determined in blood samples is a reliable index of concentrations of active PGI_2 in circulating blood might not be valid.[24] Therefore, further work is necessary to clearly establish the routes of catabolism of both PGI_2 and 6-keto $PGF_{1\alpha}$ in the human circulation and to determine if there is an effective level of circulating PGI_2 in healthy man at rest or during exercise. 6-Keto $PGF_{1\alpha}$ is a stable metabolite of PGI_2 and its concentration is higher than that of PGI_2 in circulating blood. In the present investigation we studied the effect of 6-keto $PGF_{1\alpha}$ on the action of various bronchoconstrictor and bronchodilator agents in guinea pig tracheal strips. Male Hartley strain guinea pigs, weighing 150 to 200 g were sacrificed. Their tracheal strips were suspended in bioassay glass funnels and superfused with Krebs-Henseleit solution, pH 7.4, at 37°C saturated with oxygen and carbon dioxide (95:5, v/v) as previously described.[17]

Figure 9 shows dose-response curves of 6-keto $PGF_{1\alpha}$ and isoproterenol in isolated perfused guinea pig tracheal strips. It is obvious from this figure that the relaxation response of 6-keto $PGF_{1\alpha}$ is 1/100 or less that of isoproterenol. Figure 10A shows effect of 6-keto $PGF_{1\alpha}$ on serotonin- and $PGF_{2\alpha}$-induced contractile responses in guinea pig tracheal strips. Serotonin (250 ng/mℓ)- and $PGF_{2\alpha}$ (250 ng/mℓ)-induced contractile responses were attenuated dose dependently with continuous infusion of 6-keto-$PGF_{1\alpha}$. In the same way acetylcholine (250 ng/mℓ)-, histamine (250 ng/mℓ)-, and bradykinin (250 ng/mℓ)-induced contractile responses were attenuated dose dependently with continuous infusion of 6-keto $PGF_{1\alpha}$. Figure 10B shows effect of 6-keto $PGF_{1\alpha}$ on various bronchodilating agents. Isoproterenol (5 ng/mℓ)-, salbutamol (5 ng/mℓ)-, and PGE_2 (50 ng/mℓ)-induced relaxation responses were potentiated dose dependently with continuous infusion of 6-keto $PGF_{1\alpha}$. These results may suggest that 6-keto $PGF_{1\alpha}$, a stable metabolite of prostacyclin, has not only a bronchodilating effect by itself, but also has an attenuating effect on the action of bronchoconstricting agents and a potentiating effect on the action of bronchodilating agents.

VII. EFFECT OF LEUKOTRIENES ON AIRWAY SMOOTH MUSCLE

Leukotrienes, which are derived from arachidonic acid and have similar chemical structures to the PGs, have recently been shown to contain most of the biological activity previously attributed to SRS-A (LTC_4, D_4, and E_4).

A. Effect of Leukotriene C_4 and D_4 on Isolated Perfused Guinea Pig Tracheal Strips[25]

In general, leukotrienes with SRS-A activity (LTC_4, LTD_4, and LTE_4) contract smooth muscle, whereas LTB_4 and HETEs (hydroperoxy eicosatetraenoic acids) are chemotactic. They give rise to an infiltration of inflammatory cells. LTC_4 and LTD_4

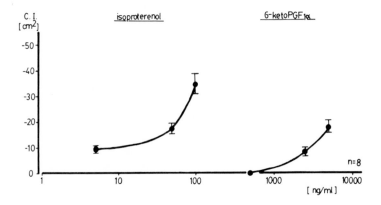

FIGURE 9.   Dose-response curves of 6-keto PGF_{1a} and isoproterenol in guinea pig tracheal strips.

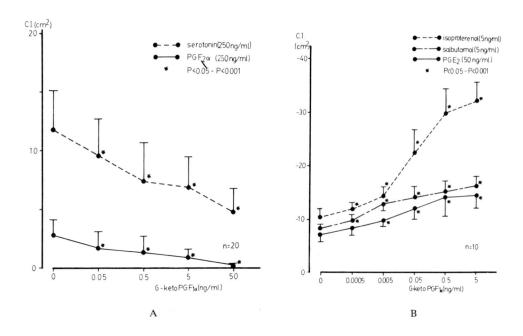

A   B

FIGURE 10.   Effect of 6-keto PGF_{1a} on various bronchoconstricting and bronchodilating agents in isolated perfused guinea pig tracheal strips.

produce an appreciable contraction of human bronchial smooth muscle preparations in vitro at concentrations as low as $10^{-8} M$.[26] In this respect they are approximately 1000 times more potent than histamine. In the present investigation we tried to explore the effect of synthetic LTC_4 and LTD_4 on isolated perfused guinea pig tracheal strips. Male Hartley strain guinea pigs weighing 200 to 250 g were sacrificed. Guinea pig tracheal strips were removed and suspended in bioassay glass funnels and superfused with Krebs-Henseleit solution at $37°C$, saturated with oxygen and carbon dioxide (95:5, v/v), and contraction of tissues was detected by an isotonic transducer and displayed on a polyrecorder as previously described.[17]

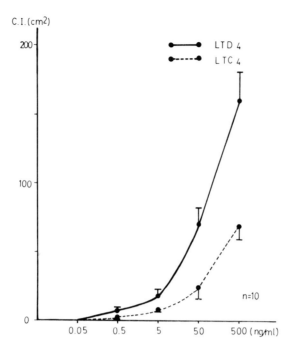

FIGURE 11. Dose-response curves of LTC_4 and LTD_4 in guinea pig tracheal strips.

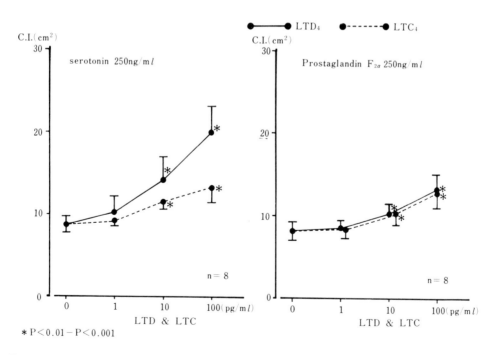

FIGURE 12. The effects of different doses of LTC_4 and LTD_4 on serotonin- and $PGF_{2\alpha}$ -induced contractile responses in guinea pig tracheal strips.

Figure 11 shows dose-response curves of LTC_4 and LTD_4 in isolated perfused guinea pig tracheal strips. LTC_4 and LTD_4 elicited contractile responses in guinea pig tracheal strips dose dependently. It is obvious from this figure that LTD_4-induced contractile responses were almost 10 times bigger than those induced by LTC_4. Figure 12 shows effects of different doses of LTC_4 and LTD_4 on serotonin (250 ng/mℓ)- and $PGF_{2\alpha}$ (250 ng/mℓ)-induced contractile responses in guinea pig tracheal strips. It is obvious from this figure that serotonin- and $PGF_{2\alpha}$-induced contractile responses were potentiated dose dependently with continuous infusion of LTC_4 and LTD_4. This potentiating effect of LTD_4 on serotonin-induced contractile responses was bigger than that of LTC_4 at doses of 10 pg/mℓ and 100 pg/mℓ. In the same way, acetylcholine- and histamine-induced contractile responses were potentiated dose dependently with continuous infusion of LTC_4 and LTD_4. The above results may suggest that LTC_4 and LTD_4 have not only powerful bronchoconstrictive actions by themselves, but also have attenuating effects on various bronchoconstrictive agents. It also suggests that they play an important role in pathological conditions such as bronchial asthma or anaphylactic shock.

B. Effects of Leukotriene C_4, D_4, and E_4 on Canine Airway and Pulmonary Circulation in Anesthetized Dogs[27]

The effects of leukotrienes on the microvasculature are complex. In guinea pigs LTD_4 dilates, whereas LTC_4 constricts the small blood vessels of the skin.[28] After intravenous injection in guinea pigs, leukotrienes C_4 and D_4 induce some of the features of systemic anaphylaxis such as arterial hypotension,[28] impaired left ventricular performance,[29] and reduced coronary arterial blood flow.[29]

The present investigation was conducted to explore the effect of LTC_4, LTD_4, and LTE_4 using anesthetized dogs. Fifteen mongrel dogs were anesthetized with sodium pentobarbital (25 mg/kg). The hemithorax was opened under artificial respiration. Catheters were inserted into the pulmonary artery trunk and left femoral artery, and pulmonary artery pressure (P_{PA}), femoral artery pressure (P_{SYST}), and tracheal pressure (P_{TR}) were measured using pressure transducers. Figure 13 shows an actual record of changes in P_{TR} and P_{SYST} after the intravenous infusion of LTD_4, LTC_4, and LTE_4 in an anesthetized dog. Intravenous infusions of LTD_4 and LTC_4 elicited the marked increase of P_{TR} and the prolonged decrease of P_{SYST}, while LTE_4 elicited almost no change. Figure 14 is the summary of the above results showing the percent change of maximum P_{TR} after intravenous infusions of various drugs (1 μg/kg) in anesthetized dogs. The percent changes of maximum P_{TR} induced by histamine, LTD_4, LTC_4, and LTE_4 were significantly lower than those induced by $PGF_{2\alpha}$. The percent changes of maximum P_{TR} induced by histamine and LTD_4 were almost the same, whereas those induced by LTC_4 were significantly lower than those induced by LTD_4. The percent changes of P_{TR} induced by LTE_4 were much lower than those induced by histamine, LTD_4, and LTC_4.

VIII. ANAPHYLACTIC RELEASE OF HISTAMINE AND SRS-A FROM GUINEA PIG LUNG TISSUES AND ITS MODULATION BY PROSTAGLANDINS[30]

Histamine and SRS-A are released during anaphylactic reactions. It has been postulated that a variety of sympathomimetic amines are capable of inhibiting the immunological release of histamine from passively sensitized human lung.[31] Furthermore, antigen-induced release of histamine from peripheral leukocytes was inhibited by both a beta-adrenergic agent and a methylxanthine.[32] Their effect was attributed to increases in cellular levels of cyclic AMP (cAMP). The present investigation was conducted to clarify the regulatory mechanism of anaphylactic release of histamine and SRS-A from guinea pig lung tissues by preincubating them with various drugs. Male Hartley strain guinea pigs weighing 250 to 300 g were used. The lung tissue was dissected free of pleura, cartilage, and large vessels and was minced into fragments (30 to 50 mg). The

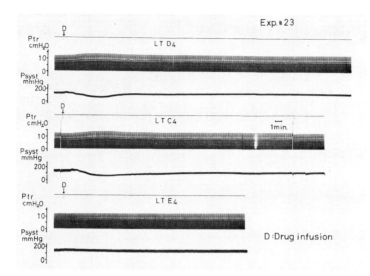

FIGURE 13.   Effect of leukotriene C_4, D_4, and E_4 (1 $\mu g/m\ell$) on tracheal and systemic blood pressure in an anesthetized dog.

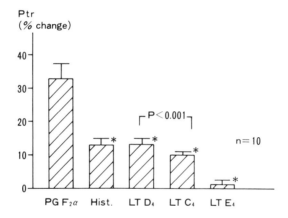

FIGURE 14.   Percent changes of maximum tracheal pressure after intravenous infusion of various drugs (1 $\mu g/kg$) in anesthetized dogs. (*$p < 0.001$, compared with % change of P_{TR} by $PGF_{2\alpha}$ infusion).

lung fragments were divided into approximately 500 mg replicates. The replicates were suspended in 24 mℓ of gamma globulin solution, diluted 1:4 in Krebs-Henseleit solution, and incubated at 37°C for 3 to 4 hr bubbling with oxygen and carbon dioxide (95:5, v/v). Histamine and SRS-A released from the lung tissue were quantitated by the bioassay method, the former on the guinea pig ileum (GPI) and the latter on the GPI with continuous infusion of a mixture of mepyramine maleate (100 ng/mℓ) and scopolamine hydrobromide (100 ng/mℓ). Figure 15 shows the schema of the tissue bioassay system. The lung fragments were put on a mesh stretched over a glass funnel. Histamine, ovalbumen (challenging antigen), and mixture of blockers were infused by an infusion pump. The amount of SRS-A was expressed as International Units; one unit of SRS-A is the dose which causes the same size of contraction of GPI as 5 ng of histamine.

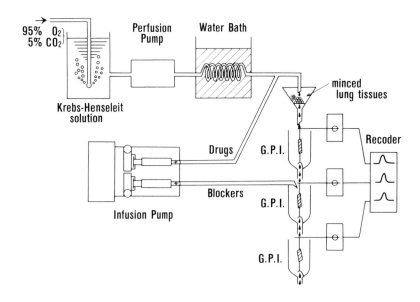

FIGURE 15.   The schema of tissue bioassay system.

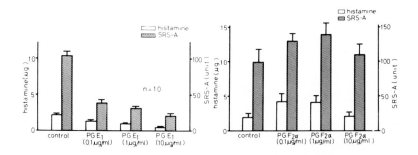

FIGURE 16.   The anaphylactic release of histamine and SRS-A from passively sensitized guinea pig lung fragments (wet weight is 500 mg) and its modulation by preincubating with various doses of PGE_1 and $PGF_{2\alpha}$.

Figure 16 shows the anaphylactic release of histamine and SRS-A from passively sensitized guinea pig lung fragments preincubated with various doses of PGF_1 (left side) and $PGF_{2\alpha}$ (right side). It is obvious from this figure that the release of histamine and SRS-A was decreased dose dependently by preincubating the lung fragments with PGE_2, and that the release of histamine and SRS-A was increased by preincubating with $PGF_{2\alpha}$.

In the same way, the release of histamine and SRS-A from lung fragments was inhibited by preincubating them with PGF_2, PGA_1, $PGF_{1\alpha}$, PGI_2, 6-keto $PGF_{1\alpha}$, isoproterenol, aminophylline, and cAMP, while it was accelerated by preincubating them with PGD_2, TXB_2, $PGF_{1\beta}$, and cGMP.

Figure 17 shows the schema of chemical mediator release modulation by various drugs and by endogenous vasoactive substances. PGE_1, PGE_2, β-adrenergic agonist, xanthine derivatives, PGI_2, and 6-keto $PGF_{1\alpha}$ induce the increase of intracellular cAMP, and inhibit generation and/or release of chemical mediators. Alpha-adrenergic agonist induces decrease of cAMP and accelerates generation and/or release of chemical mediators. On the other hand, cholinergic stimulant, histamine, serotonin, and $PGF_{2\alpha}$ induce increase of cGMP and accelerate generation and/or release of chemical

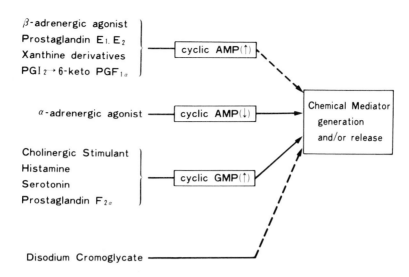

FIGURE 17.   Modulation of chemical mediator release (straight line arrow, acceleration; dotted line arrow, inhibition).

mediators. Dissodium cromoglycate inhibits directly generation and/or release of chemical mediators.

IX. METABOLIC AND BIOCHEMICAL ASPECTS OF BRONCHIAL ASTHMA

There is no agreed definition of the word "asthma". Usually a definition in terms of function has been used. Hence, asthma will be defined as a condition characterized by partial obstruction of the airways and reversible with time, either spontaneously or as a result of treatment. This failure to arrive at a precise definition of asthma is clearly a reflection of our failure to understand the basic pathogenetic mechanisms that lead to this syndrome. Those of us at the bench tend to view asthma as the result of chemical mediators released from tissue mast cells which either directly or through vagus nerve stimulation lead to contraction of tracheobronchial smooth muscle.[33]

Figure 18 is the schema that depicts the regulation of tonus in tracheobronchial smooth muscle. Among the chemical mediators released from lung mast cells histamine, serotonin, and SRS-A increase, while heparin[34] decreases the tonus of tracheobronchial smooth muscle. ACTH, glucocorticoid, sympathetic nerve stimulation, plasma epinephrine, PGE_2, PGI_2, and 6-keto PGF_{1a} decrease, while vagus nerve stimulation, PGF_{2a}, PGD_2, TXA_2, TXB_2, and bradykinin increase the tonus of bronchial smooth muscle.

Figure 19 is the schema that depicts the metabolic and biochemical aspects of bronchial asthma. Among the chemical mediators released from lung mast cells, histamine, PGF_{2a}, SRS-A, and serotonin elicit bronchoconstriction, i.e., an asthmatic attack, while heparin inhibits bronchoconstriction. If bronchoconstriction does occur, it induces hypoxemia, and hypoxemia in turn accelerates chemical mediator release. On the other hand, hypoxemia causes pulmonary hypertension, and pulmonary hypertension accelerates generation and release of PGI_2 from the pulmonary arterial wall. PGI_2 inhibits the rise of pulmonary artery pressure, PGI_2 and 6-keto PGF_{1a} inhibit the chemical mediator release, and the latter inhibits the bronchoconstriction induced by various bronchoconstrictors. Serotonin that is released from mast cells causes platelet aggregation. TXA_2 generated and released from aggregated platelets causes bronchoconstriction and chemical mediator release together with TXB_2.

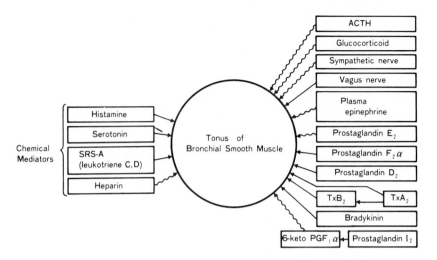

FIGURE 18.   Regulation of tonus in tracheobronchial smooth muscle (straight line arrow, increase of metabolic process; wavy line arrow, decrease).

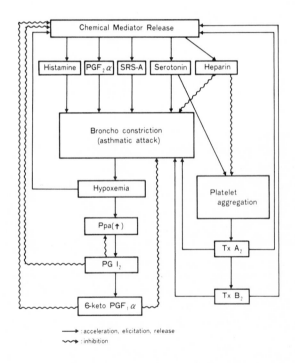

FIGURE 19.   Metabolic and biochemical aspects of bronchial asthma.

REFERENCES

1. Kunze, H. and Vogt, W., Significance of phospholipase A for prostaglandin formation, *Ann. N.Y. Acad. Sci.,* 180, 123, 1971.
2. Bell, R. L., Kennerly, D. A., Staford, N., and Majerus, P. W., in *Proc. Natl. Acad. Sci. U.S.A.,* 76, 3238, 1979.
3. Samuelsson, B., Prostaglandins and thromboxanes, in *Recent Progress in Hormone Research*, Ramwell, P. W., Ed., Academic Press, New York, 1977, 239.
4. Moncada, S. and Vane, J. R., Pharmacology and endogenous roles of prostaglandin endoperoxides, thromboxane A_2 and prostacyclin, *Pharmacol. Rev.,* 30, 293, 1979.
5. Stone, K. J. and Hart, M., Inhibition of renal PGE_2 9-ketoreductase in rabbit kidney, *Prostaglandins*, 12, 197, 1976.
6. Hansen, H. S., 15-hydroxyprostaglandin dehydrogenase. A review, *Prostaglandins*, 12, 647, 1976.
7. Johnson, R. A., Morton, D. R., Kinner, J. H. et al., The chemical characterization of prostaglandin X (prostacyclin), *Prostaglandins*, 12, 915, 1976.
8. Wong, P. Y.-K., McGiff, J. C., Cagen, L., Malik, K. U., and Sunn, F. F., Metabolism of prostacyclin in the rabbit kidney, *J. Biol. Chem.,* 254, 12, 1979.
9. Roberts, L. J., II, Sweetman, B. J., Payne, A., and Oates, J. A., Metabolism of thromboxane B_2 in man. Identification of the major urinary metabolites, *J. Biol. Chem.,* 252, 7415, 1977.
10. Sheard, P., The effect of prostaglandin E_1 on isolated bronchial muscle from man, *J. Pharm. Pharmacol.,* 20, 232, 1968.
11. Main, I. H. M., The inhibitory actions of prostaglandins on respiratory smooth muscle, *Br. J. Pharmacol. Chemother.,* 22, 511, 1964.
12. Sweatman, W. J. F. and Collier, H. O. J., Effects of prostaglandins on human bronchial muscle, *Nature (London)*, 217, 69, 1968.
13. Dawson, W., Lewis, R. L., McMahon, R. E., and Sweatman, W. J. F., Potent bronchoconstrictor activity of 15-keto prostaglandin $F_{2\alpha}$, *Nature (London)*, 250, 331, 1974.
14. Mathé, A. A., Hedquist, P., Holmgren, A., and Svanborg, N., in *Adv. Biosci.,* 9, 241, 1972.
15. Horton, E. W. and Jones, R. L., Prostaglandins A_1, A_2 and 19-hydroxy A_1; their actions on smooth muscle and their inactivation on passage through the pulmonary and hepatic portal vascular beds, *Br. J. Pharmacol.,* 37, 705, 1969.
16. Ishihara, Y., Sugiyama, Y., Hsu, L.-H., Izumi, T., Hayashi, R., and Kitamura, S., Comparison of the effect of PGD_2 and $PGF_{2\alpha}$ on guinea pig tracheal strips, *Jpn. J. Thorac. Dis.,* 18, 634, 1980.
17. Kitamura, S., Ishihara, Y., Sugiyama, Y., Izumi, T., Hayashi, R., Hsu, L.-H., and Kosaka, K., Effect of ipratropium bromide on the action of bronchoactive agents, *Arzneim. Forsch.,* 32, 128, 1982.
18. Kitamura, S., Ishihara, Y., Sugiyama, Y., and Hsu, L.-H., Effect of prostaglandins E_1, E_2, D_2, $F_{2\alpha}$ and I_2 on the canine airways and pulmonary vascular bed, *Jpn. J. Thorac. Dis.,* 17, 560, 1979.
19. Kitamura, S., Suzuki, K., Ishihara, Y., and Kosaka, K., Comparative responses of various parts of tracheo-bronchial tree to bronchoactive agents, *Jpn. J. Thorac. Dis.,* 20, 264, 1982.
20. Ishihara, Y., Kitamura, A., and Takaku, F., Effect of 6-keto prostaglandin $F_{1\alpha}$, the main metabolite of prostacyclin, on guinea pig tracheal strips, *Clin. Res.,* 30, 1983.
21. Dusting, G. J., Moncada, S., and Vane, J. R., Disappearance of prostacyclin in the circulation of the dog, *Br. J. Pharmacol.,* 62, 414, 1977.
22. Gimeno, M. J., Sterin-Borda, L., Borda, E. S., Lazzari, M. A., and Gimeno, A. L., Human plasma transforms prostacyclin (PGI_2) into a platelet antiaggregatory substance which contracts isolated bovine coronary arteries, *Prostaglandins*, 19, 907, 1980.
23. Blasko, G., Nemesanszky, E., Szabo, G., Stadler, I., and Palos, L. A., The effect of PGI_2 and PGI_2 analogues with increased stability on platelet cAMP content and aggregation, *Thromb. Res.,* 17, 673, 1980.
24. Moncada, S., Biological importance of prostacyclin, *Br. J. Pharmacol.,* 76, 3, 1982.
25. Ishihara, Y. and Kitamura, S., Effect of leukotriene C_4 and D_4 on isolated guinea pig tracheal strips, *Jpn. J. Thorac. Dis.,* 20, 391, 1982.
26. Hanna, C. J., Bach, M. K., Pare, P. D., and Schellenberg, R. R., Slow reacting substances (leukotrienes) contract human airway and pulmonary vascular smooth muscle *in vitro*, *Nature (London)*, 290, 343, 1981.
27. Ishihara, Y., Kitamura, S., and Terao, S., Effects of leukotriene C_4, D_4 and E_4 on canine airway and pulmonary circulation in anesthetized dogs, *Jpn. J. Thorac. Dis.,* in press.
28. Drazen, J. M., Austen, K. F., Lewis, R. A., Clark, D. A., Goto, G., Marfat, A., and Corey, E. J., Comparative airway and vascular activities of leukotrienes C and D *in vivo* and *in vitro*, *Proc. Natl. Acad. Sci. U.S.A.,* 77, 4354, 1980.

29. Levi, R., SRS-A, leukotrienes and immediate hypersensitivity reactions of the heart, in *Proc. Symp. Leukotrienes and Other Lipoxygenase Prod.*, Samuelsson, B. and Paoletti, R., Eds., Raven Press, New York, 1982, in press.
30. Kitamura, S., Ishihara, Y., and Hattori, Y., Anaphylactic release of histamine and slow reacting substance of anaphylaxis (SRS-A) from guinea-pig lung and its modulation by prostaglandins, *Jpn. J. Med.*, 17, 3, 1978.
31. Assem, E. S. K. and Schild, H. O., Inhibition by sympathomimetic amines of histamine release induced by antigen in passively sensitized human lung, *Nature (London)*, 224, 1028, 1969.
32. Lichtenstein, L. M. and Margolis, A., Histamine release *in vitro* inhibition by catecholamines and methylxanthines, *Science*, 161, 902, 1968.
33. Lichtenstein, L. M., Mediators and mechanism of their release, *Chest*, 73, 919, 1978.
34. Ishihara, Y. and Kitamura, S., Effect of heparin Na on the action of various bronchoconstrictors in guinea pig tracheal strips, *Tohoku J. Exp. Med.*, 133, 61, 1981.

Chapter 18

PROSTAGLANDINS AND RELATED COMPOUNDS AS POTENTIAL OCULAR THERAPEUTIC AGENTS

Laszlo Z. Bito

TABLE OF CONTENTS

I. INTRODUCTION

The rabbit eye exhibits a characteristic set of responses to mechanical or chemical trauma consisting of miosis, breakdown of the blood-aqueous barrier, transient ocular hypertension, and iridial hyperemia. This so-called ocular irritative response greatly complicates most experimental procedures that require cannulation or other manipulation of the eye. In a search for the mediator(s) of this response, Ambache[1] extracted a smooth muscle stimulating substance from irides, which he called irin. Irin was first described as an ether-soluble unsaturated hydroxy-fatty acid(s).[2,3] It was also found in the aqueous humor of rabbits after paracentesis of the anterior chamber and in anterior chamber perfusates after various forms of stimulation and irritation of the iris.[4] Subsequently, irin was reported to contain both E and F prostaglandins (PGs),[5-7] although it is most likely that this extract contained a variety of other, as yet unidentified substances.

Because of this early association of PGs with the ocular irritative response, it is not surprising that when pure preparations of PGs became available for biomedical research, primary emphasis was placed on attempts to reproduce the signs of ocular irritation with exogenous PGs and to demonstrate a role for PGs in ocular inflammation. It has indeed been shown repeatedly that PGs, in high enough doses and especially when introduced intracamerally into cannulated rabbit eyes, do have ocular irritative effects and do produce some signs of ocular inflammation. Although these observations, together with most others on the effects of steroidal and nonsteroidal anti-inflammatory (NSAI) agents, were derived from experiments on rabbits and could not be consistently repeated on other species (especially primates), the generalization that PGs are important mediators of ocular inflammation became widely accepted.

II. RELEVANT LITERATURE AND THE SCOPE OF THIS CHAPTER

Several reviews have been published on the general role of PGs in ocular pathophysiology;[8-11] it is not the purpose of this chapter to review the voluminous literature on this rapidly expanding field. Rather, in keeping with the general theme of this book, we will re-evaluate the validity of the generalization that PGs have primarily undesirable or detrimental effects on the eye. We will also explore published results that have been or can be interpreted as evidence for the beneficial roles of PGs in ocular tissues or demonstrate the potential utility of PGs in ocular therapeutics.

Several dozen publications serve as the basis for the general conclusion that PGs are important ocular hypertensive agents and primary mediators of ocular inflammation. Some of these are well designed and well presented studies in which results were interpreted in the light of the best information available at the time they were written. However, our understanding of the arachidonic acid cascade has greatly broadened over the last decade, and we now know that PGs are just one subgroup in a large but still incompletely understood family of compounds generally referred to as the eicosanoids. Many other papers have serious shortcomings; in some, conclusions are made without the inclusion of numerical data, while in others, data are given without statistical analyses or without descriptions of the methods used for the measurements. In many publications the authors themselves have stated, sometimes categorically, sometimes parenthetically, that the described results could not be obtained consistently, yet these papers are quoted in the literature without mention of such precautionary statements. An attempt has been made here to indicate some of the shortcomings of such papers. Since such shortcomings may in some cases be open to interpretation, the interested reader should refer to the original papers.

The basic tenet of this chapter is that as a result of the early association of PGs with

Table 1
STUDIES OF OCULAR TISSUES OF RABBITS AND OTHER SPECIES THAT
HAVE BEEN SHOWN TO SYNTHESIZE PGs OR TXA$_2$ (OR ITS INITIAL
BREAKDOWN PRODUCT, TXB$_2$) FROM ENDOGENOUS OR ADDED
PRECURSORS

Tissue	PGE$_1$	PGE$_2$	PGF$_{1\alpha}$	PGF$_{2\alpha}$	PGD$_2$	PGI$_2$	TXA$_2$ or B$_2$
Conjunctiva	12	12—22	12	12,13,17 18,21,22	12,13,17, 18,21,22	12,13,18 21,22	12,17,18, 21—23
Cornea	12	12,16,17,24	12	12,17	12,17	12	12,17
Sclera		17		17	17		17
Lens	25	17,26	25	17	17	17	
Anterior uvea	12,25	12—18,20—22, 24,27—32	12,25	12,13,17, 18,21,22, 28—32	12,13,17, 18,21,22, 28—32	12,13,17, 18,22,26 30—33	12,13,17, 18,21—23 23,28—32
Posterior uvea		17		17	17	26	17
Retina	25	16,26	25				

the ocular irritative response and inflammation, most of the experiments done during the late 1960s and early 1970s were oriented toward elucidating the role of PGs in these phenomena. Since the studies were designed to test irritative or inflammatory effects, doses of PGs or PG precursors sufficient to cause such effects were used, and the anticipated effects were indeed found in most cases. The sheer bulk of this research led to the acceptance of some concepts which should now be re-evaluated, and the possibility that PGs have beneficial, protective effects on the eye and visual functions should be explored.

III. THE EFFECTS OF PG ON OCULAR TISSUES

A. The Cornea and Conjunctiva

Several publications demonstrate that preparations of cornea and conjunctiva can synthesize PGs (Tables 1 and 2). In vitro chloride (Cl) transport across the epithelium of the amphibian cornea was shown to be stimulated by PGs at concentrations of 10^{-6} M to 10^{-5} M[35,36] and this Cl transport was inhibited by meclofenamic acid, an inhibitor of PG synthesis.[37] Cl transport contributes to the maintenance of normal hydration of the amphibian cornea[36,38] and hence, presumably, to the maintenance of corneal transparency. Although such Cl transport also occurs across the epithelium of the rabbit cornea,[39] the maintenance of partial dehydration of the mammalian cornea seems to be primarily due to fluid transport by its endothelium.[40] In a discussion of a paper by Paterson and Eck,[41] Dickstein stated without reference to experimental evidence that PGs do not affect the corneal endothelium. Thus, although PGs appear to play a beneficial role in the maintenance of corneal transparency in amphibians, a similar role for PGs in mammalian corneas remains to be elucidated.

The role of PGs in corneal wound healing and other repair processes also remains unresolved. Topical application of low doses of PGs to the rabbit eye elicited the entry of polymorphonuclear leukocytes (PMNs) into the tear fluid, presumably from the conjunctiva.[42] Low doses of indomethacin (5 mg/kg) administered systemically to rabbits after removal of the corneal epithelium also stimulated leukocytic invasion of the tear fluid; however, higher doses inhibited this repsonse[42,43] and topical treatment with cyclooxygenase inhibitors affected the rate of corneal re-epithelialization.[44] Prednisolone and flurbiprofen have been reported to slow postoperative corneal wound healing, indicating that PGs may facilitate the healing process;[45] however, topical application

Table 2
A REVIEW OF THE RATES OF SYNTHESIS OF SOME PGs AND OTHER EICOSANOIDS BY THE ANTERIOR
UVEA AND CONJUNCTIVA IN VITRO

Species	Tissue, prep.	Units	PGE_2	$PGF_{2\alpha}$	PGD_2	PGI_2	TXB_2	Exogenous AA added	Ref.
Bovine	AU, whole	μg/g Tissue	0.91 ± 0.09[a]					0	27
Rabbit	AU, microsomal	ng/mg Protein	117 ± 11[a]					10 μg/mℓ	16
	Conj, microsomal		205 ± 28[a]					10 μg/mℓ	16
	AU, chopped	pmol/5 min	1.5 ± 0.4	0.4 ± 0.1				?	29
	AU, whole	μg/gWW	2.20[a]					0	24
	AU, microsomal	ng/mg Protein	190[a]					10 μg/mℓ	24
	AU, microsomal		1.6	1.6	0.7	1.1	2.1	?	17
	Conj, microsomal		0.6		0.8	0.2	0.3	?	17
	AU, chopped	% Conversion	3.2 ± 0.7	4.0 ± 0.5	1.6 ± 0.4	1.6 ± 0.2	1.8 ± 0.5	Trace	18
	Conj, chopped		7.6 ± 0.6	4.7 ± 0.2	2.2 ± 0.2	4.8 ± 0.8	4.5 ± 0.4	Trace	18
	AU, microsomal		0.4 ± 0.13[b]	0.65 ± 0.39[b]	0.61 ± 0.10[b]		1.69 ± 1.12	Trace	31
	AU, chopped	μg/g Tissue	0.5[a]					0	20
	Conj, chopped		0.17[a]					0	20

Note: AU, anterior uvea; Conj, conjunctiva.

[a] PGE_2-like activity as determined by bioassay.

[b] Mean ± standard deviation.

of indomethacin solution for 2 weeks had no effect on the tensile strength of corneal wounds in rabbits.[46]

Daily topical application of high concentrations (5.5 mM) of PGE$_2$ to the corneal surface of cats during most of a 9-month treatment period caused no corneal damage that could be attributed to direct PG effects on this tissue.[47] Shorter term experiments with other PGs on cats and rhesus monkeys also showed no evidence of adverse corneal effects. Thus, currently available evidence indicates that PGs do not have a deleterious effect on the cornea, although they may be involved in the regulation of processes required for corneal transparency and repair.

B. The Anterior Uvea

The fact that the anterior uvea is capable of forming PGs and other autacoids has been especially well documented (Table 1). Unfortunately, the rate of eicosanoid production, given by different laboratories (in some cases even by the same laboratory for different tissues or species), is difficult (if not impossible) to compare, since the method of tissue preparation, the concentrations of substrate and co-factors, duration and condition of incubation, as well as the expression of the measurements vary from study to study (Table 2). Furthermore, in some studies 8,11,14-eicosatrienoic acid has been used as a substrate instead of arachidonic acid, leading to the synthesis of PGE$_1$ and PGF$_{1\alpha}$.[12,17,25] It seems most unlikely that this precursor is available in mammalian tissues from endogenous sources in amounts sufficient to form significant amounts of these PGs. Thus, earlier reports such as the one identifying PGE$_1$ in the aqueous during experimental uveitis[48] should be re-evaluated.

Most studies on PG synthesis by ocular tissues were done on rabbits (Table 1) and only a few comparative studies on this subject are available. Using the production of HHT as an index, the highest cyclooxygenase activity was found in irides of rabbits and guinea pigs, followed by dogs > cats > monkeys.[49] It is also of interest that the monkey iris was found to produce some four times more 12-HETE than HHT. Although the particular species of monkey used was not given and the authors themselves are somewhat cautious with their conclusions,[49] these findings suggest that in at least some primates the anterior uvea has a very limited capacity to synthesize cyclooxygenase products as compared to other species or to the amount of lipoxygenase products formed by this tissue.

Kulkarni et al.,[22] in a comparison of anterior uveal cyclooxygenase activity, found the highest activity in the rabbit, followed by cat > dog > human > bovine. Although the microsomal fraction of human irides produced only negligible amounts of cyclooxygenase products from added arachidonic acid, this preparation was capable of converting PGH$_2$ to PGs at a rate similar to irides of other species, including rabbits.[32] Other species differences, such as an unusually high production of PGI$_2$ by bovine irides, were also noted.[22,33] While there appears to be considerable quantitative and even some qualitative differences among mammalian species in iridial cyclooxygenase and lipoxygenase activities, it is reasonable to conclude that in all mammals the anterior uvea is capable of producing some eicosanoids, and hence it is most likely that the arachidonic acid cascade plays a physiological role in the anterior segment of the eye.

Effects on the anterior uvea frequently attributed to PGs include vascular changes that lead to iridial hyperemia, breakdown of the blood-aqueous barrier which allows the entry of plasma proteins into the aqueous humor and hence the development of anterior chamber flare, changes in the secretory activity of the ciliary processes, and constriction of the iris sphincter that leads to pupillary miosis. The first three of these effects are important components of the ocular inflammatory response and will be discussed under that topic (see Section V). Pupillary miosis will be discussed in Section VI.

C. The Lens

Microsomal fractions of rabbit lenses did not produce PGs under conditions that yielded significant PG production by other ocular tissues,[17] although some production of 5-HETE was found in lens fragments that were taken from rabbits pretreated for 14 days with ethynyl estradiol.[50] Cultured cells of chicken lens capsular epithelium did not release PGs into the tissue culture medium[51] under conditions similar to those that yielded measurable PG release by epithelial, endothelial, and stromal cells of the cornea.[52] Thus, it appears that the normal lens has little or no capacity to synthesize eicosanoids and it is unlikely that this organ has important PG-mediated physiological systems.

It has been reported that incubation of mouse or rat lenses in the presence of PGE_1 or $PGF_{1\alpha}$ reduced galactose uptake[53] and incubation of rabbit lenses for 20 hr in media containing PGE_1, PGE_2, or $PGF_{2\alpha}$ markedly increased their Na:K ratio.[41] One brief report[54] indicates that PGE_1 can affect the rate of cell division and/or DNA synthesis in the capsular epithelium of cultured rat lenses. However, in all of these studies, such effects were only observed when extremely high PG concentrations ($>10^{-4}$ M) were used, although one study using a slightly lower but still very high concentration of 10^{-4} M found PGs to stimulate cation transport of rabbit lenses and render them less sensitive to Ca^{++} deprivation,[41,55] effects that must be regarded as beneficial rather than detrimental to this organ. Even in the inflamed eye in which PG concentrations were greatly elevated, the level of PGs did not exceed 10^{-6} M in the aqueous humor[48,56] and the lens itself produced little or no PGs. It is most unlikely that the lens would ever be exposed in vivo to the high concentrations of PGs typically used in these in vitro studies. On the basis of this evidence, we can only conclude, therefore, that PGs do not appear to play an important role in the physiological processes of the lens and cannot be expected to have an adverse effect on this organ under in vivo conditions.

It must be noted, however, that most of these studies were done on lenses of non-accommodating species such as rabbits, rats, or mice. The possibility that lenses of primates, which undergo frequent and extensive deformation, are capable of eicosanoid production should be investigated. It is interesting to note in this regard that there is a report indicating that in an accommodating species (the chick), lipoxygenase pathways may be involved in the initiation of in vitro lens fiber cell differentiation;[51] however, even in this species there was no evidence that PGs were synthesized by the capsular epithelium.[51]

The apparently unique absence of a physiologically significant PG system in the lens may be the result of one of the unusual characteristics of this organ. The avascularity of the lens is unlikely to account for the absence of a PG system since the cornea is also largely avascular, yet it can synthesize PGs and respond to relatively low doses of PGs (see Section IIIA). While most lens cells (sometimes incorrectly called lens fibers) are devoid of nuclei and virtually all other organelles, cortical lens cells, and cells of the capsular epithelium have normal intracellular organelles, yet these cells also lack PG synthesizing capacity and show no detectable responses to physiological levels of PGs. Therefore, the absence of a PG system in the lens is most likely due to another unique characteristic of this organ, its lack of innervation. This suggests that either the development or the unmasking of the PG system may require some neuronal influences. A better understanding of the reasons for the apparent lack of a PG system is this highly cellular organ can be expected to greatly advance our understanding of the development and the function of the PG system and its dependence on, and interactions with, other regulatory systems of the body.

D. The Retina

Superfusion of isolated toad retinas with Ringer's solution containing 50 $\mu g/m\ell$ ($\sim$

1.5×10^{-4} *M)* $PGF_{2\alpha}$ has been shown to cause depolarization of rods, while superfusion with PGE_1 caused hyperpolarization.[57] The concentration of PGs used was, however, much higher than that usually required to produce biological effects.

Since the retina is part of the CNS, its basic enzymatic activities are likely to be similar to those of the brain in which PG-synthesizing capacity has been well demonstrated.[58,59] The retina of the rabbit indeed has been reported to produce PG-like biological activity,[16] and more recently Kulkarni and Eakins[26] stated that the bovine retina produces PGE_2 when incubated with PGH_2, but does not generate PGI_2 or TXB_2 under similar conditions. A full report on these findings has not yet been published. It is surprising that while many papers have been published on the capacity of the anterior uvea and conjunctiva to synthesize various eicosanoids (Table 1), the production of eicosanoids by the mammalian retina remains controversial. The fact that intravitreal injection of arachidonic acid caused a depression of the B-wave amplitude similar to that caused by intravitreal injection of PGE_1 or PGE_2, and that this effect was prevented by pretreatment with indomethacin,[60] suggest that the retina has physiologically significant cyclooxygenase activity.

This and similar in vivo studies[61,62] have also demonstrated that PGEs, but not PGFs, can affect the electrical activity of the retina in vivo. While reported alterations in the ERG could be explained primarily by effects on Muller cell function, inhibition of the visually evoked response following intravitreal injection of PGE_1 indicates that the neuronal activity of the retina and its output to the brain are also affected by PGEs.[60,62] However, no effects were found with intravitreal injecton of similar doses of $PGF_{2\alpha}$, and even PGEs had appreciable effects only when large doses (0.7 to 1.6 mg per eye) were injected into the vitreous body of animals that had been pretreated with a PG transport inhibitor.[60-62]

PGs can indeed be expected to play important roles in the normal physiological processes of the retina, since these autacoids modulate synaptic transmission;[63,64] however, the absorptive transport of PG across the blood-retinal barrier system (see Section IV) seems to be more than sufficient to prevent PGs from accumulating in the extracellular fluids of the retina at levels that could cause pathological effects.[65] Thus, PGs are unlikely to have any adverse effects on the retina since such adverse effects clearly require a very high local PG concentration that cannot be achieved as long as these transport processes function normally. While a direct role for PGs in the development of cystoid macula edema has been postulated based on the loss of PG transport capacity,[66] it does not necessarily imply that PGs are the causative agent. In fact, the possibility that PGs have beneficial effects on the retina, such as in some degenerative retinal diseases or in retinal ischemia, should be investigated.

IV. PROTECTION AGAINST THE INTRAOCULAR ACCUMULATION OF PGS

It has been shown that PGs are accumulated by the anterior uvea in vitro[67,68] and intravitreally injected PGE_1 disappears from the eye more rapidly than simultaneously injected sucrose, an inert substance of essentially identical molecular weight.[69] Since the basic plasma membrane is completely impermeable to E and F PGs,[70] the transfer of PGs across the tight-junctional epithelial membranes such as the blood-ocular and blood-brain barriers requires special "carrier-mediated" transport processes.

The existence of such a process[71] and its role in the removal of PGs from the extracellular fluids of the brain,[72] in the pulmonary and renal metabolism, and/or excretion of PGs and their metabolites has been well documented over the past decade and this field was recently reviewed.[73] The physiological need for the ocular PG transport system was underscored by the demonstration that intraocular tissues, as is the case in the brain, have little or no capacity to metabolize or inactivate PGs.[74,75]

Recently, the retinal choroid was found to have a PG-accumulating capacity similar to that of the anterior uvea.[73] In vivo studies on the rate of loss of PGs from the vitreous support this finding.[61] This is an important consideration in that the choroid, specifically the choroidal epithelium (frequently, but incorrectly referred to as the retinal pigment epitheium), plays an important role in maintaining the chemical homeostasis of the retina.[65] Thus in the eye, the termination of the action of PGs and the prevention of their accumulation is dependent on the above-described transport system.

PGs are unlikely to exert a pathological effect on the retina, unless the absorptive PG transport processes across the blood-ocular barriers are saturated, inhibited, or damaged. In vitro and in vivo studies indicate that saturation of the PG transport process requires PG concentrations of the order of 10^{-4} M, an increase in PG concentration of at least several thousand-fold over the normal level.[72,76,77] This transport mechanism is, in fact, unlikely to be saturated even at pathophysiological PG levels; however, severe and/or prolonged uveitis was found to have a long-lasting and possibly permanent inhibitory effect on anterior uveal PG transport capacity.[78] It should be noted that the PG transport system is part of the larger class of organic acid transport systems. Thus, the possibility that severe intraocular inflammation renders the eye vulnerable to the accumulation of PGs and other organic acids must be considered, since such mechanisms may play an important role in the etiology of some ocular disorders.

V. THE ROLE OF PGs IN THE OCULAR IRRITATIVE RESPONSE AND INFLAMMATION

It has been well documented that excessive stimulation of the iris or irritation of the ocular surface, or even the facial area surrounding the eye causes a set of ocular responses in rabbits. The irritant may be a chemical agent, such as nitrogen mustard (NM) or formaldehyde; mechanical or surgical trauma, including paracentesis of the anterior chamber; or radiant energy such as X-ray, infrared, or even visible light of high intensity (laser beam, for example). Many aspects of the ocular irritative response are similar to the inflammatory response observed clinically or after the introduction of a foreign protein or bacterial endotoxin into the vitreous body of experimental animals. The typical components of the ocular inflammatory response are acute elevation of intraocular pressure (IOP), frequently followed by an episode of ocular hypotony; the development of flare in the anterior chamber, presumably due to breakdown of the blood-aqueous barrier; engorgement of, and leakage of fluorescein from iridial blood vessels;[79,80] strong atropine-resistant pupillary constriction; invasion of intraocular compartments by leukocytes; degranulation of mast cells;[81] loss of secretory and absorptive transport functions of the ciliary processes;[78,82] and ultimately, permanent damage to intraocular tissues.

Some forms of irritation, such as simple paracentesis of the anterior chamber, cause only one or two of these responses. Some authors appear to advocate a distinction between the ocular irritative response and the ocular inflammatory response on the basis of the presence or absence of some response, such as leukocytic infiltration, or on the basis of the presumed mediation of the response by a neurogenic mechanism, as opposed to PGs. For example, the sharp NM-induced rise in IOP and breakdown of the blood-aqueous barrier in rabbits were initially thought not to be mediated by PGs;[9] in addition, the initial rise in IOP is not associated with leukocyte infiltration. Thus, on both of these accounts, the reaction of the rabbit eye to NM was regarded as an irritative response. It was later shown, however, that the first phase of this response, which has been studied by most investigators, is followed by a second rise in IOP that is not only accompanied by a further increase in protein concentration, but also by cellular invasion of the anterior chamber.[83,84] Hence, this must be regarded as a true inflammatory response. Furthermore, although the first phase is apparently mediated by a neurogenic mechanism (possibly the release of substance P or other neuropeptides), many aspects of the second phase can be blocked, or at least reduced by PG synthesis inhibitors. This suggests that this second phase is mediated or at least potentiated indirectly by PGs or related eicosanoids.[83]

Thus, in some cases, the "irritative response" may simply be an early phase of the inflammatory process. Even a true inflammatory process may therefore appear to be a simple irritative response if the observation period is kept short, as is done in most experiments because the cannulated rabbit eye deteriorates rapidly. Thus, making a sharp distinction between irritative and inflammatory responses may be counterproductive; it is, however, necessary to make some distinction between different phases of the inflammatory response.

In at least some forms of ocular inflammation the initial phase is mediated by a neurogenic mechanism rather that PGs. The role of PGs in the rest of the inflammatory response is more difficult to evaluate. The overwhelming number of experiments that serve as the basis of the concept that PGs are the mediators of ocular inflammation were done on rabbits only (Table 3). It has since been shown that the rabbit is not typical of mammals in general in its ocular responses to irritation,[160,163] and as was described above (Section III. B) this species has a much more active cyclooxygenase system than most other species. Furthermore, much of the work was done before the existence of the many biologically active arachidonic acid derivatives was generally known, and before the species differences in the ocular arachidonic acid cascade were fully appreciated. Eakins[9] listed four lines of evidence supporting the conclusion that PGs are the mediators of ocular inflammation. The interpretation of each of these lines of evidence has recently been reassessed in view of our present understanding of the arachidonic cascade.[164] Such reassessment suggests that even in rabbits PGs cannot be regarded as the primary or only mediators of ocular inflammation, although the arachidonic acid cascade as a whole may play an important role in the ocular responses of the particular species. It has never been demonstrated that any PG can trigger all aspects of the inflammatory response in any species, and in primates even very high doses of PGs cannot reproduce most signs of ocular inflammation. It has been shown, for example, that the influx of leukocytes into the anterior chamber, probably the most important single aspect of ocular inflammation, is triggered by leukotrienes rather than PGs.[140] Thus, ocular inflammation is most likely mediated by several autacoids while PGs might be one of these in the rabbit; however, the importance of PGs, even in the rabbit, as mediators of ocular inflammation may have been exaggerated.

VI. REASSESSMENT OF THE ROLE OF PGs IN PUPILLARY MIOSIS

The concept that PGs are strong miotics originated with the observation that irin, an iridial extract that causes pupillary constriction[1] (see Section I) is a mixture of PGs.[6,7] It should be noted, however, that at that time, only a few of the compounds now called eicosanoids were known and the total composition of irin was not established. Even today we cannot assume that we know all members of this group. Thus, while Ambache's work is of historical significance, it should not be cited in support of the role of PGs as the primary mediators of some forms of pupillary miosis.

An earlier review of the action of PGs on the eye[9] lists five investigator teams as providing indications that PGs cause pupillary constriction,[114,116,119,121,143] and two reviewers[118,145] who concluded that PGs have no miotic effects. Only one of the five

Table 3

STUDIES THAT WERE INTERPRETED BY THE AUTHORS OR WERE
QUOTED BY OTHERS TO SUPPORT THE CONCEPT THAT PGs ARE
MEDIATORS OF THE OCULAR IRRITATIVE RESPONSE AND/OR OCULAR
INFLAMMATION

	Rabbit	Human	Other species
Demonstration of increased PG levels in aqueous humor or increased PG prod. by intraocular tissues	24, 31, 48, 85—108	109—112	
Induction by exogenous PGs or AA of 1 or more components of ocular irritative response or inflammation	92, 97, 113—142		114, 143—146
Prevention or reduction of an ocular inflammatory condition by indomethacin or other cyclooxygenase inhibitors	83, 86—97, 103—105, 113, 115, 117, 119, 121, 123—127, 132, 135, 141, 147—160	46, 111, 112, 161	144, 146, 162

reports that stated that PGs had a miotic effect dealt primarily with miosis, while the other four did not describe the methods or conditions of pupil measurement, provided no data on the extent or time course of pupillary miosis, and/or made only passing reference to miosis in their discussions.

The first of the five papers on the effects of exogenous PGs[114] refers to pupil size in its title; however, the text did not state how and when pupil size was measured, what the resting pupillary diameters were, or under what lighting conditions measurements were made. The number of eyes in which the pupil constricted was reported, but the criteria used to assess constriction were not given. While the authors conclude that the miosis observed in both cats and rabbits was due to direct stimulation of iris smooth muscle by PGs, this conclusion is hard to evaluate in the absence of actual values or description of the methods. The second paper cited in the review as demonstrating pupillary constriction in the rabbit eye induced with exogenous PGE_1, PGE_2, or $PGF_{2\alpha}$ clearly focused on IOP, and provided no data on miosis.[116] The authors stated only that PG-induced increases in IOP were frequently accompanied by pupillary constriction. As can be seen from the summary in Table 4, the majority of the papers that either report that PGs are miotic or that are used by others in support of this concept suffer from similar shortcomings.

An early paper including more detailed and precise information[170] reported that in rhesus monkeys, topical application of 10 μg of PGE_2 per eye or intracameral injection of 1 μg of PGE_2 per eye caused pupillary constriction; the actual decrease in pupil diameter was less than 0.5 mm. The sophisticated photographic method used to measure pupillary diameter showed this small change in pupil diameter to be statistically significant after topical application, but not after intracameral injection. Casey[170] also reported that topical or intracameral administration of PGE_2, even in doses that had no measurable miotic effect, reduced the pupillary dilation caused by systemic administration of atropine.

In a series of reports, van Alphen and co-workers[174-177] presented results on the effects of PGs alone and in combination with other drugs on the isolated iris sphincter and dilator, as well as on the ciliary muscle of cats, rabbits, monkeys, and man. These studies present a picture too complex to review here. PGs were found to have both contractile and relaxant effects on these muscles; for example, PGE_2 was shown to relax the isolated iris-sphincter of rabbits, while $PGF_{2\alpha}$ had a contractile effect on the iris dilator. Other workers reported that PGE_1, PGE_2, or $PGF_{2\alpha}$, in concentrations from 10^{-4} to 10^{-5} M, did not constrict the rabbit iris sphincter in vitro under conditions

Table 4
SUMMARY OF THE FINDINGS AND RELEVANT INFORMATION PRESENTED IN SOME REF. ON THE IN VIVO EFFECTS OF EXOGENOUS PGs ON THE PUPIL

Species	PG used	Statement on miosis	Revelant methods	Numerical data	Statistical evaluation	Ref.
Rabbit	E_2	Moderate to marked	No	No	No	165
	E_1, E_2, F_{1a}	Marked	Yes	Yes	No	114
	E_2	Miosis prod.	No	Yes	No	134
	E_1	Miosis prod.	Yes	Yes	Yes	133
	E_1, E_2	Miosis prod.	Yes	Yes	No	141
	E_2	Little or none	Yes	Yes	No	166
	E_1, E_2, F_{1a}, F_{2a}	Miosis prod.	No	No	No	116
	E_2	Miosis prod.	No	No	No	167
	E_2	Miosis, most cases	No	No	No	128
	$E_2, D_2, I_2,$ 6-keto-E_1, 6-keto-F_{1a}	No miosis	No	No	No	142
	E_1, E_2	No miosis	No	No	No	118
	I_2	No miosis	No	Yes	No	173
Cat	E_1, E_2, F_{1a}	Marked	Yes	No	No	114
	E_2	Slight	Yes	Yes	No	168
	F_{2a}	Strong, dose-dependent	Yes	Yes	Yes	168
	E_1, E_2	Miosis prod.	No	No	No	143
	E_2, F_{2a}	Strong, dose-dependent	Yes	Yes	Yes	169
Rhesus	E_2	Equivocal	Yes	Yes	Yes	170
	F_{2a}	Very slight	Yes	No	No	168
	E_2	Small	Yes	Yes	Yes	169
	F_{2a}	No miosis	Yes	No	No	172
Cynomolgus	E_1, E_2, F_{1a}, F_{2a}	No miosis	Yes	No	No	145
Owl monkey	F_{2a}	Miosis prod.	Yes	Yes	No	171
Human	F_{2a}	Miosis prod.	Yes	Yes	No	172

in which carbachol, substance P, bradykinin, and capsaicin produced constriction.[178] Recent experiments[179] have shown that the in vitro iris of the anterior segment of rat eyes, which shows miotic responses to cholinergic drugs or a variety of other agents,[180] exhibits little or no miotic response to exogenous PGs unless the rats are pretreated with indomethacin or flurbiprofen, or unless the tissue bath contains these PG synthesis inhibitors. It is clear, therefore, that such in vitro studies do not support the generalization that PGs are strong miotics.

More recently it was shown that intravitreal injection of PGE_2, at doses sufficient to cause iridial hyperemia, breakdown of the blood-aqueous barrier, and increases in IOP, have no miotic effect in rabbits. However, under identical conditions, as little as 0.1 μg of substance P produced significant effects, and higher doses resulted in complete pupillary constriction without producing hyperemia or anterior chamber flare;[181] however, PGE_2 potentiated the miotic effects of substance P in these experiments. It is possible, therefore, that some of the miotic effects of PGs reported in early studies were due to such potentiation of the miotic effects of other autacoids, such as substance P, that were released into ocular compartments as a result of the trauma caused by cannulation and/or other manipulations of the eye.

Topical application of PGF_{2a} in the range of 0.1 to 1000 μg per eye caused a dose-dependent miosis in cats, with maximum pupillary constriction within 2 to 3 hr;[169] however, PGE_2 was found to be a much weaker miotic in this species. Doses of PGF_{2a} that caused a reduction of IOP were found to have little or no miotic effect on rhesus monkey eyes.[169]

A review of these and other findings (Table 4) clearly indicates that PGs, in general, cannot be regarded as potent miotic agents in all species, although some PGs do have a pronounced miotic effect in some species. The conclusion that PGs in general are potent miotics was based on observations of miosis that might have been due to potentiation by these PGs of the miotic effects of other autacoids released into the eye as a result of trauma to ocular tissues associated with the experimental procedures.

VII. REASSESSMENT OF THE EFFECTS OF PGs ON INTRAOCULAR PRESSURE

There are dozens of reports showing that intracameral or topical administration of PGs or arachidonic acid causes an increase in IOP in rabbits.[8,9,11] Recent studies have demonstrated, however, that even in rabbits, lower doses of topically applied PGs reduce, rather than increase IOP.[182] It should also be noted that in rabbits PG-induced ocular hypertension is associated with breakdown of the blood-aqueous barrier and therefore, the associated ocular hypertension cannot be regarded as an effect on the normal IOP control mechanisms. Because the rabbit is atypical of mammals with regard to its arachidonic acid cascade and the so-called lability of its blood-aqueous barrier,[160,163,183] we will focus this reassessment of the literature on the effects of PGs on the IOP of species other than rabbits.

Eakins[143] reported that PGE_1 and PGE_2 increased IOP in the cat, but could not reconcile this finding with a previous report by Waitzman and King[114] that there was no rise in the IOP of cats following intracameral injection of similar doses of these PGs. More recent studies indicate that the predominant effect of a variety of PGs, PG derivatives, and other eicosanoids, when topically applied to the eyes of slightly tranquilized or untranquilized cats, is a reduction rather than an increase in IOP.[168,169,184]

The effects of exogenous PGs on the IOP in several primate species have also been studied. Kelly and Starr[145] reported that intracameral injection of 10 μg of PGE_2 increased the IOP of cynomolgus monkeys by 10.2 mmHg. These authors stated, however, that "the last six monkeys . . . tested failed to respond consistently to intraocular injections of new batches of PGE_1 and PGE_2". Because the PGs used in the latter experiments were biologically active, we must conclude that intracamerally injected PGs, in doses 1000 times higher than those required in rabbits,[116] do elevate IOP in cynomolgus monkeys under some circumstances, but not consistently. The fact that IOP increases were consistently observed in their earlier, but not in their later experiments, suggests that the degree of trauma suffered by the eye during the course of cannulation may be a determining factor. Such trauma could be expected to be reduced during a series of experiments.

Topical or intracameral administration of PGE_2 is also reported to cause a rise in the IOP of rhesus monkeys;[185] however, these animals had an extremely low baseline IOP (apparently below 9 mmHg), probably due to the use of ketamine HCl, sodium pentobarbitol, and sodium thiamylal to gain anesthesia. Thus, even in the PG-treated eyes, the highest mean IOP reported was 16 mmHg, a value that is well within the normal IOP range for this species.[186] We, therefore, cannot conclude from these experiments that PGs produce a pathological rise in the IOP of rhesus monkeys as they do in rabbits. In fact, one interpretation of these results is that in rhesus monkeys PGs facilitate the return of normal IOP after it was reduced to below normal by anesthetic agents. The fact that Casey[185] observed an increased outflow facility in the PG-treated eye despite an increased IOP remains to be explained, but suggests that under some conditions PGs may have a dual effect on the eye.

In contrast to such reports, topical application of even relatively high doses of PGE_2 or $PGF_{2\alpha}$ to the uncannulated eyes of unanesthetized rhesus monkeys was found to have a predominantly hypotensive rather than hypertensive effect (see Section VIII). An increased IOP was observed only occasionally and only for very brief periods of time[168,169] and may have been due to local irritation and/or to the potentiation by PGs of the hypertensive effects of some other mediators that are released by local irritation. It should be noted that PGF_{2a} also reduced IOP in normal owl monkeys and in one glaucomatous owl monkey.[171] These observations suggest that in most species, especially in primates (but with the notable exception of rabbits), the predominant effect of PGs on the IOP of normal, uncannulated eyes is hypo-, rather then hypertensive.

VIII. EICOSANOIDS AS POTENTIAL ANTIGLAUCOMA AGENTS

The visual loss associated with chronic glaucoma is the result of damage to the ganglion cell axons in the optic nerve head caused by increased IOP resulting from an increased resistance to the outflow of aqueous humor. An ideal drug for the treatment of glaucoma would be one that when administered on a regular but acceptable schedule maintains reduced IOP by causing a prolonged reduction in outflow resistance without adverse local or systemic side effects. Unfortunately, none of the currently used drugs fulfill these criteria. Timolol and diamox reduce IOP by reducing aqueous production, thereby also reducing delivery of nutrients to and removal of metabolic wastes from avascular ocular tissues such as the lens and the cornea that depend on normal flow of aqueous humor for all their metabolic exchanges.[65] The drugs that act by decreasing outflow resistance, such as pilocarpine and carbachol, are strong miotics and therefore can seriously diminish night vision and cause severe, and sometimes painful ciliary spasms.

Studies on trained, unanesthesized cats have demonstrated that long-term reduction in IOP can be achieved with PGs.[168] During a 9-month treatment period, the reduction in the IOP of the treated eyes of 6 cats was maintained as long as PGE_2 was administered topically at least once a day. Shorter term experiments indicated that PGF_{2a} is also an effective ocular hypotensive in both cats and rhesus monkeys.[168,169] Neither E- nor F-type PGs had a physiologically significant miotic effect, or other obvious adverse effect on the rhesus eye, although PGF_{2a}, but not PGE_2, was found to be a potent miotic in cats.

In these experiments, precautions were not taken to minimize the drainage of the topically applied solutions into the lacrimal canal; nevertheless, no systemic side effects were observed. During the 9-month treatment period, all 3 females in a group of 6 cats conceived, bore, and nursed apparently healthy kittens.[47] This is not surprising, since PGs are known to be virtually quantitatively inactivated during one passage through the lungs, then further metabolized, and excreted by the kidneys via highly active transport systems.[73,187,188] Thus, PGs that reach the general circulation through the conjunctiva or the lacrimal canal would not be expected to reach most organ systems in their active form. Local side effects were also moderate — suprisingly so, considering that these PGs were applied to the eye without special formulation, and that tonometry was performed at frequent intervals.[168]

Single applications of PGF_{2a} also reduced IOP in normal owl monkeys,[171] although in this species (probably because of its very small body size) systemic effects were evident. An especially striking reduction of IOP was observed in one eye of an owl monkey that exhibited IOP in the range of 47 to 50 mmHg for several months and responded to topical applications of pilocarpine with a further increase in IOP. The pressure in this eye, which apparently had an angle recession glaucoma of unknown origin, was reduced dramatically after a single topical application of 1 mg of PGF_{2a}. It remained within the normal range of 13 to 16 mmHg for several days, after which it gradually returned toward the pretreatment glaucomatous level.[171] This IOP reduction in primates is presumably due (at least in part) to an increased outflow facility since the outflow facility was reported to be increased by PGs in rhesus monkeys even under conditions that increased, rather than decreased IOP (see also Section VI);[185] however, the mechanism by which such increase in outflow facility is achieved remains obscure.

Pilocarpine was shown to increase outflow facility in cynomolgus monkeys via its effect on the ciliary muscle,[189] presumably by asserting tension on the outflow region via its tendon, the scleral spur. Such a mechanism is unlikely to offer a general explanation for the effects of PGs since PGs which have no miotic effects are unlikely to constrict the ciliary muscles; furthermore, cats do not have a well-developed scleral spur. We must, therefore, consider the possibility that PGs have a direct effect on the cells of the trabecular meshwork and/or more distal regions of the outflow channels. It is interesting to note that the trabecular endothelial cells in culture were shown to produce PGE_2 and $PGF_{2\alpha}$ and to respond to exogenous PGs with an increase in intracellular cAMP concentration.[190,191] The possibility that PGs increase uveo-scleral outflow should also be investigated.

Topical application of single, very low doses of $PGF_{2\alpha}$ also reduced IOP in rabbits. This IOP reduction was also associated with an increased outflow facility; however, the margin between hypo- and hypertensive doses of topically applied $PGF_{2\alpha}$ is very small in this species.[182] Furthermore, reduced IOP could not be maintained in rabbits during 5 days of repeated $PGF_{2\alpha}$ applications because of the development of tachyphylaxis that could not be overcome by increasing the $PGF_{2\alpha}$ dose. In fact, higher doses caused an increase in the IOP of these PG-treated rabbit eyes.[168]

A comparison of 15 eicosanoids and 2 currently used antiglaucoma agents (carbachol and timolol) demonstrated that some PG derivatives can be found, such as the esters of $PGF_{2\alpha}$, that are not only more effective ocular hypotensive agents than $PGF_{2\alpha}$ itself, but that are more effective than any currently used antiglaucoma agent.[184] Clearly, considerably more work will be required to identify the eicosanoid or eicosanoid derivative best suited for long-term maintenance of reduced IOP in glaucoma patients and to find the formulation of this drug that provides the greatest ocular comfort and the fewest side effects. While much work remains to be done, currently available evidence indicates that the eicosanoids must be considered as a new class of potential antiglaucoma agents.

IX. SUMMARY AND CONCLUSIONS

Currently available information indicates that the anterior uvea in most species is capable of forming PGs and related autacoids, and that the retina and cornea but not the lens also contain physiologically significant cyclooxygenase activity. These ocular tissues have no mechanism for metabolizing PGs to inactive forms, but an active organic acid transport system normally maintains the PG concentration within the eye at a very low level.

The effects of PGs on the mammalian cornea are not well established, but the observed effects on vertebrate corneas can be characterized as beneficial rather than detrimental. Attempts to demonstrate adverse PG effects on the lens led to the use of much higher concentrations of PGs than could ever be expected to occur in the local environment of this organ that has no demonstrable PG-synthesizing capacity of its own. Although similarly high concentrations of PGs affect retinal function in vitro, adverse effects on retinal electrical activity could only be demonstrated in vivo when PG transport had been inhibited prior to intravitreal injection of very high doses of PGE_1 or PGE_2. Even under such conditions, $PGF_{2\alpha}$ had no adverse effect on the electrical activity of the *in situ* retina. It is reasonable to conclude, therefore, that at physiological or even elevated levels, PGs have no harmful effects on the cornea, lens, or retina and may, in fact, have some beneficial effects on some of these tissues.

In contrast, literally dozens of publications have indicated that the anterior uvea is adversely affected by PGs. Reported effects include iridial hyperemia, pupillary miosis, and breakdown of the blood-aqueous barrier, which leads to the accumulation of proteins in the anterior chamber and a sustained rise in IOP. Virtually all studies that showed these effects involved cannulated rabbit eyes, in spite of the fact that cannulation itself can have such consequences. Furthermore, these findings have been generalized to other species, although substantial evidence now indicates that the rabbit eye is atypical among mammalian eyes in its sensitivity to ocular irritation or trauma, as well as in its pathophysiological responses to PGs. In fact, the responses of rabbit and primate eyes to mechanical or chemical irritation appear to represent opposite extremes of the mammalian spectrum.[192] While attempts have been made to show that PGs play a similar role in the irritative and inflammatory responses of eyes of other species, the six or so papers on the ocular responses of cats and primates to PGs are generally contradictory. Moreover, there is no evidence that at concentrations that may occur in the eye under normal or pathological conditions, PGs could have an effect on primate eyes similar to their demonstrated adverse effects on cannulated rabbit eyes.

Clearly, the first two decades of research on the ocular effects of PG were prejudiced by the assumption that PGs are the mediators of the ocular irritative response and inflammation. In order to reproduce some of the signs of ocular inflammation, most studies utilized preparations, such as the (cannulated) rabbit eye, that are especially vulnerable to (further) irritation or trauma. It is now time to focus our attention on the elucidation of the role of PGs in the normal physiology of ocular tissues. Such studies will require experimental designs and techniques much more sophisticated than those used when PG doses were simply increased until easily recognizable adverse effects were noted. Only an understanding of the role of PGs and other eicosanoids in the normal functions of ocular tissues will allow us to assess the true potential of this new class of compounds and its derivatives in ocular therapeutics. The demonstration that repeated topical application of PGs to eyes of species other than rabbits can maintain a reduced IOP should be regarded as just the first step in this direction.

REFERENCES

1. Ambache, N., Properties of irin, a physiological constituent of the rabbit's iris, *J. Physiol. (London)*, 135, 114, 1957.
2. Ambache, N., Further studies on the preparation, purification and nature of irin, *J. Physiol. (London)*, 146, 255, 1959.
3. Ambache, N., Prolonged erythema produced by chromatographically purified irin, *J. Physiol. (London)*, 160, 3P, 1962.
4. Ambache, N., Kavanagh, L., and Whiting, J., Effect of mechanical stimulation on rabbit's eyes: release of active substance in anterior chamber perfusates, *J. Physiol. (London)*, 176, 378, 1965.
5. Anggard, E. and Samuelsson, B., Smooth muscle stimulating lipids in sheep iris. The identification of prostaglandin $F_{2\alpha}$. Prostaglandins and related factors 21, *Biochem. Pharmacol.*, 13, 281, 1964.
6. Ambache, N., Brummer, H. C., Rose, J. G., and Whiting, J., Thin-layer chromatography of spasmogenic unsaturated hydroxy-acids from various tissues, *J. Physiol. (London)*, 185, 77P, 1966.
7. Waitzman, M. B., Bailey, W. R., and Kirby, C. G., Chromatographic analysis of biologically active lipids from rabbit irides, *Exp. Eye Res.*, 6, 130, 1967.
8. Eakins, K. E., Ocular effects, in *The Prostaglandins*, Vol. 1, Ramwell, P. W., Ed., Plenum Press, New York, 1973, 219.
9. Eakins, K. E., Prostaglandin and non-prostaglandin mediated breakdown of the blood-aqueous barrier, *Exp. Eye Res. (Suppl.)*, 25, 483, 1977.
10. Waitzman, M. B., Possible new concepts relating prostaglandins to various ocular functions, *Surv. Ophthalmol.*, 14, 301, 1970.

11. Podos, S. M. and Sugar, A., The use of nonsteroidal antiinflammatory drugs in ocular conditions, in *Ocular Therapeutics*, Srinivasan, D., Ed., Masson Publishing, New York, 1980, chap. 9.

12. Kass, M. A., Holmberg, N., and Needleman, P., Prostaglandin synthesis by microsomes of rabbit ocular tissues, *Invest. Ophthalmol. Vis. Sci. (Suppl.)*, 162, 1978.

13. Bhattacherjee, P., Kulkarni, P. S., and Eakins, K. E., "In vitro" formation of prostaglandins, prostacyclin and thromboxane-A_2 by rabbit ocular tissues, *Ophthalmic Res.*, 10, 321, 1978.

14. Ku, E. C., Signor, C., and Eakins, K. E., Antiinflammatory agents and inhibition of ocular prostaglandin synthetase, in *Advances in Prostaglandin and Thromboxane Research*, Vol. 2, Samuelsson, B. and Paoletti, R., Eds., Raven Press, New York, 1976, 819.

15. Bhattacherjee, P. and Eakins, K. E., A comparison of the inhibitory activity of compounds on ocular prostaglandin biosynthesis, *Invest. Ophthalmol.*, 13, 967, 1974.

16. Bhattacherjee, P. and Eakins, K. E., Inhibition of the prostaglandin synthetase systems in ocular tissues by indomethacin, *Br. J. Pharmacol.*, 50, 227, 1974.

17. Kass, M. A. and Holmberg, N. J., Prostaglandin and thromboxane synthesis by microsomes of rabbit ocular tissues, *Invest. Ophthalmol. Vis. Sci.*, 18, 166, 1979.

18. Bhattacherjee, P., Kulkarni, P. S., and Eakins, K. E., Metabolism of arachidonic acid in rabbit ocular tissues, *Invest. Ophthalmol. Vis. Sci.*, 18, 172, 1979.

19. Srinivasan, B. D. and Kulkarni, P. S., The effect of indomethacin (Indo), flurbiprofen (F) and prednisolone acetate on conjunctival prostaglandin (PG) biosynthesis and polymorphonuclear leukocyte (PMN) release following corneal injury, *Invest. Ophthamol. Vis. Sci. (Suppl.)*, 228, 1980.

20. Kulkarni, P. S. and Srinivasan, B. D., Effect of topical and intraperitoneal indomethacin on the generation of PGE_2-like activity in rabbit conjunctiva and iris-ciliary body, *Exp. Eye Res.*, 33, 121, 1981.

21. Kulkarni, P. S., Bhattacherjee, P., and Eakins, K. E., Biosynthesis of prostaglandins, prostacyclin and thromboxane-A_2 from ^{14}C-arachidonic acid in rabbit ocular tissues, *Pharmacologist*, 20, 233, 1978.

22. Kulkarni, P. S., Fleisher, L., and Srinivasan, B. D., Comparison of arachidonic acid metabolism in ocular tissues of various species, *Curr. Eye Res.*, 3, 447, 1984.

23. Bhattacherjee, P., Kulkarni, P. S., and Eakins, K. E., Differential inflammatory effects of arachidonic acid on rabbit conjunctiva and iris: a possible role of lipoxygenase in the conjunctival response, in *Advances in Prostaglandin and Thromboxane Research*, Vol. 8, Samuelsson, B., Ramwell, P. W., and Paoletti, R., Eds., Raven Press, New York, 1980, 1727.

24. Bhattacherjee, P. and Phylactos, A., Increased prostaglandin synthetase activity in inflamed tissues of the rabbit eye, *Eur. J. Pharm.*, 44, 75, 1977.

25. Van Dorp, D. A., Jouvenaz, G. H., and Struijk, C. B., The biosynthesis of prostaglandin in pig eye iris, *Biochim. Biophys. Acta*, 137, 396, 1967.

26. Kulkarni, P. S. and Eakins, K. E., Generation of prostacyclin-like activity from prostaglandin endoperoxides by bovine ocular tissues, *Pharmacologist*, 19, 149, 1977.

27. Posner, J., Prostaglandin E_2 and the bovine sphincter pupillae, *Br. J. Pharmacol.*, 49, 415, 1973.

28. Kass, M. A. and Holmberg, N., Prostaglandin product synthesis by microsomes of inflamed rabbit ciliary body-iris, *Invest. Ophthalmol. Vis. Sci. (Suppl.)*, 220, 1980.

29. Engstrom, P., Dunham, E. W., and Cameron, J. D., Phenylephrine-stimulated prostaglandin release from rabbit iris-ciliary body in vitro, *Invest. Ophthalmol. Vis. Sci. (Suppl.)*, 20, 33, 1981.

30. Engstrom, P. and Dunham, E. W., Alpha-adrenergic stimulation of prostaglandin release from rabbit iris-ciliary body in vitro, *Invest. Ophthalmol. Vis. Sci.*, 22, 757, 1982.

31. Kass, M. A., Holmberg, N. J., and Smith, M. E., Prostaglandin and thromboxane synthesis by microsomes of inflamed rabbit ciliary body-iris, *Invest. Ophthalmol. Vis. Sci.*, 4, 442, 1981.

32. Kulkarni, P. S., Synthesis of cyclooxygenase products by human anterior uvea from cyclic prostaglandin endoperoxide (PGH_2), *Exp. Eye Res.*, 32, 197, 1981.

33. Kulkarni, P. S., Eakins, H. M. T., Saber, W. L., and Eakins, K. E., Microsomal preparations of normal bovine iris-ciliary body generate prostacyclin-like but not thromboxane-A_2-like activity, *Prostaglandins*, 14, 689, 1977.

34. Kulkarni, P. S. and Eakins, K. E., The enzymatic conversion of prostaglandin endoperoxide to thromboxane-A_2-like activity by human iris microsomes, *Prostaglandins*, 14, 601, 1977.

35. Beitch, B. R., Beitch, I., and Zadunaisky, J. A., Chloride transport activation by prostaglandins in the frog cornea, *Fed. Proc. Fed. Am. Soc. Exp. Biol.*, 37, 245, 1973.

36. Beitch, B. R., Beitch, I., and Zadunaisky, J. A., The stimulation of chloride transport by prostaglandins and their interaction with epinephrine, theophylline, and cyclic AMP in the corneal epithelium, *J. Membrane Biol.*, 19, 381, 1974.

37. Bentley, P. J. and McGahan, M. C., A pharmacological analysis of chloride transport across the amphibian cornea, *J. Physiol. (London)*, 325, 481, 1982.

38. Zadunaisky, J. A. and Lande, M. A., Active chloride transport and control of corneal tranparency, *Am. J. Physiol.*, 221, 1837, 1971.

39. Klyce, S. D., Neufeld, A. H., and Zadunaisky, J. A., The activation of chloride transport by epinephrine and D_β cyclic-AMP in the cornea of the rabbit, *Invest. Ophthalmol.*, 12, 127, 1973.
40. Maurice, D. M., The location of the fluid pump in the cornea, *J. Physiol. (London)*, 221, 43, 1972.
41. Paterson, C. A. and Eck, B. A., Influence of prostaglandins on cation movement in the lens, *Exp. Eye Res.*, 15, 767, 1973.
42. Srinivasan, B. D. and Kulkarni, P. S., The role of arachidonic acid metabolites in the mediation of the polymorphonuclear leukocyte response following corneal injury, *Invest. Ophthalmol. Vis. Sci.*, 19, 1087, 1980.
43. Srinivasan, B. D. and Kulkarni, P. S., Polymorphonuclear leukocyte response: inhibition following corneal epithelial denudation by steroidal and nonsteroidal anti-inflammatory agents, *Arch. Ophthalmol.*, 99, 1085, 1981.
44. Srinivasan, B. D. and Kulkarni, P. S., The effect of steroidal and non-steroidal anti-inflammatory agents on corneal re-epithelialization, *Invest. Ophthalmol. Vis. Sci.*, 20, 688, 1981.
45. Miller, D., Gruenberg, P., Miller, R., and Bergamini, M. V. W., Topical flurbiprofen or prednisolone. Effect on corneal wound healing, *Arch. Ophthalmol.*, 99, 681, 1981.
46. Mochizuki, M., Sawa, M., and Masuda, K., Topical indomethacin in intracapsular extraction of senile cataract, *Jpn. J. Ophthalmol.*, 21, 215, 1977.
47. Bito, L. Z., Srinivasan, B. D., Baroody, R. A., and Schubert, H., Noninvasive observations on eyes of cats after long-term maintenance of reduced intraocular pressure by topical application of prostaglandin E_2, *Invest. Ophthalmol. Vis. Sci.*, 24, 376, 1983.
48. Eakins, K. E., Whitelocke, R. A. F., Perkins, E. S., Bennett, A., and Unger, W. G., Release of prostaglandins in ocular inflammation in the rabbit, *Nature (London) New Biol.*, 239, 248, 1972.
49. Williams, R. N., Bhattacherjee, P., and Eakins, K. E., Biosynthesis of lipoxygenase products by ocular tissues, *Exp. Eye Res.*, 36, 397, 1983.
50. Guivernau, M., Terragno, A., Dunn, M. W., and Terragno, N. A., Estrogens induce lipoxygenase derivative formation in rabbit lens, *Invest. Ophthalmol. Vis. Sci.*, 23, 214, 1982.
51. Zelenka, P. S. and Beebe, D. C., Phospholipid methylation and arachidonic acid metabolism during in vitro lens fiber cell differentiation, *Invest. Ophthalmol. Vis. Sci. (Suppl.)*, 22, 152, 1982.
52. Guivernau, M., Dunn, M., Terragno, A., and Terragno, N. A., Arachidonic acid metabolism in normal and deepithelializated cornea, *Invest. Ophthalmol. Vis. Sci. (Suppl.)*, 20, 159, 1981.
53. Waitzman, M. B., Kuck, J. F. R., Jr., and Woods, W. D., Effect of prostaglandins (PGs) on galactose uptake by lenses and on adenylate cyclase of isolated lens cells, *Fed. Proc. Fed. Am. Soc. Exp. Biol.*, 31, 384, 1972.
54. Von Sallman, L. and Grimes, P., Inhibition of cell division in rat lenses by prostaglandin E, *Invest. Ophthalmol.*, 15, 27, 1976.
55. Paterson, C. A. and Eck, B. A., Prostaglandin E_1 and the ocular lens, *Ophthalmic Res.*, 2, 246, 1971.
56. Eakins, K. E., Release of prostaglandin-like activity in ocular inflammation, in *Prostaglandins and cAMP*, Kahn, R. H. and Lands, W. E., Eds., Academic Press, New York, 1973, 211.
57. Lipton, S. A., Rasmussen, H., and Dowling, J. E., Electrical and adaptive properties of rod photoreceptors in *Bufo marinus*. II. Effects of cyclic nucleotides and prostaglandins, *J. Gen. Physiol.*, 70, 771, 1977.
58. Christ, E. J. and van Dorp, D. A., Comparative aspects of prostaglandin biosynthesis in animal tissues, *Biochim. Biophys. Acta*, 270, 537, 1972.
59. Wolfe, L. S., Coceani, F., and Pace-Asciak, C., Brain prostaglandins and studies of the action of prostaglandins on the isolated rat stomach, in *Prostaglandins, Nobel Symposium 2*, Bergstrom, S. and Samuelsson, B., Eds., Almqvist & Wiksell, Stockholm, 1967, 265.
60. Siminoff, R. and Bito, L. Z., The effects of prostaglandins and arachidonic acid on the electroretinogram: evidence for functional cyclooxygenase activity in the retina, *Curr. Eye Res.*, 1, 635, 1982.
61. Bito, L. Z. and Wallenstein, M. C., Transport of prostaglandins across the blood-brain and blood-aqueous barriers and the physiological significance of these absorptive transport processes, *Exp. Eye Res. (Suppl.)*, 25, 229, 1977.
62. Wallenstein, M. C. and Bito, L. Z., The effects of intravitreally injected prostaglandin E_1 on retinal function and their enhancement by a prostaglandin-transport inhibitor, *Invest. Ophthalmol. Vis. Sci.*, 17, 795, 1978.
63. Gustafsson, L. E., Studies on modulation of transmitter release and effector responsiveness in autonomic cholinergic neurotransmission, *Acta Physiol. Scand. (Suppl.)*, 489, 1, 1980.
64. Hedqvist, P., Gustafsson, L., Hjendahl., P., and Svanborg, K., Aspects of prostaglandin action on autonomic neuroeffector transmission, in *Advances in Prostaglandin and Thromboxane Research*, Vol. 8, Samuelsson, B., Ramwell, P. W., and Paoletti, R., Eds., Raven Press, New York, 1980, 1245.
65. Bito, L. Z. and DeRousseau, C. J., Transport functions of the blood-retinal barrier system and the micro-environment of the retina, in *The Blood-Retinal Barriers*, Cunha-Vaz, J. G., Ed., Plenum Press, New York, 1980, 133.

66. Tennant, J. L., Is cystoid macular edema reversible by oral indocin, yes or no? in *Current Concepts in Cataract Surgery; Selected Proceedings of the Fourth Biennial Cataract Surgical Congress,* Emery, J. M. and Paton, D., Eds., C. V. Mosby, St. Louis, 1976.

67. Bito, L. Z., Accumulation and apparent active transport of prostaglandins by some rabbit tissues in vitro, *J. Physiol. (London),* 221, 371, 1972.

68. Bito, L. Z., Comparative study of concentrative prostaglandin accumulation by various tissues of mammals and marine vertebrates and invertebrates, *Comp. Biochem. Physiol.,* 43A, 65, 1972.

69. Bito, L. Z. and Salvador, E. V., Intraocular fluid dynamics. III. The site and mechanism of prostaglandin transfer across the blood intraocular fluid barriers, *Exp. Eye Res.,* 14, 233, 1972.

70. Bito, L. Z. and Baroody, R. A., Impermeability of rabbit erythrocytes to prostaglandins, *Am. J. Physiol.,* 229, 1580, 1975.

71. Bito, L. Z., Saturable, energy-dependent, transmembrane transport of prostaglandins against concentration gradients, *Nature (London),* 256, 134, 1975.

72. Bito, L. Z., Davson, H., and Hollingsworth, J. R., Facilitated transport of prostaglandins across the blood-cerebrospinal fluid and blood-brain barriers, *J. Physiol. (London),* 256, 273, 1976.

73. Bito, L. Z., Eicosanoid transport systems: their mechanism, physiological roles and inhibitors, in *CRC Handbook of the PGs and Related Lipids,* Willis, A. L., Ed., CRC Press, Boca Raton, Fla., in press.

74. Eakins, K. E., Atwal, M., and Bhattacherjee, P., Inactivation of prostaglandin E_1 by ocular tissues in vitro, *Exp. Eye Res.,* 19, 141, 1974.

75. Bito, L. Z. and Baroody, R., Concentrative accumulation of ^{3}H-prostaglandins by some rabbit tissues in vitro: the chemical nature of the accumulated ^{3}H-labelled substances, *Prostaglandins,* 7, 131, 1974.

76. Bito, L. Z., Davson, H., and Salvador, E. V., Inhibition of in vitro concentrative prostaglandin accumulation by prostaglandins, prostglandin analogues and by some inhibitors of organic anion transport, *J. Physiol. (London),* 256, 1976.

77. DiBenedetto, F. E. and Bito, L. Z., The kinetics and energy dependence of prostaglandin transport processes. I. In vitro studies on the rate of $PGF_{2\alpha}$ accumulation by the rabbit anterior uvea, *Exp. Eye Res.,* 30, 175, 1980.

78. Bito, L. Z., The effects of experimental uveitis on anterior uveal prostaglandin transport and aqueous humor composition, *Invest. Ophthalmol.,* 13, 959, 1974.

79. Whitelocke, R. A. F. and Eakins, K. E., Vascular changes in the anterior uvea of the rabbit produced by prostaglandins, *Arch. Ophthalmol.,* 89, 495, 1973.

80. Whitelocke, R. A. F., Eakins, K. E., and Bennett, A., Acute anterior uveitis and prostaglandins, *Proc. R. Soc. Med.,* 5, 429, 1973.

81. Segawa, K. and Smelser, G. K., Electron microscopy of experimental uveitis, *Invest. Ophthalmol.,* 8, 497, 1969.

82. Bito, L. Z., The physiology and pathophysiology of intraocular fluids, *Exp. Eye Res. (Suppl.),* 25, 273, 1977.

83. Camras, C. B. and Bito, L. Z., The pathophysiological effects of nitrogen mustard on the rabbit eye. I. The biphasic intraocular pressure response and the role of prostaglandins, *Exp. Eye Res.,* 30, 41, 1980.

84. Camras, C. B. and Bito, L. Z., The pathophysiological effects of nitrogen mustard on the rabbit eye. II. The inhibition of the initial hypertensive phase by capsaicin and the apparent role of substance P, *Invest. Ophthalmol. Vis. Sci.,* 19, 423, 1980.

85. Eakins, K. E., Whitelocke, R. A. F., Perkins, E. S., Bennett, A., and Unger, W. G., Release of prostaglandins into the aqueous humour in experimental immunogenic uveitis, *Exp. Eye Res.,* 14, 174, 1972.

86. Perkins, E. S., Unger, W. G., and Bass, M., The role of prostaglandin in the ocular responses to laser irradiation of the iris, *Exp. Eye Res.,* 17, 394, 1973.

87. Miller, J. D., Eakins, K. E., and Atwal, M., The release of PGE_2-like activity into aqueous humor after paracentesis and its prevention by aspirin, *Invest. Ophthalmol.,* 12, 939, 1973.

88. Jaffe, B. M., Podos, S. M., and Becker, B., Indomethacin blocks arachidonic acid-associated elevation of aqueous humor prostaglandin E, *Invest. Ophthalmol.,* 12, 621, 1973.

89. Cole, D. F. and Unger, W. G., The involvement of prostaglandin in ocular trauma, *Exp. Eye Res.,* 17, 395, 1973.

90. Cole, D. F. and Unger, W. G., Prostaglandins as mediators for the responses of the eye to trauma, *Exp. Eye Res.,* 17, 357, 1973.

91. Unger, W. G., Perkins, E. S., and Bass, M. S., The response of the rabbit eye to laser irradiation of the iris, *Exp. Eye Res.,* 19, 367, 1974.

92. Unger, W. G., Cole, D. F., and Hammond, B., Disruption of the blood-aqueous barrier following paracentesis in the rabbit, *Exp. Eye Res.,* 20, 255, 1975.

93. Paterson, C. A. and Pfister, R. R., Prostaglandin-like activity in the aqueous humor following alkali burns, *Invest. Ophthalmol.,* 14, 177, 1975.

94. Paterson, C. A., Paterson, E. F., and Eakins, K. E., The effects of experimental ocular acid burns, *Invest. Ophthalmol. Vis. Sci. (Suppl.)*, 163, 1978.

95. Floman, N. and Zor, U., Mechanism of steroid action in ocular inflammation: inhibition of prostaglandin production, *Invest. Ophthalmol. Vis. Sci.*, 16, 69, 1977.

96. Unger, W. G. and Bass, M. S., Prostaglandin and nerve-mediated response of the rabbit eye to argon laser irradiation of the iris, *Ophthalmologica*, 175, 153, 1977.

97. Masuda, K., Izawa, Y., and Mishima, S., Breakdown of the blood: aqueous barrier and prostaglandins, *Bibl. Anat.*, 16, 99, 1977.

98. Bhattacherjee, P., Stimulation of prostaglandin synthetase activity in inflamed ocular tissue of the rabbit, *Exp. Eye Res.*, 24, 215, 1977.

99. Unger, W. G., Effect of unilateral sympathectomy on the ocular response of the rabbit eye to laser irradiation of the iris, *Trans. Ophthalmol. Soc. U. K.*, 97, 674, 1977.

100. Unger, W. G., Cole, D. F., and Bass, M. S., Prostaglandin and neurogenically mediated ocular response to laser irradiation of the rabbit iris, *Exp. Eye Res.*, 25, 209, 1977.

101. Rahi, A., Bhattacherjee, P., and Misra, R., Release of prostaglandins in experimental immune-complex endophthalmitis and phacoallergic uveitis, *Br. J. Ophthalmol.*, 62, 105, 1978.

102. Bhattacherjee, P. and Butler, J. M., Responses of the sympathetically denervated rabbit eye to intravitreal or intravenous injection of Shigella endotoxin, *Exp. Eye Res.*, 28, 611, 1979.

103. Unger, W. G., Prostaglandin mediated inflammatory changes induced by α-adrenoceptor stimulation in the sympathectomised rabbit eye, *Albrecht von Graefes Arch. Klin. Exp. Ophthalmol.*, 211, 289, 1979.

104. Paterson, C. A., Eakins, K. E., Paterson, E., Jenkins, R. M., II, and Ishikawa, R., The ocular hypertensive response following experimental acid burns in the rabbit eye, *Invest. Ophthalmol. Vis. Sci.*, 18, 67, 1979.

105. Yamauchi, H., Iso, T., Iwao, J., and Iwata, H., The role of prostaglandins in experimental ocular inflammations, *Agents Actions*, 9, 280, 1979.

106. Unger, W. G., Butler, J. M., and Morsi, E. E. A., Shigella endotoxin-induced ocular inflammation in the normal and sensory denervated rabbit eye, *Albrecht von Graefes Arch. Klin. Exp. Ophthalmol.*, 214, 39, 1980.

107. Unger, W. G., Butler, J. M., and Cole, D. F., Prostaglandin and increased sensitivity of the sympathetically denervated rabbit eye to laser-induced irritation of the iris, *Exp. Eye Res.*, 32, 699, 1981.

108. Rosenbaum, J. T., Perez, H. D., Goldyne, M. E., Howes, E. L., Webster, R. O., and Goldstein, I. M., Endotoxin tolerance inhibits endotoxin induced increases in levels of prostaglandin E$_2$ and chemotactic activity in the rabbit eye, *Arthritis Rheum. (Suppl.)*, 25, S99, 1982.

109. Eakins, K. E., Whitelocke, R. A. F., Bennett, A., and Martenet, A. C., Prostaglandin-like activity in ocular inflammation, *Br. Med. J.*, 3, 452, 1972.

110. Masuda, K., Izawa, Y., and Mishima, S., Prostaglandins and uveitis: a preliminary report, *Jpn. J. Ophthalmol.*, 17, 166, 1973.

111. Masuda, K., Izawa, Y., and Mishima, S., Prostaglandins and glaucomatocyclitic crisis, *Jpn. J. Ophthalmol.*, 19, 368, 1975.

112. Kremer, M., Baikoff, G., and Charbonnel, B., The release of prostaglandins in human aqueous humor following intraocular surgery. Effect of indomethacin, *Prostaglandins*, 23, 695, 1982.

113. Tolman, E. L., Partridge, R., Myers, T. O., and Birnbaum, J. E., Inhibition of prostaglandin-mediated ocular inflammatory responses by 4-biphenyl-acetic acid, *Invest. Ophthalmol.*, 15, 1005, 1976.

114. Waitzman, M. B. and King, C. D., Prostaglandin influences on intraocular pressure and pupil size, *Am. J. Physiol.*, 212, 329, 1967.

115. Beitch, B. R. and Eakins, K. E., The actions of various prostaglandins on intraocular pressure, *Fed. Proc. Fed. Am. Soc. Exp. Biol.*, 28, 678, 1969.

116. Beitch, B. R. and Eakins, K. E., The effects of prostaglandins on the intraocular pressure of the rabbit, *Br. J. Pharmacol.*, 37, 158, 1969.

117. Bethel, R. A. and Eakins, K. E., Antagonism by polyphloretin phosphate of the intraocular pressure rise induced by prostaglandin and formaldehyde in the rabbit eye, *Fed. Proc. Fed. Am. Soc. Exp. Biol.*, 30, 626, 1971.

118. Starr, M. S., Further studies on the effect of prostaglandin on intraocular pressure in the rabbit, *Exp. Eye Res.*, 11, 170, 1971.

119. Bethel, R. A. and Eakins, K. E., The mechanism of the antagonism of experimentally induced ocular hypertension by polyphloretin phosphate, *Exp. Eye Res.*, 13, 83, 1971.

120. Kass, M. A., Podos, S. M., Moses, R. A., and Becker, B., Prostaglandin E$_1$ and aqueous humor dynamics, *Invest. Ophthalmol.*, 11, 1022, 1972.

121. Chiang, T. S. and Thomas, R. P., Consensual ocular hypertensive response to prostaglandin, *Invest. Ophthalmol.*, 11, 169, 1972.

122. Chiang, T. S., Effects of epinephrine and progesterone on the ocular hypertensive response to intravenous infusion of prostaglandin A$_2$, *Prostaglandins*, 4, 415, 1973.

123. Neufeld, A. H. and Sears, M. L., The site of action of prostaglandin E_2 on the disruption of the blood-aqueous barrier in the rabbit eye, *Exp. Eye Res.*, 17, 445, 1973.

124. Whitelocke, R. A. F. and Eakins, K. E., A comparison of some derivatives of phloretin as prostaglandin antagonists, *Exp. Eye Res.*, 17, 395, 1973.

125. Zink, H. A., Podos, S. M., and Becker, B., Inhibition by imidazole of the increase in intraocular pressure induced by topical prostaglandin E, *Nature (London) New Biol.*, 245, 21, 1973.

126. Podos, S. M., Becker, B., and Kass, M. A., Prostaglandin synthesis, inhibition, and intraocular pressure, *Invest. Ophthalmol.*, 12, 426, 1973.

127. Podos, S. M., Becker, B., and Kass, M. A., Indomethacin blocks arachidonic acid-induced elevation of intraocular pressure, *Prostaglandins*, 3, 7, 1973.

128. Takats, S., Jobst, C., and Szilvassy, H., Effect of prostaglandin E_2 on aqueous humor flow in the rabbit eye, *Albrecht von Graefes Arch. Klin. Exp. Ophthalmol.*, 190, 221, 1974.

129. Green, K. and Podos, S. M., Antagonism of arachidonic acid-induced ocular effects by Δ^1-tetrahydrocannabinol, *Invest. Ophthalmol.*, 13, 422, 1974.

130. Cole, D. F., The site of breakdown of the blood-aqueous barrier under the influence of vaso-dilator drugs, *Exp. Eye Res.*, 19, 591, 1971.

131. Green, K. and Kim, K., Pattern of ocular response to topical and systemic prostaglandin, *Invest. Ophthalmol.*, 14, 36, 1975.

132. Conquet, P., Plazonnet, B., and Le Douarec, J. C., Arachidonic acid-induced elevation of intraocular pressure and anti-inflammatory agents, *Invest. Ophthalmol.*, 14, 772, 1975.

133. Butler, J. M. and Hammond, B., Neurogenic responses of the eye to injury. Effect of sensory denervation on the response of the rabbit eye to bradykinin and prostaglandin E_1, *Trans. Ophthalmol. Soc. U.K.*, 97, 668, 1977.

134. Bengtsson, E., The effect of theophylline on the breakdown of the blood-aqueous barrier in the rabbit eye, *Invest Ophthalmol. Vis. Sci.*, 16, 636, 1977.

135. Podos, S. M., Effect of dipyridamole on prostaglandin-induced ocular hypertension in rabbits, *Invest. Ophthalmol. Vis. Sci.*, 18, 646, 1979.

136. Masunaga, J., Effects of prostaglandin on the blood-ocular barriers. II. Effects on the blood-retinal barrier, *Acta Soc. Ophthalmol. Jpn.*, 84, 1746, 1980.

137. Unger, W. G. and Grierson, I., Morphologic changes in the rabbit iridic processes following noxious stimulation of the eye, *Ophthalmic Res.*, 12, 134, 1980.

138. Masunaga, J., Effects of prostaglandin on the blood-ocular barriers. I. Effects on the blood-aqueous barrier, *Acta Soc. Ophthalmol. Jpn.*, 84, 427, 1980.

139. Kulkarni, P. S. and Srinivasan, B. D., Comparative effects of intravitreal cyclooxygenase products on intraocular inflammation, *Invest. Ophthalmol. Vis. Sci. (Suppl.)*, 20, 32, 1981.

140. Bhattacherjee, P., Hammond, B., Salmon, J., Stepney, R., and Eakins, K. E., Chemotactic response to some arachidonic acid lipoxygenase products in the rabbit eye, *Eur. J. Pharmacol.*, 73, 21, 1981.

141. Mandahl, A. and Bill, A., Ocular responses to antidromic trigeminal stimulation, intracameral prostaglandin E_1 and E_2, capsaicin and substance P, *Acta Physiol. Scand.*, 112, 331, 1981.

142. Kulkarni, P. S. and Srinivasan, B. D., The effect of intravitreal and topical prostaglandins on intraocular inflammation, *Invest. Ophthalmol. Vis. Sci.*, 23, 383, 1982.

143. Eakins, K. E., Increased intraocular pressure produced by prostaglandins E_1 and E_2 in the cat eye, *Exp. Eye Res.*, 10, 87, 1970.

144. Van Alphen, G. W. H. M. and Wilhelm, P., Effect of prostaglandins on the blood-aqueous barrier of the perfused cat eye, *Invest. Ophthalmol. Vis. Sci.*, 17, 60, 1978.

145. Kelly, R. G. M. and Starr, M. S., Effects of prostaglandins and a prostaglandin antagonist on intraocular pressure and protein in the monkey eye, *Can. J. Ophthalmol.*, 6, 205, 1971.

146. Stetz, D. E. and Bito, L. Z., The insensitivity of the chicken eye to the inflammatory effects of X-rays in contrast to its sensitivity to other inflammatory agents, *Invest. Ophthalmol. Vis. Sci.*, 17, 412, 1978.

147. Cole, D. F., Formaldehyde-induced ocular hypertension: the effects of polyphloretin phosphate and (+)-catechin, *Exp. Eye Res.*, 19, 533, 1974.

148. Chavis, R. M., Vygantas, C. M., and Vygantas, A., Experimental inhibition of prostaglandin-like inflammatory response after cryotherapy, *Am. J. Ophthalmol.*, 82, 310, 1976.

149. Howes, E. L., Jr. and McKay, D. G., The effects of aspirin and indomethacin on the ocular response to circulating bacterial endotoxin in the rabbit, *Invest. Ophthalmol.*, 15, 648, 1976.

150. Bengtsson, E., The effect of polyphloretin phosphate on the aqueous flare reponse to α-melanocyte stimulating hormone, *Acta Ophthalmol.*, 55, 976, 1977.

151. Perkins, E. S., Prostaglandins and ocular trauma, *Adv. Ophthalmol.*, 34, 149, 1977.

152. Kottow, M. H. and Seligman, L. J., Consensual reactions to anterior chamber paracentesis in the rabbit, *Am. J. Ophthalmol.*, 85, 392, 1978.

153. Al-Ghadyan, A., Mead, A., and Sears, M., Increased pressure after paracentesis of the rabbit eye is completely accounted for by prostaglandin synthesis and release plus pupillary block, *Invest. Ophthalmol. Vis. Sci.*, 18, 361, 1979.

154. Camras, C. B. and Bito, L. Z., Nitrogen mustard-induced ocular inflammation in the rabbit eye: the biphasic IOP response and the role of prostaglandins, *Invest. Ophthalmol. Vis. Sci. (Suppl.)*, 14, 1979.

155. Haddad, R., Grabner, G., and Braun, F., Die Blockade sekundarer Drucksteigerungen nach Cyclokryocoagulation, *Albrecht von Graefes Arch. Klin Exp. Ophthalmol.*, 210, 225, 1979.

156. Haddad, R., Grabner, G., and Braun, F., Cyclocryokoagulation. Sequelae of induced alterations and effect of a prostaglandin-inhibitor on the breakdown of the blood-aqueous barrier, *Albrecht von Graefes Arch. Klin. Exp. Ophthalmol.*, 214, 129, 1980.

157. Kulkarni, P. S., Bhattacherjee, P., Eakins, K. E., and Srinivasan, B. D., Anti-inflammatory effects of betamethasone phosphate, dexamethasone phosphate and indomethacin on rabbit ocular inflammation induced by bovine serum albumin, *Curr. Eye Res.*, 1, 43, 1981.

158. Haddad, R., Grabner, G., Strasser, G., and Braun, F., Mediation of the ocular response to cyclocryocoagulation, *Albrecht von Graefes Arch. Klin. Exp. Ophthalmol.*, 216, 219, 1981.

159. Oosterhuis, J. A., van Haeringen, N. J., Glasius, E., van Delft, J. L., and Swart-van den Berg, M., The effect of indomethacin on the anterior segment of the eye after paracentesis, *Doc. Ophthalmol.*, 50, 303, 1981.

160. Bito, L. Z. and Klein, E. M., The role of the arachidonic acid cascade in the species-specific X-ray-induced inflammation of the rabbit eye, *Invest. Ophthalmol. Vis. Sci.*, 22, 579, 1982.

161. Hillman, J. S., Frank, G. J., and Kheskani, M. B., Flurbiprofen and human intraocular inflammation, in *Advances in Prostaglandin and Thromboxane Research*, Vol. 8, Samuelsson, B., Ramwell, P. W., and Paoletti, R., Eds., Raven Press, New York, 1980, 1723.

162. Spinelli, H. M. and Krohn, D. L., Inhibition of prostaglandin-induced iritis. Topical indoxole vs. indomethacin therapy, *Arch. Ophthalmol.*, 98, 1106, 1980.

163. Klein, E. M. and Bito, L. Z., Species variations in the pathophysiologic responses of vertebrate eyes to a chemical irritant, nitrogen mustard, *Invest. Ophthalmol. Vis. Sci.*, 24, 184, 1983.

164. Bito, L. Z., Prostaglandins, other eicosanoids, and their derivatives as potential antiglaucoma agents, in *Applied Pharmacology in the Medical Treatment of the Glaucomas*, Drance, S. M. and Neufeld, A. H., Eds., Grune & Stratton, New York, 1984.

165. Mandahl, A. and Bill, A., Effects of substance P, PGE_2, and capsaicin on the pupillary sphincter, modification by tetrodotoxin, *Acta Physiol. Scand.*, 109, 26A, 1980.

166. Bhattacherjee, P., Release of prostaglandin-like substances by Shigella endotoxin and its inhibition by non-steroidal anti-inflammatory compounds, *Br. J. Pharmacol.*, 54, 489, 1975.

167. Macri, F. J. and van Alphen, G. W. H. M., The effects of prostaglandins on aqueous humor dynamics, *Prostaglandins*, 20, 179, 1980.

168. Bito, L. Z., Draga, A., Blanco, J., and Camras, C. B., Long-term maintenance of reduced intraocular pressure by daily or twice daily topical application of prostaglandins to cat or rhesus monkey eyes, *Invest. Ophthamol. Vis. Sci.*, 24, 312, 1983.

169. Stern, F. A. and Bito, L. Z., Comparison of the hypotensive and other ocular effects of prostaglandins E_2 and $F_{2\alpha}$ on cat and rhesus monkey eyes, *Invest. Ophthalmol. Vis. Sci.*, 22, 588, 1982.

170. Casey, W. J., The effect of prostaglandin E_2 on the rhesus monkey pupil, *Prostaglandins*, 6, 243, 1974.

171. Camras, C. B. and Bito, L. Z., Reduction of intraocular pressure in normal and glaucomatous primate (*Aotus trivirgatus*) eyes by topically applied prostaglandin $F_{2\alpha}$, *Curr. Eye Res.*, 1, 205, 1981.

172. Zajacz, M., Torok, M., and Mocsary, P., Effect on human eye of prostaglandin and a prostaglandin analogue used to induce abortion, *IRCS Med. Sci.*, 4, 316, 1976.

173. Wizemann, A., Ebinger, G., Krey, H., and Wizemann, V., Biphasic action of prostacyclin on intraocular pressure, *Ophthalmologica*, 184, 204, 1982.

174. Crawford, C. G., van Alphen, G. W. H. M., Cook, H. W., and Lands, W. E. M., The effect of precursors, products and product analogs of prostaglandin cyclooxygenase upon iris sphincter muscle, *Life Sci.*, 23, 1255, 1978.

175. Van Alphen, G. W. H. M. and Angel, M. A., Activity of prostaglandin E, F, A and B on sphincter, dilator and ciliary muscle preparation of the cat eye, *Prostaglandins*, 9, 157, 1975.

176. Van Alphen, G. W. H. M., Wilhelm, P. B., and Eisenfeld, P. W., The effect of prostaglandins on the isolated internal muscles of the mamalian eye, including man, *Doc. Ophthalmol.*, 42, 397, 1977.

177. Wilhelm, P. B. and van Alphen, G. W. H. M., Potentiation of PG effects on the intraocular muscles of the cat by inhibition of PG synthesis, *Doc. Ophthalmol.*, 42, 417, 1977.

178. Zhang, S. Q., Butler, J. M., Ohara, K., and Cole, D. F., Sensory neural mechanisms in contraction of the isolated sphincter pupillae: the role for substance P and the effects of sensory denervation on the responses to miotics, *Exp. Eye Res.*, 35, 43, 1982.

179. Bito, L. Z., Unpublished data, 1982.

180. Bito, L. Z., Baroody, R. A., Backerman, A., The mechanism of peptidergic miosis. I. The structural basis of miotic potency among biologically active polypeptides, *Curr. Eye Res.*, 1, 559, 1982.

181. Bito, L. Z., Nichols, R. R., and Baroody, R. A., A comparison of the miotic and inflammatory effects of biologically active polypeptides and prostaglandin E₂ on the rabbit eye, *Exp. Eye Res.*, 34, 325, 1982.

182. Camras, C. B., Bito, L. Z., and Eakins, K. E., Reduction of intraocular pressure by prostaglandins applied topically to the rabbit eye, *Invest. Ophthalmol. Vis. Sci. (Suppl.)*, 57, 1977.

183. Bito, L. Z. and Klein, E. M., The unique sensitivity of the rabbit eye to X-ray-induced ocular inflammation, *Exp. Eye Res.*, 33, 403, 1981.

184. Bito, L. Z., Comparison of the ocular hypotensive efficacy of eicosanoids and related compounds, *Exp. Eye Res.*, 38, 181, 1984.

185. Casey, W. J., Prostaglandin E₂ and aqueous humor dynamics in the rhesus monkey eye, *Prostaglandins*, 8, 327, 1974.

186. Bito, L. Z., Merritt, S. Q., and DeRousseau, C. J., Intraocular pressure of rhesus monkeys *(Macaca mulatta)*, *Invest. Ophthalmol. Vis. Sci.*, 18, 785, 1979.

187. Bito, L. Z., Baroody, R. A., and Reitz, M. E., Dependence of pulmonary prostaglandin metabolism on carrier-mediated transport processes, *Am. J. Physiol.*, 232, E382, 1977.

188. Bito, L. Z. and Baroody, R. A., Comparison of renal prostaglandin and p-aminohippuric acid transport processes, *Am. J. Physiol.*, 234, F80, 1978.

189. Kaufman, P. L. and Barany, E. H., Loss of acute pilocarpine effect on outflow facility following surgical disinsertion and retrodisplacement of the ciliary muscle from the scleral spur in the cynomolgus monkey, *Invest. Ophthalmol.*, 15, 793, 1976.

190. Weinreb, R. N., Mitchell, M., and Polansky, J., Prostaglandin synthesis by human trabecular cells. Inhibitory effect of dexamethasone, *Invest. Ophthalmol. Vis. Sci. (Suppl.)*, 24, 136, 1983.

191. Polansky, J. R., Bloom, E., Weinreb, R. N., and Alvarado, J. A., Evaluation of hormone responses in cultured human trabecular cells, *Invest. Ophthalmol. Vis. Sci. (Suppl.)*, 273, 1980.

192. Bito, L. Z., Species differences in the responses of the eye to irritation and trauma: A hypothesis of divergence in ocular defense mechanisms, and the choice of experimental animals for eye research, *Exp. Eye Res.*, 39, 807, 1984.

Chapter 19

SCHIZOPHRENIA

David F. Horrobin

TABLE OF CONTENTS

I. INTRODUCTION

When considering the possibility that a group of substances such as the prostaglandins (PGs) may play a role in a clinical syndrome (e.g., schizophrenia), the following questions should be raised:

1.   Is what is known about schizophrenia and about the basic biochemistry and physiology of the PGs consistent with the possibility that an abnormality of PG metabolism might be involved in the disease?
2.   Is there any indirect evidence from the clinical spectrum of the disease that points to the possibility that PGs may be involved in schizophrenia?
3.   Is there any direct evidence of the participation of a PG abnormality in schizophrenia?
4.   What are the current specific hypotheses which can be proposed with regard to PGs and schizophrenia?

II. BACKGROUND

A. Schizophrenia

Schizophrenia is the most serious psychiatric illness and in the Western world schizophrenics occupy about one third of all hospital beds. Opinion has long been deeply divided as to whether schizophrenia has a psychological cause rooted in environmental experience or, on the other hand, a biological cause rooted in faulty biochemistry. Most authorities now seem convinced that the substrate on which schizophrenia develops is biological, but that when, how, and even whether that substrate is expressed as psychiatric illness depends on social and psychological factors. The most persuasive evidence is genetic.[1] All major studies have observed an increased susceptibility to schizophrenia among the close relatives of schizophrenics. Children of schizophrenics adopted at birth into nonschizophrenic families are much more likely to develop schizophrenia than are children of nonschizophrenics. Identical twin studies indicate a high rate of concordance for schizophrenia even when the twins are raised apart, but the concordance is by no means 100%, indicating a substantial effect of environmental factors.

Therefore, it seems that there is a constitutional susceptibility to schizophrenia. If, as most believe, all genes express themselves in biochemical terms, then schizophrenia must have biochemical roots. Thus, it is not inherently improbable that PGs may have a role to play.

B. Prostaglandins

The PGs are derived from dietary essential fatty acids (EFA) and it would be inappropriate to discuss the PGs without outlining the vital roles of their precursors. The metabolic pathways are shown in outline in Figure 1. Dihomogammalinolenic acid (DGLA) is the precursor for 1 series PGs, arachidonic acid (AA) for the 2 series PGs, and eicosapentaenoic acid (EPA) for the 3 series PGs. The brain is exceptionally rich in EFA, with the fatty acid fractions of important phospholipids containing 30 to 60% of EFA.[2] There are large amounts of AA and much smaller, though still substantial amounts of DGLA. EPA does not appear to be present except in trace amounts, but the longer chain EFA derived from EPA, notably 22:6n-3, are present in abundance. The EFA, being highly unsaturated, are key determinants of membrane fluidity and hence of the functioning of such important nervous system entities as receptors. While the EFA function as PG precursors is undoubtedly important in the brain, it is highly unlikely to be the only EFA function. EFA, quite independently of their roles as PG precursors, are likely to play important parts in brain physiology and biochemistry.

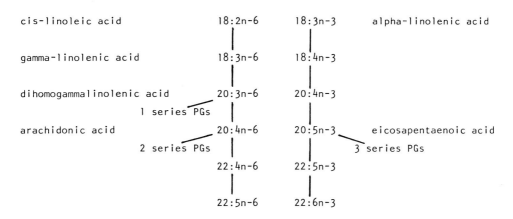

FIGURE 1. Outline of the pathways of PG formation from the essential fatty acids of the n-6 and n-3 series. The first number (18,20,22) refers to the number of carbon atoms in the molecule; the second (2,3,4,5,6) refers to the number of double bonds interrupting the carbon chain; the third (n-3, n-6) refers to the position of the first double bond from the methyl end of the molecule.

The major EFA in the Western diet is linoleic acid, but there are substantial amounts of arachidonic acid, notably in meat and dairy products. The n-3 fatty acids are present in much smaller amounts in the usual Western diet. Alpha-linolenic acid is present in moderate quantities in some more "primitive" diets, while EPA and 22:6n-3 are present in abundance in marine oily fish. Fatty acids readily cross the blood-brain barrier,[3-5] and changes in the dietary intake of EFA produce surprisingly rapid changes in the rates of PG formation in the brain.[6] This is true even though total brain EFA levels may change little, indicating that brain PG formation may depend on as yet unidentified pools of EFA precursors, which are in close equilibrium with dietary EFA intake. There is therefore the possibility that different diets may have substantial effects on the rates of PG formation in the brain.

PG can be produced in large amounts by the brain and are present in cerebrospinal fluid (CSF).[4,5,7] Although most attention has been paid to PGs of the 2 series, 1 series PGs are also present in amounts more than sufficient to exert physiological effects.[6]

Many experiments have shown that PGs can modulate nerve conduction, release of neurotransmitters, and post-synaptic actions of transmitters. PGE_1 had a biphasic effect on the speed and amplitude of action potentials in isolated neurons; low concentrations enhanced transmission whereas high concentrations inhibited it.[8] Such "bell-shaped" dose-response curves are characteristic of many PG actions, with the result that it is impossible to say that a particular PG has this or that effect. The PGs may have quite different effects depending on the concentration and all too few experiments have systematically tested a wide variety of doses. PGs have complex effects on neurotransmitter release, which seem to differ with the PG, the concentration, and the tissue.[9-11] PGs interact with neurotransmitters in many different tissues in many different ways to modulate postsynaptic transmitter actions.[12-15] Thus, there is ample evidence that PGs have effects on fundamental neurophysiology, which are compatible with their also having effects on behavior. Horton[16,17] was the first to show that PGs do, in fact, have profound effects on the behavior of animals, and this observation has been confirmed by others.[18-20]

Conversely there is also an abundance of evidence that neurotransmitters and neuromodulating drugs can regulate PG synthesis and actions. This is true of biogenic amines,[21] opioids,[22,23] melatonin,[24] and various psychotropic drugs.[25] While drugs known to inhibit PG synthesis in other tissues can have similar effects on the brain, extraordinarily high doses are required.[26] It is therefore unlikely that the doses of non-steroidal anti-inflammatory (NSAI) drugs used in clinical practice will have any major effect on brain PG synthesis. It is often not appreciated that monoamine oxidase inhibitors are as potent in their inhibition of PG synthesis as of oxidase function. It is possible that the monoamine oxidase inhibitors may have more specific and potent actions on brain PGs than do aspirin and drugs related to it.[27,28]

In view of the current widespread view that schizophrenia is a disorder of dopamine metabolism or action, interactions between PGs and dopamine are of particular interest. PGE_2 and analogues in animal models had anti-dopaminergic effects similar to the atypical antipsychotic clozapine, rather than like those of the conventional neuroleptic drugs.[12] Inhibition of PG synthesis significantly decreased the effect of the dopamine-blocking agent, metaclopramide, on prolactin secretion.[13] This suggests that a cyclooxygenase product modulates the effects of antipsychotic drugs on prolactin, an action which is believed to closely mirror the effects of these drugs on schizophrenic behavior. PGE_1 and dopamine had antagonistic effects on cyclic AMP (cAMP) in neuroblastoma cells.[14] PGE_1 and inhibition of synthesis of dopamine and other amines by 60H-dopamine had similar effects on sleep in animals.[18] Dopamine and PGE_1 had antagonistic effects on vascular smooth muscle.[29]

The basic biochemistry and physiology of the PGs and EFA are therefore not inconsistent with the possibility that the EFA and PGs could be involved in major psychiatric disorders.

III. PROSTAGLANDIN INVOLVEMENT IN SCHIZOPHRENIA

A. Indirect Evidence

There are several indirect pieces of evidence which suggest that PGs may be involved in schizophrenia. These relate to the observations that phenomena or diseases known to be associated with altered PG formation may be different in schizophrenics than in normal individuals. These indirect items of evidence have previously been reviewed in some detail.[29-32] The main items are

1. Rheumatoid arthritis (RA) and schizophrenia, both very common, are almost mutually exclusive. Patients with both diseases do exist, but they are very unusual, whereas they ought to be common.[33,34] Since PG production is undoubtedly enhanced in RA, there is the possibility that the rheumatoid patients' freedom from schizophrenia may be associated with a PG abnormality.

2. PGs play important roles in local inflammatory responses and in pain. Schizophrenics are resistant to the local inflammatory response to histamine,[30,35] to the febrile effects of typhoid vaccine,[30] and to a wide variety of painful stimuli.[36] Their blood pressure and pupillary reactions fail to react normally to pain.[30] Again these observations hint at the possibility of a PG abnormality in schizophrenics.

3. PGs are known to affect intestinal motility. Schizophrenics have greatly reduced intestinal motility.[37]

4. The diuretic response to furosemide can be inhibited by blockers of PG synthesis. This effect is much reduced in schizophrenics.[38]

5. Almost all effective antischizophrenic drugs stimulate prolactin secretion as a result of their dopamine-blocking effects. Prolactin is an effective stimulator of PG formation, especially that of PGE_1. It appears to act by mobilizing DGLA.[39,40] The consistency of the antischizophrenic effect of drugs which are able to block the pituitary dopamine receptors that control prolactin secretion is the strongest evidence of dopamine involvement in schizophrenia. However,

since the drugs also enhance prolactin secretion and hence PG synthesis, the evidence from the actions of these drugs cannot be used to distinguish between the effects of dopamine blockade, prolactin secretion, or PG synthesis on the schizophrenic process.

6. Clozapine, an antipsychotic which is unusual both in its effectiveness and its weak effect on prolactin, behaves as a PG agonist both in in vitro pharmacological studies and in behavioral tests on animals.[12,31]

7. Very high doses of NSAI drugs which inhibit PG synthesis may occasionally produce achizoid psychotic reactions.[41,42]

8. There is an abundance of evidence, reviewed by Lipper and Werman,[43] that schizophrenia may remit during a febrile illness. PG levels in the brain may rise during fever.[44] On the other hand, in a small minority of schizophrenics, febrile illness is associated with exacerbation of a schizophrenic episode.

9. Niacin flushing seems to be caused by increased formation of PGEs in response to high doses of the niacin form of vitamin B_3.[46,47] This "side effect" of administration of high-dose niacin seems to be much less common in schizophrenics than in normal individuals and restoration of normal flushing in response to niacin is associated with clinical improvement.[48,49]

None of these items is hard evidence of PG involvement in schizophrenia. Each point is merely a straw in the wind; however, there are a surprising number of straws, most of them pointing to some form of deficit of PG synthesis or action in schizophrenics. As with the basic biochemistry of PGs, there is nothing which is incompatible with the general concept that PGs may be involved in schizophrenia, and much that is in support of that concept.

B. Direct Evidence

In the final analysis, only direct studies of the concentrations or effects of EFA and PGs can be used to demonstrate or refute the idea of PG involvement in schizophrenia. There have been a number of such direct studies.

With regard to the EFA, Obi and Nwanze[50] reported that alpha-linolenic acid (18:3n-3) levels were exceptionally high in schizophrenics. In unpublished studies my group has been unable to confirm this; however, the Nigerian population studied by Obi almost certainly has a relatively high alpha-linolenic acid intake, whereas our Western population is likely to have negligible intake of this EFA. If there were a defect in alpha-linolenic acid metabolism, this might therefore be more apparent in a Nigerian than in a Western population. Obi's work hints at the possibility that schizophrenics may be unable to metabolize alpha-linolenic acid normally. Hitzemann and Garver[51] reported that linoleic and DGLA levels were unusually low in red blood cell phospholipids from schizophrenics, whereas AA levels were exceptionally high. This observation raises the possibility that schizophrenics convert dietary LA to AA with unusual rapidity.

Abdulla and Hamadah,[52] in a remarkable study which has been largely ignored, showed that PGE_1 formation from DGLA in platelets taken from schizophrenics off drugs was resistant to ADP stimulation. PGE_1 formation in platelets from depressed patients was below normal and in those from manic patients was above normal, but in both cases there was a normal dose-response curve to ADP. Schizophrenics, in contrast, totally failed to raise PGE_1 formation in the presence of ADP. At maximal ADP concentrations, the difference between the highest rate of PGE_1 formation in the schizophrenics and the lowest rate of formation in the nonschizophrenics was more than eight times the range of values within either group. There is no more striking, clear cut, or statistically significant observation in the whole of biological psychiatry. At this time in unpublished studies my group has been able to confirm that PG formation in platelets from schizophrenics is indeed resistant to ADP stimulation. I am therefore reasonably confident that the Abdulla observations are valid, and that if they can be understood and followed to their ultimate origin we shall be very close to finding the biochemical basis for schizophrenia.

Mathé et al.[53] reported that while thromboxane (TX) B_2 levels were normal in CSF from schizophrenics, PGE levels were significantly elevated. Their immunoassay did not distinguish between PGE_1 and PGE_2, and thus it is impossible to say whether the abnormality was related to 1 or 2 series PGs.

There have also been indications that PG action is abnormal in schizophrenics. Two independent groups have confirmed that the platelet cAMP response to PGE_1 is significantly reduced in schizophrenics.[54-56] Agents acting via receptors seem to fall into two classes, those in which the agonist induces tissue responsiveness and those in which agonist exposure reduces responsiveness. PGE_1 seems to come into the former class, since in EFA-deficient animals in which PG formation is reduced, cAMP responsiveness to PGE_1 is also reduced.[57,58] Thus, the observations of reduced platelet sensitivity to PGE_1 are fully compatible with the observation of Abdulla that PGE_1 formation in platelets from schizophrenics is below normal.

In summary, the direct evidence relating to PGs, EFA, and schizophrenia suggests that there is a defect in the formation of PGE_1 in platelets; there is an excess of a PGE in CSF; there are deficiencies of LA and DGLA in red cell phospholipids, coupled with an excess of AA; there may be defective metabolism of alpha-linolenic acid; and the response of platelet cAMP to PGE_1 is reduced.

C. Therapeutic Trials

A number of therapeutic trials point to the possible involvement of EFA and/or PGs in schizophrenia, but none is conclusive since each has alternative explanations.

The great majority of antischizophrenic drugs block dopamine receptors and increase the secretion of prolactin and hence the formation of 1 series PGs. The effectiveness of these drugs is compatible with any one of three hypotheses. They may work because of the dopamine-receptor blockade, the raised prolactin levels, or enhanced PG formation. It is unfortunate that this drug evidence has been used almost exclusively to support the concept of dopamine involvement in schizophrenia. It is certainly compatible with such a concept, but it is equally compatible with the other two ideas.

Penicillamine and penicillin both appear to be able selectively to increase the formation of 1 series PGs.[58,59] Both also do many other things. Both have been shown in placebo-controlled studies to be modestly effective in treating schizophrenics.[60,61]

Administration of the PG precursor, gamma-linolenic acid, in the form of evening primrose oil (Efamol) had little effect alone; however, in combination with the PG synthesis stimulators captopril,[62] niacin,[49] or penicillin,[63] uncontrolled studies indicated that gamma-linolenic acid has therapeutic effects.

Niacin does appear to have an antischizophrenic effect when given in high doses to some patients.[64] Niacin is a potent stimulator of PGE synthesis.

High doses of alpha-linolenic acid appear to have an antischizophrenic effect.[65] If as suggested by Obi's work, alpha-linolenic metabolism is defective in schizophrenia, large doses may help to overcome the defect.

D. Hypotheses

Two hypotheses were originally put forward with regard to PG involvement in schizophrenia:

1.   Schizophrenia is associated with a general excess of PG synthesis.[45] The main supporting evidence offered was the association between fever (and therefore

possibly enhanced brain PG synthesis) in a small minority of schizophrenics and the effects of PGs on animal behavior. This view is compatible with the high levels of PGE in CSF, and possibly with the high AA levels in red cell phospholipids, but not with the low PGE_1 levels in platelets and with most of the indirect evidence.

2. Schizophrenia is associated with a generalized deficit in PG synthesis.[30] The main evidence was the prolactin stimulation of PG synthesis, the many pieces of indirect evidence suggesting a PG deficit in schizophrenics, notably their resistance to pain and inflammation. This is compatible with the low PGE_1 formation in platelets, but not with the high PGE levels in CSF. It may be compatible with the high AA levels in red cell phospholipids. A high level of AA could indicate a failure of conversion of AA to PGs (compatible with this second hypothesis) or excessive availability of AA for PG formation (compatible with the first hypothesis).

It seems to me that both these original hypotheses, while heuristically valuable at the time they were presented, are now incompatible with the evidence. A synthesis of the available evidence might be made along the following lines[29,66,67]:

1. In any successful hypothesis the PGs and EFA must be considered together. EFAs have independent effects quite apart from their roles as PG precursors. A primary EFA abnormality would lead to changes both in PG formation and in these independent effects. A primary PG abnormality, by either depleting EFA or allowing them to accumulate abnormally, would also lead to changes in the independent EFA actions.

2. In any successful hypothesis the low level of PGE_1 formation from DGLA must be taken into account since it seems the most solidly established of all the direct evidence and is supported by the abnormal cAMP responses to PGE_1. Less certainly established, but worthy of serious consideration are the low LA and DGLA and high AA levels in membrane phospholipids, which may indicate unusually rapid conversion of LA to AA. Also potentially important is the observation that alpha-linolenic acid metabolism may be defective. It will be essential to establish whether the high PGE levels in CSF are due to PGE_1, E_2, or both.

These biochemical phenomena could be produced in a variety of different ways. My current working hypothesis is that the clinical syndrome of schizophrenia is akin in many ways to the clinical syndrome of fever. Fever may be caused by a wide range of different microorganisms and now that fever is reasonably well understood, more attention is paid to the underlying infection than to the precise characteristics of the fever itself. I suspect that the clinical syndrome of schizophrenia may be caused by several different underlying biochemical mechanisms. If and when these can be identified, we shall begin to lose interest in schizophrenia except as an indication that something is wrong, and we shall concentrate on the underlying biochemistry. My hypotheses as to the major possible biochemical causes of schizophrenia are as follows:

1. The enzymes which metabolize EFA normally have a higher affinity for the n-3 acids than the n-6 acids. As a result, there is substantial competition between the two series of EFA and alpha-linolenic acid is normally metabolized more rapidly than is linoleic acid. A mutation that changed the affinity of the enzyme sequence would have the effect of leading to the accumulation of alpha-linolenic acid and to the rapid conversion of LA to AA.[67] Such a mutation cannot, of course, be directly simulated but it can be indirectly approximated by feeding animals a diet containing only n-6 and no n-3 EFA. This diet will remove the competition to the

LA metabolic pathway normally afforded by the alpha-linolenic acid series. In such animals, LA and DGLA levels are reduced, while AA levels are elevated, apparently due to more rapid transmission of n-6 acids along the pathway.[67] This fatty acid pattern is similar to that found in red cell phospholipids from human schizophrenics and would be compatible with reduced formation of 1 series PGs and increased formation of 2 series PGs.

2. The Abdulla experiments suggest that there may be a selective deficit in the formation of 1 series PGs. This will lead to reduced formation of PGE_1 and a reduced sensitivity to PG modulation of cAMP levels. There are many possible factors which could exert such a selective effect. A major candidate must be an opioid, since opioids are able to inhibit the conversion of DGLA to PGE_1.[23,59]

3. Prolactin seems to selectively stimulate the mobilization of DGLA from membrane phospholipids. The success of prolactin-stimulating drugs suggests that there is in schizophrenics a factor which inhibits this process or an absence of a natural factor which stimulates this reaction. One candidate is melatonin, whose levels seem to be low in schizophrenics and whose secretion, like that of prolactin, may be enhanced by psychotropic drugs.[68,69] Schizophrenia seems to be exceptionally rare in congenitally blind individuals in whom melatonin levels are elevated from birth.[29]

IV. CONCLUSIONS

Research on the possible roles of EFA and PGs in schizophrenia is in its infancy. The basic biochemistry and physiology, the indirect evidence from clinical observations, the direct evidence from PG and EFA measurements, and the clinical trial results all suggest that this is a line of research which is worth pursuing vigorously. It offers completely new directions in schizophrenia research, an area which has stagnated because of the obsession with the dopamine hypothesis and reluctance to discard that hypothesis in the face of contrary experimental evidence. There are likely to be many unexpected twists and turns in the story. I predict that schizophrenia (like fever) will prove to have several different basic causes, that some of these causes will have their roots in EFA and PG metabolism, and that as with fever, understanding of the causes will lead to cures.

REFERENCES

1. Heston, L. L., The genetics of schizophrenia and schizoid disease, *Science,* 167, 249, 1970.
2. Svennerholm, L., Distribution and fatty acid composition of phosphoglycerides in normal human brain, *J. Lipid Res.,* 9, 570, 1968.
3. Dhopeshwarkar, G. A. and Mead, J. F., Fatty acid uptake by the brain, *Biochim. Biophys. Acta,* 210, 250, 1970.
4. Galli, C., Dietary essential fatty acids, polyunsaturated fatty acids and prostaglandins in the central nervous system, *Adv. Prostaglandin Thromboxane Res.,* 4, 181, 1978.
5. Galli, C., Galli, G., Spagnuolo, C. et al., Dietary essential fatty acids, brain polyunsaturated fatty acids and prostaglandin biosynthesis, *Adv. Exp. Med. Biol.,* 83, 561, 1977.
6. Hassam, A. G., Willis, A. L., Denton, J. P. et al., The effect of essential fatty acid deficient diet on the levels of prostaglandins and their fatty acid precursors in the rabbit brain, *Lipids,* 14, 78, 1979.
7. Wolfe, L. S., Some facts and thoughts on the biosynthesis of prostaglandins and thromboxanes in brain, *Adv. Prostaglandin Thromboxane Res.,* 4, 215, 1978.
8. Horrobin, D. F., Durand, L. G., and Manku, M. S., Prostaglandin E_1 modifies nerve conduction and interferes with local anaesthetic action, *Prostaglandins,* 14, 103, 1977.
9. Hedqvist, P., Basic mechanisms of prostaglandin action on autonomic neurotransmission, *Ann. Rev. Pharmacol. Toxicol.,* 17, 259, 1977.

10. Reimann, W., Steinhauer, H. B., Hedler, L. et al., Effect of prostaglandins D_2, E_2 and F_2 alpha on catecholamine release from slices of rat and rabbit brain, *Eur. J. Pharmacol.*, 69, 421, 1981.

11. Shimizu, T., Mizuno, N., Amano, T. et al., Prostaglandin D_2, a neuromodulator, *Proc. Natl. Acad. Sci. U.S.A.*, 76, 6231, 1979.

12. Bloss, J. L. and Singer, G. H., Neuropharmacological and behavioral evaluation of prostaglandin E_2 and 11-thiol-11-desoxy-prostaglandin E_2 in the mouse and rat, *Psychopharmacology*, 57, 295, 1978.

13. Golub, M. S., Sowers, J. R., Eggena, P. et al., Effect of PG inhibition on the prolactin, renin and aldosterone responses to dopamine antagonism, *Metabolism*, 31, 740, 1982.

14. Blosser, J. C., Myers, P. R., and Shain, W., Neurotransmitter modulation of prostaglandin E_1 stimulated increases in cyclic AMP, *Biochem. Pharmacol.*, 27, 1167, 1978.

15. Manku, M. S., Mtabaji, J. P., and Horrobin, D. F., Effects of prostaglandins on baseline pressure and responses to noradrenaline in a perfused rat mesenteric artery preparation, *Prostaglandins*, 13, 701, 1977.

16. Horton, E. W., Actions of prostaglandins E_1, E_2 and E_3 on the central nervous system, *Br. J. Pharmacol.*, 22, 189, 1964.

17. Horton, E. W., *The Prostaglandins*, Springer-Verlag, Berlin, 1972.

18. Masek, K., Kadlecova, O., and Poschlova, N., Effect of intracisternal administration of prostaglandin E_1 on waking and sleeping in the rat, *Neuropharmacology*, 15, 491, 1976.

19. Haubrich, D. R., Perez-Cruet, J., and Reid, W. D., Prostaglandin E_1 causes sedation and increases 5-hydroxytryptamine turnover in the rat brain, *Br. J. Pharmacol.*, 48, 80, 1973.

20. Segarnick, D. J., Cordasco, D. M., and Rotrosen, J., Biochemical and behavioral interactions between prostaglandin E_1 and alcohol, in *Clinical Uses of Essential Fatty Acids*, Horrobin, D. F., Ed., Eden Press, Montreal, 1983.

21. Schaefer, A., Komlos, M., and Seregi, A., Effects of biogenic amines and psychotropic drugs on endogenous prostaglandin biosynthesis in the rat brain homogenates, *Biochem. Pharmacol.*, 27, 213, 1978.

22. Collier, H. O. J., McDonald-Gibson, W. J., and Saeed, S. A., Apomorphine and morphine stimulate prostaglandin biosynthesis, *Nature (London)*, 252, 56, 1974.

23. Horrobin, D. F., Possible roles of prostaglandins in mediating opioid actions, in *Endorphins and Opiate Antagonists in Psychiatric Research*, Shah, N. S. and Donald, A. G., Eds., Plenum Press, New York, 1982.

24. Horrobin, D. F., The regulation of prostaglandin biosynthesis, *Med. Hypotheses*, 6, 687, 1980.

25. Janicke, U. and Forster, W., Effects of imipramine, chlorpromazine and promazine treatment on the in vivo prostaglandin biosynthesis of rabbit brain and renal medulla, *Pharmacol. Res. Comm.*, 9, 501, 1977.

26. Abdel-Halim M. S., Sjoquist, B., and Änggård, E., Inhibition of prostaglandin biosynthesis in rat brain, *Acta Pharmacol. Toxicol.*, 43, 266, 1978.

27. Lambert, B. and Jacquemin, C., Synergic effect of insulin and prostaglandin E_1 on stimulated lipolysis, *Prostaglandins Med.*, 5, 375, 1980.

28. Fjalland, B., Influence of various substances on prostaglandin biosynthesis by guinea pig chopped lung, *J. Pharm. Pharmacol.*, 28, 683, 1976.

29. Horrobin, D. F., Schizophrenia: reconciliation of the dopamine, prostaglandin, and opioid concepts and the role of the pineal, *Lancet*, 1, 529, 1979.

30. Horrobin, D. F., Schizophrenia as a prostaglandin deficiency disease, *Lancet*, 1, 936, 1977.

31. Horrobin, D. F., Ally, A. I., Karmali, R. A. et al., Prostaglandins and schizophrenia: further discussion of the evidence, *Psychol. Med.*, 8, 43, 1978.

32. Horrobin, D. F., The roles of prostaglandins and prolactin in depression, mania and schizophrenia, *Postgrad. Med. J.*, 53(Suppl. 4), 160, 1977.

33. Osterberg, E., Olhagen, B., and Wetterberg, L., Schizophrenia and rheumatoid arthritis, *Lancet*, 1, 1367, 1977.

34. Gattaz, W. F., Kasper, S., Ewald, R. W. et al., Arthropathies and schizophrenia, *Lancet*, 2, 536, 1980.

35. Lucy, J. D., Histamine tolerance in schizophrenia, *AMA Arch. Psychiatry*, 71, 629, 1954.

36. Gowdy, J. M., Headaches after lumbar puncture and insensitivity to pain in psychiatric patients, *N. Engl. J. Med.*, 301, 110, 1979.

37. Lechin, F. and van der Dijs, B., Intestinal pharmacomanometry and glucose tolerance: evidence for two antagonistic dopaminergic mechanisms in the human, *Biol. Psych.*, 16, 969, 1981.

38. Patino, R., Mateo, I., Fuentenebro, F. et al., Reduction of indomethacin inhibition of natriuretic furosemide effect in schizophrenia: a preliminary report, *IRCS J. Med. Sci.*, 7, 544, 1979.

39. Horrobin, D. F., Cellular basis of prolactin action, *Med. Hypotheses*, 5, 599, 1979.

40. Manku, M. S., Horrobin, D. F., Karmazyn, M. et al., Prolactin and zinc effects on rat vascular reactivity: possible relationship to dihomogammalinolenic acid and to prostaglandin synthesis, *Endocrinology*, 104, 774, 1979.

41. Turner, P., Schizophrenia as a prostaglandin deficiency disease, *Lancet,* 1, 1058, 1977.
42. Thornton, T. L., Delirium after sulindac, *JAMA,* 243, 1630, 1980.
43. Lipper, S. and Werman, D. S., Schizophrenia and intercurrent physical illness: a critical review of the literature, *Compr. Psychiatry,* 18, 11, 1977.
44. Feldberg, W. and Gupta, K. P., Pyrogen fever and prostaglandin-like activity in the cerebrospinal fluid, *J. Physiol. (London),* 228, 41, 1973.
45. Feldberg, W., Possible association of schizophrenia with a disturbance in prostaglandin metabolism: a physiological hypothesis, *Psychol. Med.,* 6, 359, 1976.
46. Andersson, R. G. G., Aberg, G., Brattsand, R. et al., Studies on the mechanism of flush induced by nicotinic acid, *Acta Pharm. Toxicol.,* 41, 1, 1977.
47. Eklund, B., Kaijser, L., Nowack, J. et al., Prostaglandins contribute to the vasodilatation induced by nicotinic acid, *Prostaglandins,* 17, 821, 1979.
48. Hoffer, A., Safety, side effects and relative lack of toxicity of nicotinic acid and nicotinamide, *Schizophrenia,* 1, 78, 1969.
49. Horrobin, D. F., Niacin flushing, prostaglandin E and evening primrose oil. A possible objective test for monitoring therapy in schizophrenia, *J. Orthomol. Psych.,* 9, 33, 1980.
50. Obi, F. O. and Nwanze, E. A. C., Fatty acid profiles in mental disease. I. Linolenate variations in schizophrenia, *J. Neurol. Sci.,* 43, 447, 1979.
51. Hitzemann, R. J. and Garver, D. L., Abnormalities in membrane lipids associated with deficiencies in lithium counterflow, Society of Biological Psychiatry, New Orleans, June, 1981.
52. Abdulla, Y. H. and Hamadah, K., Effect of ADP on PGE formation in blood platelets from patients with depression, mania and schizophrenia, *Br. J. Psychiatry,* 127, 591, 1975.
53. Mathé, A. A., Sedvall, G., Wiesel, F. A. et al., Increased content of immunoreactive prostaglandin E in cerebrospinal fluid of patients with schizophrenia, *Lancet,* 1, 16, 1980.
54. Rotrosen, J., Miller, A. D., Mandio, D. et al., Reduced PGE_1-stimulated ^{3}H-cAMP accumulation in platelets from schizophrenics, *Life Sci.,* 23, 1989, 1978.
55. Rotrosen, J., Miller, D., Mandio, D. et al., Prostaglandins, platelets and schizophrenia, *Arch. Gen. Psych.,* 37, 1047, 1980.
56. Kafka, M. S., Van Kammen, D. P., and Bunney, W. E., Reduced cyclic AMP production in the blood platelets from schizophrenic patients, *Am. J. Psychiatry,* 136, 685, 1979.
57. Vincent, J. E., Melai, A., Bonta, I. L. et al., Comparison of the effects of prostaglandin E_1 on platelet aggregation in normal and essential fatty acid deficient rats, *Prostaglandins,* 5, 369, 1974.
58. Horrobin, D. F., *Prostaglandins: Physiology, Pharmacology and Clinical Significance,* Eden Press, Montreal, 1978.
59. Horrobin, D. F., Regulation of prostaglandin biosynthesis, *Med. Hypotheses,* 6, 687, 1980.
60. Nicolson, G. A., Greiner, A. C., McFarlane, W. J. G. et al., Effect of penicillamine on schizophrenic patients, *Lancet,* 1, 344, 1966.
61. Chouinard, G., Annable, L., and Horrobin, D. F., An antipsychotic action of penicillin in schizophrenia, *IRCS J. Med. Sci.,* 6, 187, 1978.
62. Parmigiania, P., Evening primrose oil (Efamol) and captopril in schizophrenia: a preliminary report, in *Clinical Uses of Essential Fatty Acids,* Horrobin, D. F., Ed., Eden Press, Montreal, 1983.
63. Vaddadi, K. S., Penicillin and evening primrose oil in schizophrenia, *Prostaglandins Med.,* 2, 77, 1979.
64. Osmond, H. and Hoffer, A., Massive niacin treatment in schizophrenia, *Lancet,* 1, 316, 1962.
65. Rudin, D. O., The major psychoses and neuroses as omega-3 essential fatty acid deficiency syndrome, *Biol. Psychiatry,* 16, 837, 1981.
66. Horrobin, D. F., Prostaglandins and schizophrenia, *Lancet,* 1, 706, 1980.
67. Horrobin, D. F. and Huang, Y.-S., Schizophrenia: the role of abnormal essential fatty acid and prostaglandin metabolism, *Med. Hypotheses,* in press.
68. Smith, J. A., Mee, T. J. X., and Barnes, J. L. C., Elevated melatonin serum concentrations in psychiatric patients treated with chlorpromazine, *J. Pharm. Pharmacol.,* Suppl. 1, 30, 1977.
69. Ferrier, I. N., Johnstone, E. C., Crow, T. J. et al., Melatonin/cortisol ratio in psychiatric illness, *Lancet,* 1, 1070, 1982.

Index

INDEX

A

Granulocyte-macrophage colony stimulating factor, 53
Group B streptococcal sepsis, 68
Guinea pig lung, 14
Guinea pig skin, 14—15

H

Hamster cheek pouch, 14—16
Headache, 152—153, 166
Heart, 6
Helper cell, 114
Hematopoiesis, 45—55
Hemiplegia, 152
Hemodialysis, 149, 170, 178
Hemolytic uremic syndrome (HUS), 151, 154
Hemoperfusion, 170
Hemorrhage, 69
Hemorrhagic shock, 66—67
Hemostasis, 94, 132
Heparin, 94, 118—119, 121—123, 149—150, 152, 170, 172, 174—178, 194, 216
    tracheobronchial smooth muscle, 227
Herpes simplex virus type 1 (HSV), 21
5-HETE, 6, 17, 19, 34—35, 236
    inhibition of lymphocyte transformation, 75
12-HETE, 34—35
High density lipoproteins (HDL), 132—140, 200
Histamine, 14, 20, 68, 112, 203, 219, 221—222, 224
    anaphylactic release, 224—227
    inhibition of smooth muscle contraction, 214
    local inflammatory response to, 256
    tracheobronchial smooth muscle, 227
Histocompatibility matching, 113
HLA-DR antigen expression, 47—51
Homeostatic mechanisms, 46
Homotypic aggregation, 96
Host defense against infection, 18
Host defense mechanisms, 22
Host defenses, 74—75
Host-tumor interaction, 82
Host-vs.-graft reactions, 116
12-HPETE, 19, 34—35, 37, 102
15-HPETE, 14, 34—35, 76, 97, 100
5-HT, 152—153
Human alveolar macrophages, 17—18
Human blood mononuclear leukocytes, 18
Human blood PMNL, see PMNL
Human fetal adrenal tissue, 38
Human fetal liver, 34
Human interleukin (IL) 2, 115
Human leukemic cells, 74
Human lung fibroblasts, 4
Human PMNL, 16
Humoral factors, 94
Humoral immunity, 83, 115
Hyaline membrane disease, 31
Hydergine, 150
Hydralazine, 204

Hydrochlorothiazide, 202
Hydrocortisone, 121
Hydrolases, 69
Hydroperoxides, 132, 185
15-Hydroperoxy arachidonic acid (15-HPAA), 198
5S-Hydroperoxy-eicosatetraenoic acid, see 5-HPETE
Hydroxy acids, 17
5(S)-Hydroxy-6,8,11,14-eicosatetraenoic acid, see 5-HETE
12S-Hydroxy-5,8,10,14-eicosatetranenoic acid, see 12-HPETE
3-Hydroxy-3-methylglutaryl CoA reductase, 134
15-Hydroxy-PG dehydrogenase, 201, 214
5-Hydroxy-tryptamine, 69
Hyperacute allograft rejection, 149
Hyperacute rejection, 113—114, 119
Hyperaggregability of platelets, 92
Hypercalcemia, 8, 76, 82, 84, 86
Hypercholesterolemia, 135, 139
Hypermetabolism, 193
Hyperplasia, 75
Hypersensitivity reactions, 7, 14, 22
Hypertension, 146, 197—212
Hypometabolism, 193
Hypoperfusion, 193
Hypotension, 153
Hypotonia, 185
Hypovolemic shock, 66—67
Hypoxemia, 227
Hypoxia, 112

I

Ia-antigen expression, 52
Ia-like antigens, 46—47
Ibuprofen, 4
Idiopathic pulmonary artery stenosis, 149
Imidazole, 5—6, 67, 102, 198
Immune functions, see Immunology
Immune response, leukotrienes as modulators of, 20—21
Immune system, modulation of, 82
Immunity, 74—75
Immunologic reactivity, 83
Immunological effects, breast cancer, 83
Immunology, transplantation, 115—117
Immunosuppression, 75, 113—114, 117, 124
Indomethacin, 4, 20—21, 51, 76—77, 84, 86, 116, 121, 137, 241
    basal PRA levels, 203—204
    cyclooxygenase activity, inhibition of, 198
    cyclooxygenase/lipoxygenase pathway, 187
    hypertension, 200
    immune response, 75
    lymphocyte proliferation, 74
    patent ductus arteriosus management, 30
    sodium retention, 199
Infiltration, 69

Sodium salicylate, 121
S-phase of cell cycle, 47
Spironolactone, 203
Spleen, 4, 6
SRS-A, 7, 14, 19, 214, 221, 224—227
SRS of anaphylaxis, see SRS-A
Steal hypothesis, 102—103
Stem cells, 46
Steroid hormones, see Steroids
Steroids, 7, 31, 39, 82, 113—114, 117, 120—121,
    138, 194
Stomach, 4, 6, 31
Streptozotocin, 61
Stroke, 187, 192
Substance P, 239, 241
Succinyl choline chloride, 216
Sulfasalazine, 201
Sulfinpyrazone, 123
Suloctidil, 200
Superoxide dismutase (SOD), 187, 189
Superoxide radicals, 187
Superoxides, 185
Suppressor cells, 21, 116
Suppressor lymphocytes, 20
Sympathetic nervous system, 203
Sympathomimetic amines, 224
Synovial fluid, 21
Synthesis, leukotrienes, 17—20
Synthetases, 214
Systemic arterial pressure, 68
Systemic lupus erythematosus (SLE), 151
Systemic vascular resistance, 66

T

T cell-derived suppressor (PITSβ), 116
T cells, 83, 115—116
Tensile strength of corneal wounds, 235
Tetraphorbol acetate, 75
Theophylline, 97, 201
Thin layer chromatography (TLC), 31
Thrombangiitis obliterans, 148, 165—166
Thrombin, 146, 200
Thrombocytopenia, 68, 92—93
β-Thromboglobulin, 96, 153, 171—173,
    177—178, 198
Thrombosis, 69, 94, 100, 103
Thrombotic microangiography, 151, 154
Thrombotic thrombocytopenic purpura (TTP),
    151, 154
Thromboxane, 16, 66—67, 83
    arachidonic acid via cyclooxygenase pathway,
        4—7
    immune system, 75
    tumor metastasis, 94
Thromboxane A$_2$ (TXA$_2$), 4, 5, 7, 68—69, 132,
    146, 152
Thromboxane B$_2$ (TXB$_2$), 5, 7
Thromboxane synthetase inhibitor OKY-1581, 21

Thromboxane synthetase inhibitors, 102—103,
    147
Thrombus, 92
Thymocytes, 83
Timolol, 243
T lymphocytes, 20, 53, 74
α-Tocopherol, 194
Tonometry, 243
Trachea, 14
Tracheal muscle, 215
Tracheal smooth muscle, 221
Tracheal strips, 221—224
Tracheobronchial smooth muscle, 227
Tracheobronchial tree, 219—221
Transient cerebral oligemia, 185—187
Transient ischemic attacks (TIA), 152, 187, 189,
    192—193
Transient oligemia, 184
Transplantable tumors, 92
Transplantation, 111—128
    acute rejection, 113—114, 120—123
    chronic rejection, 113, 115, 123
    early organ function, 113
    hyperacute rejection, 113—114, 119
    immunology, 115—117
    inhibition of immune functions, 115—116
    neoplasia, 114
    organ preservation, 112—114, 118—119
    organ procurement, 112, 114, 117—118
    platelets, role of, 114—115
    stimulation of immune functions, 116—117
    therapeutic uses in, 117—123
    xenograft rejection, 114, 119
Tranylcypromine, 116, 198
Trauma, 4, 238, 245
Traumatic shock, 66—67, 146
Triglycerides, 132—134
Trypsin, 200
TSH, 59
T suppressor cell, 117
Tumor cell extravasation, 92
Tumor cell-induced platelet aggregation (TCIPA),
    94—96
Tumor cell-induced platelet release reaction
    (TCIPR), 96—97
Tumor cells, 84
Tumor cell surface topology, 96—97, 100
Tumor growth, 82
Tumor metastasis, 91—110
Tumor virus, 85
Typhoid vaccine, 256

U

U54701, 102
Ubiquinone 50 (coenzyme Q10), 189
UK 37248-01, 200
Umbilical artery, 9
Umbilical circulation, 28—29
Unstable angina pectoris, 147, 150—151, 154